FUNDAMENTALS OF
EMERGENCY ULTRASOUND

FUNDAMENTALS OF
EMERGENCY ULTRASOUND

JOHN P. McGAHAN, MD

Professor and Vice Chair of Academic Affairs
Director of Abdominal Fellowship
Department of Radiology
UC Davis Health
Sacramento, California

MICHAEL A. SCHICK, DO

Associate Professor
Director of Technology-Enabled Active Learning
Emergency Medicine
UC Davis Health
Sacramento, California

LISA D. MILLS, MD

Director of Emergency Medicine Ultrasound; Professor
Emergency Medicine
UC Davis Health
Sacramento, California

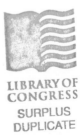

ELSEVIER

Elsevier
1600 John F. Kennedy Blvd.
Ste 1600
Philadelphia, PA 19103-2899

FUNDAMENTALS OF EMERGENCY ULTRASOUND

ISBN: 978-0-323-59642-8

Notice

Practitioners and researchers must always rely on their own experience and knowledge in evaluating and using any information, methods, compounds or experiments described herein. Because of rapid advances in the medical sciences, in particular, independent verification of diagnoses and drug dosages should be made. To the fullest extent of the law, no responsibility is assumed by Elsevier, authors, editors or contributors for any injury and/or damage to persons or property as a matter of products liability, negligence or otherwise, or from any use or operation of any methods, products, instructions, or ideas contained in the material herein.

Library of Congress Control Number: 2019943476

Content Strategist: Cathleen Sether
Content Development Specialist: Mary Hegeler
Publishing Services Manager: Shereen Jameel
Senior Project Manager: Kamatchi Madhavan
Design Direction: Bridget Hoette

Printed in China

Last digit is the print number: 9   8   7   6   5   4   3   2   1

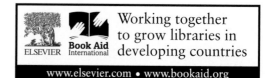

Dedicated to my grandchildren, Gabriela, Brianna, Ava, Mia, Delaney, Lucia, Brian, and Jude, and to all those throughout the world who are learning and helping others through the use of ultrasound to improve patient care.
John P. McGahan

To my wife Elisa; my children Oliver and Maya; and my mentors, colleagues, trainees, and patients who inspire me every day.
Michael A. Schick

Thank you to my husband, Trevor, for his forever support.
Lisa D. Mills

PREFACE

Diagnostic ultrasound is the most common cross-sectional imaging modality used worldwide. Sonography provides real-time clinical data and is now seen as essential in the care of critically ill patients. It is utilized by not only multiple physician specialties but also midlevel providers, nurses, and prehospital health care workers.

This text is a true collaboration from more than 50 experts and is unique in that the collaboration spans a multitude of medical specialties. Our text is organized into anatomic regions from head to toe in which sonography is useful in evaluating the emergent patient. We begin with a fundamental concept chapter discussing physics, artifacts, and techniques, which is followed by chapters that cover the emergent patient. Areas in which ultrasound has had a well-established indication in both adult and pediatric patients are covered and expanded upon. We begin with head and neck ultrasound, including the intracranial exam of the infant. From there we explore the use of ultrasound for emergent applications, including trauma, echocardiography, lung ultrasound, important considerations in resuscitation, and shortness of breath and chest pain. Included within the abdomen is the evaluation of the liver, gallbladder, pancreas, kidney, and bowel. We review the use of emergent ultrasound for the male and female pelvis, including its use in pregnancy emergencies. Extremity evaluation includes the use of musculoskeletal ultrasound and sonography of the soft tissues. We cover cutting-edge techniques, including key ultrasound-guided procedures and selected nerve blocks.

Chapters are organized in such a way that ultrasound anatomy and technique are explored first. We then review specific abnormalities and disease states occurring within each anatomic region and emphasize the ultrasound features of different diseases encountered in emergent situations. For instance, in a patient with right upper quadrant pain, we first review the sonographic features of cholelithiasis and cholecystitis. After, we review the other sonographic findings of disease processes that may be encountered in patients with right upper quadrant pain. Multiple tables are included to help expand differential diagnoses. Numerous figures are used to demonstrate specific ultrasound features of different disease states. Real-time clips are provided throughout the text as learning tools for both the novice and the advanced learner.

Our aim was to produce a comprehensive text that serves as an accessible reference and teaching tool for the use of ultrasound in critical and emergent situations. We hope readers find that the topics and techniques covered here enhance their patient care and are helpful in their daily practice.

John P. McGahan
Michael A. Schick
Lisa D. Mills

CONTRIBUTORS

Kenton L. Anderson, MD
Director of Emergency Ultrasound Research
Department of Emergency Medicine
Stanford University
Palo Alto, California

Orode Badakhsh, MD
Department of Anesthesiology and Pain Medicine
UC Davis Health
Sacramento, California

Cristiana Baloescu, MD, MPH
Clinical Instructor
Department of Emergency Medicine
Yale University School of Medicine
New Haven, Connecticut

Christopher M. Beck, MD
Emergency Medicine
UC Davis Health
Sacramento, California

Michael J. Campbell, MD
Associate Professor
UC Davis Cancer Center
Sacramento, California

Gabriel S. Espinoza, MD
Resident Physician
University of California San Francisco
Zuckerberg San Francisco General Hospital
San Francisco, California

Ghaneh Fananapazir, MD
Associate Professor
Radiology
UC Davis Health
Sacramento, California

Eugenio O. Gerscovich, MD
Clinical Professor of Radiology
UC Davis Health
Sacramento, California

Kenn Ghaffarian, DO
Director of Emergency Ultrasound
Department of Emergency Medicine
Jefferson Northeast
Philadelphia, Pennsylvania

Laleh Gharahbaghian, MD
Director Emeritus of Emergency
    Ultrasound
Department of Emergency Medicine
Stanford University
Palo Alto, California

Alicia A. Gingrich, MD
UC Davis Health
Sacramento, California

Ryan Horton, MD
Attending Physician
Emergency Medicine
Dell Seton Medical Center at the
    University of Texas
Austin, Texas

Drew Jones, MD
Ultrasound Director
Advent Health
East Orlando, Florida

Kenneth M. Kelley, MD, FACEP
Associate Professor
Department of Emergency Medicine
UC Davis Health
Sacramento, California

Deborah S. Kim, MD
Co-director Emergency Ultrasound
Kaiser Permanente, South Sacramento
Sacramento, California

Deborah Kimball, MD, MBA
Department of Emergency Medicine
Cook County Hospital
Chicago, Illinois

Kara M. Kuhn-Riordon, MD
Assistant Clinical Professor, Neonatology
Department of Pediatrics
UC Davis Health
Sacramento, California

David Li, MD
Department of Anesthesiology and Pain Medicine
UC Davis Health
Sacramento, California

Mindy Lipsitz, MD, MPH
Dartmouth-Hitchcock Medical Center
Department of Medicine
Section of Emergency Medicine
Lebanon, New Hampshire

Rachel Liu, MD
Assistant Professor
Director of Clinical Ultrasound Education
Emergency Medicine
Yale School of Medicine
New Haven, Connecticut

Viveta Lobo, MD
Director, Emergency Ultrasound
Department of Emergency Medicine
Stanford University School of Medicine
Palo Alto, California

David A. Martin, MD
Ultrasound Fellow
Highland General Hospital
Alameda Health System
Oakland, California

Christine N. McBeth, DO
Assistant professor
Emergency Medicine
UC Davis Health
Sacramento, California

Chad McCarthy, MD
Senior Resident Physician
Highland General Hospital
Alameda Health System
Oakland, California

John P. McGahan, MD
Professor and Vice Chair of Academic Affairs
Director of Abdominal Fellowship
Department of Radiology
UC Davis Health
Sacramento, California

Sarah Medeiros, MD, MPH
Assistant Professor
Director of Technology Enabled Active Learning
Emergency Medicine
UC Davis Health
Sacramento, California

Lisa D. Mills, MD
Director of Emergency Medicine Ultrasound; Professor
Emergency Medicine
UC Davis Health
Sacramento, California

Arun Nagdev, MD
Director, Emergency Ultrasound
Highland General Hospital
Alameda Health System
Oakland, California

Bjork Olafsdottir-Gardali, MD
Emergency Medicine
UC Davis Health
Sacramento, California

Kathryn H Pade, MD
Assistant Professor of Pediatrics
Division of Emergency Medicine
Rady Children's Hospital San Diego
University of California San Diego
San Diego, California

Leslie Palmerlee, MD, MPH
Assistant Professor
Emergency Medicine
UC Davis Health
Sacramento, California

William C. Pevec, MD, RVT, RPVI
Professor Emeritus
Vascular and Endovascular Surgery
UC Davis Health
Sacramento, California

Jeremiah W. Ray, MD, FACEP, CAQSM
Head Team Physician
Associate Diplomat Physician
Orthopaedic Surgery
UC Davis Health
Sacramento, California

John R. Richards, MD
Department of Emergency Medicine
UC Davis Health
Sacramento, California

John S. Rose, MD
Professor of Emergency Medicine
UC Davis Health
Sacramento, California

Deborah J. Rubens, MD, FACR
Professor of Imaging Sciences, Oncology and
    Biomedical Engineering
Associate Chair, Imaging Sciences
Associate Director for the Center for Biomedical
    Ultrasound
University of Rochester Medical Center
Rochester, New York

Thomas Ray Sanchez, MD
Pediatric Radiologist
Sutter Medical Group
Sacramento, California

Michael A. Schick, DO, MA, DIMPH, FACEP
Associate Professor
Director of Technology-Enabled Active Learning
Emergency Medicine
UC Davis Health
Sacramento, California

J. Anthony Seibert, PhD
Professor
Radiology
UC Davis Health
Sacramento, California

Simran Sekhon, MBBS
Department of Radiology
UC Davis Health
Sacramento, California

Siobhan Smith, MD
Director or Emergency Ultrasound
Department of Emergency Medicine
Kaiser Permanente Medical Group, Redwood City, CA

Zachary P. Soucy, DO, FAAEM, FACEP
Assistant Professor
Section of Emergency Medicine
Director
Emergency Ultrasound and EUS Fellowship
Dartmouth-Hitchcock Medical Center
Lebanon, New Hampshire

Rebecca Stein-Wexler, MD
Professor and Section Chief
Pediatric Radiology
Director
Global Radiology Education and Outreach
Department of Radiology
UC Davis Health
Sacramento, CA

Jeffrey L. Tanji, MD
Associate Medical Director
Sports Medicine
Orthopaedics
UC Davis Health
Sacramento, California

Leigha J. Winters
Ultrasound Fellow
Emergency Medicine
UC Davis Health
Sacramento, California

Jay Yeh, MD
Associate Professor
Medical Director
Pediatric Echocardiography
UC Davis Health
Sacramento, California

CONTENTS

VIDEO CONTENTS

Principle of Ultrasound

Physics of Ultrasound

J. Anthony Seibert

Imaging systems using ultrasound have attained a large presence as point-of-care (PoC) devices across many clinical domains over the past 10 years. The success of ultrasound for this purpose is attributed to several characteristics, including the low cost and portability of ultrasound devices, the nonionizing nature of ultrasound waves, and the ability to produce real-time images of the acoustic properties of the tissues and tissue structures in the body to deliver timely patient care, among many positive attributes. An understanding of the basic physics of ultrasound, in addition to hands-on training, practice, and development of experience are of great importance in its effective and safe use. This chapter describes the characteristics, properties, and production of ultrasound; interaction with tissues, acquisition, processing, and display of the ultrasound image; the instrumentation; achievable measurements, including blood velocity; and safety issues.

CHARACTERISTICS OF SOUND

Sound is mechanical energy that propagates through a continuous, elastic medium by the compression (high pressure) and rarefaction (low pressure) of particles that comprise it. Compression is caused by a mechanical inward deformation by an external force, such as an expanding and contracting transducer crystal composed of multiple elements in contact with the medium. During transducer surface expansion, an increase in the local pressure at contact occurs. Contraction of the crystal follows, causing a decrease in pressure. The mechanical energy imparted at the surface is transferred to adjacent particles of the medium, which travels at the speed of sound through the medium. Continuous expansion and contraction of the crystal surface by an external power source introduces energy into the medium as a series of compressions and rarefactions, traveling as a wave front in the direction of travel, known as a *longitudinal wave*, as shown in Fig. 1.1.

Wavelength, Frequency, Speed

The *wavelength* (λ) is the distance between any two repeating points on the wave (a cycle), typically measured in millimeters (mm). The *frequency* (*f*) is the number of times the wave repeats per second (s), also defined in hertz (Hz), where 1 Hz = 1 cycle/s. Frequency identifies the category of sound: less than 15 Hz is infrasound, 15 Hz to 20,000 Hz (20 kHz) is audible sound, and above 20 kHz is ultrasound. Medical ultrasound typically uses frequencies in the million cycles/*s* megahertz (MHz) range, from 1 to 15 MHz, with some specialized ultrasound applications beyond 50 MHz. The period is the time duration of one wave cycle and is equal to $1/f$. The *speed of sound, c,* is the distance traveled per unit time through a medium and is equal to the wavelength (distance) divided by the period (time). As frequency is inversely equal to the period, the product of wavelength and frequency is equal to the speed of sound, $c = \lambda f$. The speed of sound varies substantially for different materials, based on compressibility, stiffness, and density characteristics of the medium. For instance, air is highly compressible and of low density, with a relatively low speed of sound; bone is stiff and dense, with a relatively very high speed of sound; and soft tissues have compressibility and density characteristics with intermediate speeds, as listed in Table 1.1. Of importance are the average speeds for "soft tissue" (1540 m/s), fatty tissue (1450 m/s), and air (330 m/s). To relate time with depth

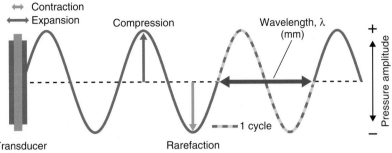

Fig. 1.1 Mechanical energy is generated from an expanding and contracting crystal in contact with a medium, introducing high-pressure (compression) and low-pressure (rarefaction) variations of the constituent particles that transfer the energy to adjacent particles as a longitudinal wave.

TABLE 1.1 Density, Speed of Sound, and Acoustic Impedance for Tissues and Materials Relevant to Medical Ultrasound			
Material	**Density (kg/m³)**	**c (m/s)**	**Z (rayls)***
Air	1.2	330	3.96×10^2
Lung	300	600	1.80×10^3
Fat	924	1450	1.34×10^6
Water	1000	1480	1.48×10^6
"Soft tissue"	1050	1540	1.62×10^6
Kidney	1041	1565	1.63×10^6
Blood	1058	1560	1.65×10^6
Liver	1061	1555	1.65×10^6
Muscle	1068	1600	1.71×10^6
Skull bone	1912	4080	7.8×10^6
PZT	7500	4000	3.0×10^7

*Acoustic impedance is the product of density and speed of sound. The rayl is the named unit, with base units of kg/m²/s. Acoustic impedance directly relates to the propagation characteristics of ultrasound in a given medium and between media.

interactions in the patient, medical ultrasound devices assume a speed of sound of 1540 m/s, despite slight differences in actual speed for the various tissues encountered. Changes in the speed of sound can affect how ultrasound travels through the tissues and may result in unexpected artifacts (see Chapter 2 on speed artifact and refraction artifact). The product of the density and speed of sound is known as the *acoustic impedance*. This characteristic of the tissues is intrinsic in the generation of ultrasound echoes, which return to the transducer to create the ultrasound image. More detail is in the next section on ultrasound interactions.

In a homogeneous medium, ultrasound frequency and speed of sound are constant. When higher ultrasound frequency is selected, the wavelength becomes shorter, giving better detail and spatial resolution along the direction of propagation. For instance, in soft tissue with a speed of 1540 m/s, a 5-MHz frequency has a wavelength in tissue of $\lambda = c / f$; 1540 m/s ÷ 5,000,000/s = 0.00031 m = 0.31 mm. A 10-MHz frequency has a wavelength = 0.15 mm (Fig. 1.2). Although higher frequencies provide better resolution, they are also more readily attenuated, and depth penetration can be inadequate for certain examinations, such as for the heart and abdomen.

Intensity

The amount of ultrasound energy imparted to the medium is dependent on the pressure amplitude variations generated by the degree of transducer expansion and contraction, controlled by the transmit gain applied to a transducer. Power is the amount of energy per unit time introduced into the medium, measured in milliwatts (mW). Intensity is the concentration of the power per unit area in the ultrasound beam, typically expressed in mW/cm². Signals used for creating images are derived from ultrasound interactions in the tissues and the returning intensity of the produced echoes. Absolute intensity depends on the method of ultrasound production and can result in heating or mechanical disruption of tissues, as discussed later in this chapter.

INTERACTIONS OF ULTRASOUND WITH TISSUES

Interactions of ultrasound are chiefly based on the acoustic impedance of tissues and result in reflection, refraction, scattering, and absorption of the ultrasound energy.

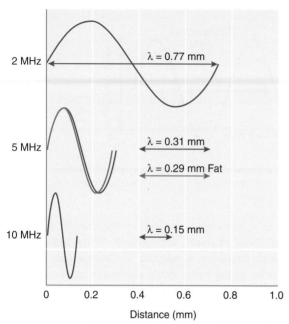

2 MHz
λ = 0.77 mm

5 MHz
λ = 0.31 mm
λ = 0.29 mm Fat

10 MHz
λ = 0.15 mm

Distance (mm)

Fig. 1.2 Wavelength and frequency are inversely proportional, determined by the speed of sound in the medium. For soft tissue, with an average speed of 1540 m/s, the wavelength is directly calculated as the speed of sound divided by the frequency in cycles/s. As frequency remains constant in different media, wavelength must change. Shown is the wavelength for a 5-MHz frequency in fat (red line), with a speed of sound of 1450 m/s.

Acoustic Impedance

Acoustic impedance, Z, is a measure of tissue stiffness and flexibility, equal to the product of the density and speed of sound: $Z = \varrho c$, where ϱ is the density in kg/m^3 and c is the speed of sound in *m/s,* with the combined units given the name *rayl,* where 1 rayl is equal to 1 kg/(m^{2}s). Air, soft tissues, and bone represent the typical low, medium, and high ranges of acoustic impedance values encountered in the patient, as listed in Table 1.1. The efficiency of sound energy transfer from one tissue to another is largely based on the differences in acoustic impedance—if impedances are similar, a large fraction of the incident intensity at the boundary interface will be transmitted, and if the impedances are largely different, most will be reflected. In most soft tissues, these differences are typically small, allowing for ultrasound travel to large depths in the patient.

Reflection

Reflection occurs when a beam is traveling perpendicular (at normal incidence or 90 degrees) to the boundary between two tissues that have a difference in acoustic impedance (Fig. 1.3A). The fraction of incident intensity I_i reflected back to the transducer (I_r) is the intensity reflection coefficient, R_I, calculated as

$$R_I = \frac{I_r}{I_i} = \left(\frac{Z_2 - Z_1}{Z_2 + Z_1}\right)^2$$

The subscripts 1 and 2 represent tissues that are proximal and distal to the boundary. The intensity transmission coefficient, T_I, is defined as the fraction of the incident intensity that is transmitted across an interface, equal to $T_I = 1 - R_I$. For a fat–muscle interface, the intensity reflection and transmission coefficients are calculated as

$$R_{I,\,(Fat \to Muscle)} = \frac{I_r}{I_i} = \left(\frac{1.71 - 1.34}{1.71 + 1.34}\right)^2 = 0.015\,;$$

$$T_{I,\,(Fat \to Muscle)} = 1 - R_{I,\,(Fat \to Muscle)} = 0.985$$

A high fraction of ultrasound intensity is transmitted at tissue boundaries for tissues that have similar acoustic impedance. For tissues with large differences of acoustic impedance, such as air-to-tissue or tissue-to-bone boundaries, most of the intensity is reflected, with no further propagation of the ultrasound pulse. At a muscle–air interface, nearly 100% of incident intensity is reflected, making anatomy unobservable beyond an air-filled cavity. Acoustic coupling gel placed between the transducer and the patient's skin is a critical part of the standard ultrasound imaging procedure to ensure good transducer coupling and to eliminate air pockets that would reflect the ultrasound. For imaging beyond lung structures, avoidance of the ribs and presence of a "tissue conduit" are necessary to achieve propagation of the pulse. When an ultrasound pulse is incident on a tissue boundary at an angle other than 90 degrees (normal incidence), the reflected ultrasound echo is directed away from the transducer and does not generate a signal.

Refraction

Refraction is a change in direction of the transmitted ultrasound pulse when the incident pulse is not perpendicular to the tissue boundary and the speeds of sound in the two tissues are different. The frequency does not change, but the ultrasound wavelength changes at the boundary due to the speed change, resulting in a redirection of the transmitted pulse, as shown in Fig. 1.3B. The angle of redirection

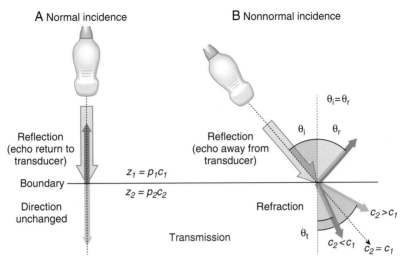

Fig. 1.3 A boundary separating two tissues with different acoustic impedances demonstrates (A) perpendicular (normal) incidence of an ultrasound wave with reflection of an echo back to the source (transducer) and transmission to greater depths in a straight line and (B) incidence of the wave at a nonperpendicular angle, with the incident angle measured relative to the normal incidence and the reflected echo at an angle opposite but equal to the incident angle. The transmitted ultrasound wave is refracted if the speed of sound is different in the two tissues, with the angle of refraction also referenced to the normal direction. Refraction angle depends on the relative speed differences and the change in the wavelength at the boundary.

is dependent on the change in wavelength; no refraction occurs when the speed of sound is the same in the two tissues or with perpendicular incidence. Because a straight-line propagation of the ultrasound pulse is assumed, misplacement of anatomy can result when refraction occurs. See Chapter 2 on ultrasound artifacts for further discussion and manifestation of this type of artifact.

Scattering

Scattering arises from objects and interfaces within a tissue that are about the size of the ultrasound wavelength or smaller. At low frequencies (1–5 MHz), wavelengths are relatively large, and tissue boundaries appear smooth or specular (mirror-like). A *specular reflector* is a smooth boundary between two media. At higher frequencies (5–15 MHz), wavelengths are smaller, and boundaries become less smooth, causing echo reflection in many directions. A *nonspecular reflector* represents a boundary that presents many different angles to the ultrasound beam, and returning echoes have significantly less intensity (Fig. 1.4). Many organs can be identified by a defined "signature" caused by intrinsic structures that produce variations in the returning scatter intensity. Scatter amplitude differences from one tissue region to

Boundary interactions

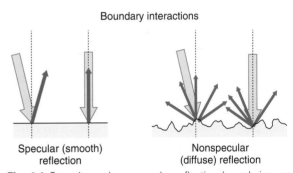

Fig. 1.4 Specular and nonspecular reflection boundaries are chiefly dependent on wavelength of the ultrasound beam and therefore frequency. Higher-frequency operation generates shorter wavelengths that are about the same size as the boundary variations, leading to nonspecular interactions and diffuse reflection patterns.

another result in corresponding brightness changes on the ultrasound display. In general, the echo signal amplitude from a tissue or material depends on the number of scatterers per unit volume, the acoustic impedance differences at interfaces, the sizes of the scatterers, and the ultrasound frequency. Higher scatter amplitude tissues are called *hyperechoic,* and lower scatter amplitude tissues are called *hypoechoic* relative to the average background signal. Scattered echo signals are more prevalent relative to specular echo signals when using higher ultrasound frequencies.

Absorption and Attenuation

Attenuation is the loss of intensity with distance traveled, caused by scattering and absorption of the incident beam. Scattering has a strong dependence on increasing ultrasound frequency. Absorption occurs by transferring energy to the tissues that result in heating or mechanical disruption of the tissue structure. The combined effects of scattering and absorption result in exponential attenuation of ultrasound intensity with distance travelled as a function of increasing frequency. When expressed in decibels (dB), a logarithmic measure of intensity, attenuation in dB/cm linearly increases with ultrasound frequency. An approximate rule of thumb for ultrasound attenuation average in soft tissue is 0.5 dB/cm times the frequency in MHz. Compared with a 1-MHz beam, a 2-MHz beam will have approximately twice the attenuation, a 5-MHz beam will have *five times* the attenuation, and a 10-MHz beam will have *ten times* the attenuation *per unit distance traveled.* Therefore higher-frequency ultrasound beams have a rapidly diminishing penetration depth (Fig. 1.5), so careful selection of the transducer frequency must be made in the context of the imaging depth needed. The loss of ultrasound intensity in decibels can be determined empirically for different tissues by measuring as a function of distance travelled in centimeters (cm) and is the attenuation coefficient, μ, expressed in dB/cm. For a given ultrasound frequency, tissues and fluids have widely varying attenuation coefficients chiefly resulting from structural and density differences, as indicated in Table 1.2 for a 1-MHz ultrasound beam.

THE ULTRASOUND SYSTEM

PoC ultrasound systems are available from many vendors and come with different features and options, which depend on acquisition capabilities, number of transducer probes, durability, software functionality, size and weight, battery longevity for handheld units, power requirements, and other considerations. Although all ultrasound systems have unique instrumentation, software, and user interfaces, common components include transducer probes, pulser, beam former, scan converter, processor, display, and user interface for instrumentation adjustments and controls.

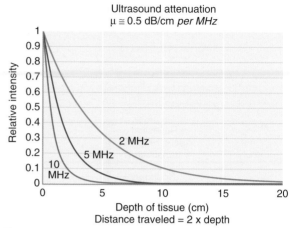

Fig. 1.5 Attenuation and relative intensity of ultrasound remaining as a function of depth for 2-, 5-, and 10-MHz beams.

TABLE 1.2 Attenuation Coefficient μ (dB/cm-MHz) for Tissues*	
Tissue	**μ (1 MHz)**
Air	1.64
Blood	0.2
Bone	7–10
Brain	0.6
Cardiac	0.52
Connective tissue	1.57
Fat	0.48
Liver	0.5
Muscle	1.09
Tendon	4.7
Soft tissue (average)	**0.54**
Water	0.0022

*For higher-frequency operation, multiply the attenuation coefficient by the frequency in MHz.

Ultrasound Transducer Operation and Beam Properties

Ultrasound is produced and detected with a *transducer array,* composed of hundreds of ceramic elements with electromechanical (piezoelectric) properties. Ultrasound transducers for medical imaging applications employ a synthetic piezoelectric ceramic, *lead–zirconate–titanate* (PZT), with a crystal structure that generates a surface charge of either negative or positive polarity when its thickness is expanded under negative pressure or

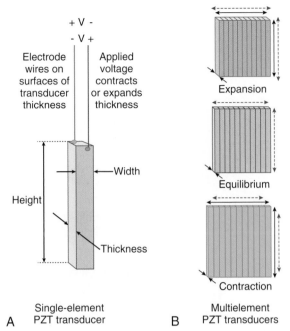

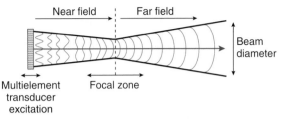

Fig. 1.7 The ultrasound beam from a surface vibration has a converging section known as the *near field*, a diverging section known as the *far field*, and a focal zone with a minimum beam diameter. In this situation, each transducer element is activated simultaneously. The perspective is looking down on the top edge of the transducer multielement array surface.

Fig. 1.6 (A) A single-element transducer is made of a synthetic lead–zirconate–titanate (*PZT*) crystal with an internal electrical dipole molecular structure that expands and contracts in thickness mode under a voltage applied to the surfaces via attached electrodes. (B) Grouped transducer elements create a surface to expand and contract in the thickness direction of the transducer crystal to introduce mechanical energy into tissues adjacent to the surface.

compressed under positive pressure due to the internal molecular crystal polarity. Surface electrodes and wires are attached to each element and multiplexed to a transmit/receive sensor that measures the surface charge variation when sensing any thickness variations. These same wires and attached electrodes generate mechanical expansion or contraction by applying a voltage of known polarity and amplitude from an external power source, as illustrated in Fig. 1.6A. By varying the applied voltage polarity at a known frequency, the crystal expands and contracts, imparting mechanical energy into the adjacent medium at the same frequency. Thus each transducer element functions either in an excitation mode to transmit ultrasound energy or in a reception mode to receive ultrasound energy. In practice, a subset of elements in a linear transducer array, or all elements in a phased transducer array, are activated, as shown in Fig. 1.6B, to create an ultrasound beam.

The surface vibration and interaction among the individual elements create a collimated beam converging in the near field with a minimum beam diameter at the focal zone depth and, with further travel, diverging into the far field, as shown in Fig. 1.7. The focal zone depth can be adjusted by introducing brief timing delays of the individual element arrays, as discussed later.

Ultrasound systems have transducer assemblies of many shapes and sizes composed of an array of PZT elements (typically 64–512) categorized into linear and phased array operation. Common to all transducers are a protective housing with a shield to prevent electrical interference, an acoustic damping block to shorten the vibrations of the piezoelectric elements, a matching layer to improve the efficiency of ultrasound wave transmission to the skin by reducing acoustic impedance differences, and a material to absorb backward-directed ultrasound energy (Fig. 1.8A).

Because the transducer array cannot simultaneously generate and detect ultrasound, a short ultrasound pulse is created in the transmit mode with a large applied voltage of 100 to 150 volts (V) with a duration equal to about a millionth of a second (1 μs), causing contraction of the transducer elements. Vibration of the crystal occurs at a natural resonance frequency dependent on its element thickness. A short ultrasound pulse is created by the attached damping block, as shown in Fig. 1.8B, which introduces a wide band of higher and lower frequencies, so that most transducers can operate at multiple transmit and receive frequencies. Immediately after excitation, the transducer elements are switched to receive mode to detect the returning ultrasound echoes generated by reflections from tissue boundaries. A receive multiplexer sensor in the ultrasound unit records the voltage signals as a function of time for further processing. Once all echoes are received from the transmit

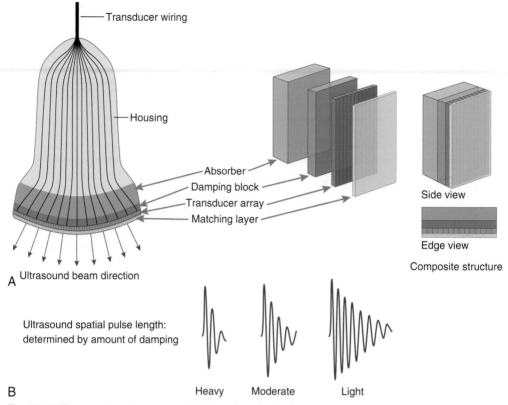

Fig. 1.8 (A) The transducer is composed of a housing, electrical insulation, and a composite of active element layers, including the PZT crystal, damping block and absorbing material on the backside, and a matching layer on the front side of the multielement array. (B) The ultrasound spatial pulse length is based on the damping material causing a ring-down of the element vibration. For imaging, a pulse of two to three cycles is typical, with a broad-frequency bandwidth, whereas for Doppler transducer elements, less damping provides a narrow-frequency bandwidth.

pulse, the process repeats along a slightly different direction to ultimately cover the volume of interest defined by the field of view (FOV).

For a given transducer, multifrequency operation allows flexibility of the sonographer to interactively choose the appropriate frequency to emphasize the spatial resolution or depth of penetration based on the examination, as shown in Fig. 1.9.

Transducer Arrays

Three basic transducer types for PoC ultrasound include linear, curvilinear, and phased arrays, as shown in Fig. 1.10. *Linear array* transducers activate a subset of elements, producing a single transmit beam at one location, and then listen for echoes in the receive mode. Within a fraction of a second, when all echoes are received from the greatest depths, the next pulse is created by activating another subelement group that is incrementally shifted along the transducer array, and the process repeats on the order of thousands of times per second to generate a rectangular image format with real-time video image capture. Linear arrays are typically composed of 256 to 512 transducer elements, are of smaller form factor, and generally operate at higher frequency ranges (5–15 MHz). Because of the higher operating frequency and limited FOV, these transducers are suitable for imaging superficial structures such as the eyes, joints, muscles, and proximal blood vessels and for performing ultrasound-guided procedures. *Curvilinear array* transducers have 256 to 512 elements in a convex geometry, with a subset of elements activated sequentially, like the linear array, producing a trapezoidal

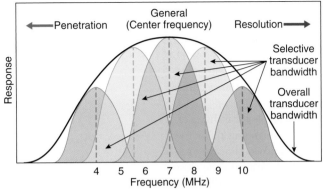

Fig. 1.9 Multifrequency transducer transmit and receive response to operational frequency bandwidths allows the operator to select an appropriate transmit and receive frequency, depending on the type of examination, type of transducer, transducer bandwidth range, and need for penetration depth (selecting a lower frequency) or spatial resolution (selecting a higher frequency). The transducer response shown has a selectable frequency range of 4 to 10 MHz.

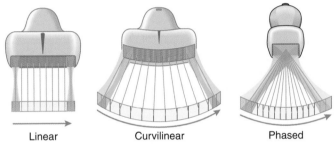

Fig. 1.10 Linear and curvilinear array transducers activate a subgroup of transducer elements, whereas phased array transducers activate all elements in the array to create a single ultrasound beam in the tissues. Rectangular, trapezoid, and sector beam areas are created, respectively. Location of the beam for linear and curvilinear operation is determined by the active element subgroup across the array, and for the phased array operation by electronic steering of the ultrasound beam. The beam sequentially moves across the field of view in one direction to produce one image frame and then repeats for real-time acquisition. This figure illustrates only a fraction of the actual number of lines acquired during acquisition.

image format with increased FOV at both proximal and distal depths. These transducers are ideal for imaging intraabdominal organs such as the liver, spleen, kidneys, and bladder. Lower frequencies (2–5 MHz) are used for depth visualization, but spatial resolution can be limited as a result. *Phased array* transducers with 64, 128, and up to 256 elements use all transducer elements in the formation of the ultrasound beam. Beam direction is determined by relatively large incremental delays for sequential excitation of elements from one side of the array to the other, effectively steering the beam in a perpendicular direction to the excitation pattern. Along a given direction, small incremental excitation delays in a concave pattern focus the beam diameter

at a predetermined depth (or depths), which is operator selectable. After excitation, beam direction, and beam formation, the phased array is placed in receive mode to listen for echoes. The sequence then repeats along a slightly different beam direction, ultimately creating a sector-shaped image format at a frame rate dependent on the number of lines, depth, and FOV. In the receive mode, returning echoes are detected by all active transducer elements used in the formation of the beam. Phased array transducers typically operate at low frequencies (1–5 MHz), have flexible selection of a narrow to wide FOV by the operator, and provide efficient two-dimensional (2D) imaging for heart and thoracic imaging requiring small acoustic windows.

Intracavitary array probes (not shown) have a convex, small footprint and operate like a linear transducer. Because of the proximity of the region to be imaged, a high-frequency range is typically used (5–8 MHz), with a wide FOV and limited range but excellent image resolution. These transducers are used in transvaginal, transrectal, and intraoral applications.

Transmit beam focusing at selectable focal distances is achieved by specific timing delays among the active transducer elements, each with a known concave excitation profile, as shown in Fig. 1.11. A focal zone close to the transducer surface is produced by initially firing the outer transducer elements in the active array and incrementally firing the inner elements to the center element with slightly longer delays using a concave excitation pattern. A more distant focal zone is achieved by reducing the delay time differences among the transducer elements with a shallow concave excitation pattern, resulting in beam convergence at a greater depth. The *beam former* in the ultrasound unit controls the excitation patterns, with the focal zone depth selectable by the operator. On some advanced ultrasound systems, multiple transmit focal zones can be selected by repeating the excitation pattern for each focal zone and melding the information from each focal zone into a composite image. This does reduce the acquisition frame rate by a factor equal to the number of focal zones set.

Spatial Resolution

In ultrasound, the visibility of image detail is determined by three separate factors: (1) in-plane resolution along the direction of beam travel, known as *axial resolution*; (2) in-plane resolution perpendicular to the direction of beam travel, known as *lateral resolution*; and (3) out-of-plane resolution perpendicular to the in-plane resolution, known as *elevational* or *slice-thickness resolution*. These constituents of spatial resolution are illustrated in Fig. 1.12.

Axial resolution represents the ability to distinctly separate closely spaced objects in the direction of the ultrasound beam. Returning echoes from adjacent boundaries to be resolved as separate are dependent on the spatial pulse length (SPL), which is the average wavelength times the number of cycles in the pulse. Because distance travelled for a pulse-echo interacting between two adjacent reflectors is twice the separation distance, echoes to be recorded as separate signals need a spacing just greater than one-half SPL. For example, a 5-MHz frequency pulse has a wavelength of 0.31 mm in

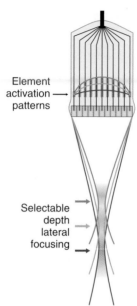

Element activation patterns

Selectable depth lateral focusing

Fig. 1.11 Focal zones can be produced at various depths in tissues by controlling the excitation timing of the transducers in a group. Shown are three different focal zones produced by the system "beam former" to activate the outer elements first, followed by successive activation of the inner elements to produce a concave excitation of the individual ultrasound pulses. This is achievable for the element subgroups in a linear/curvilinear array, as well as for all the elements in a phased array transducer.

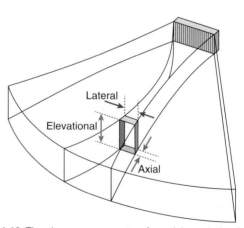

Lateral

Elevational

Axial

Fig. 1.12 The three components of spatial resolution in the ultrasound image are shown. *Axial*, along the beam direction, is constant with depth. *Lateral*, in-plane and perpendicular to the beam direction, varies substantially with depth. *Elevational*, perpendicular to the lateral and axial directions, is the slice thickness and varies with depth.

soft tissue, consisting of three cycles. The SPL is 3×0.31 = 0.93 mm, and the axial resolution is ½(0.93 mm) = 0.46 mm. A 10-MHz frequency pulse with three cycles has SPL = 0.46 mm, with axial resolution of ½(0.46) = 0.23 mm. Axial resolution is independent of depth. To achieve enhanced axial resolution, use of a higher-frequency transducer operation can be selected, but penetration depth may be compromised and inadequate.

Lateral resolution refers to the ability to resolve objects of a given size perpendicular to the beam direction and is directly dependent on the beam diameter, which varies as a function of depth and is best within the focal zone. Lateral resolution worsens proximal and distal to the focal zone. The operator can adjust the lateral focal zone typically to one depth, and in some higher-end systems at several depths within the image; however, the trade-off is a loss of temporal resolution or number of scan lines per image. Lateral resolution is typically two to three times less than axial resolution.

Elevational resolution indicates the ability to distinctly resolve acoustically generated objects represented in the slice-thickness dimension of the image, which is perpendicular to the displayed image plane. In this dimension, the beam thickness varies like the lateral beam dimension, where close to the transducer the beam thickness is large, converges over a region at mid-depth, and then diverges with continued propagation. Volume averaging causes objects close to the transducer surface or at greater depths to be not as well depicted. Slice thickness is typically the weakest measure of resolution for array transducers. The ability to vary elevational resolution is possible with sophisticated transducers, not usually found for PoC ultrasound systems.

ULTRASOUND DATA ACQUISITION

Data acquisition and image formation occur in a pulse–echo mode and are operationally dependent on creating an ultrasound pulse, listening for echoes, and constantly repeating the procedure over the acquisition event. The ultrasound pulse is intermittently produced by activating transducer elements at a rate known as the *pulse repetition frequency (PRF),* equal to the number of pulses produced per second. For data acquisition and imaging, the PRF typically ranges from 1000 to 5000 pulses/s (1–5 kHz), depending on the application, depth of echoes to be recorded, and frame rate desired, among other parameters. Usually, the PRF is automatically determined and

is dependent on the maximum image depth. Between pulses is the pulse repetition period (PRP), equal to 1/PRF, and is the time that the transducer is in receive mode to listen for returning echoes. A 2-kHz PRF has a PRP = 1/2000 s^{-1} = 0.0005 s = 0.5 ms. Within this time, an ultrasound pulse in tissue can propagate to a depth of 38.5 cm and return as an echo to the transducer before the next pulse. Thus the maximum PRF is determined by the time required for echoes from the most distant structures to reach the transducer; otherwise, these echoes can be confused with prompt echoes from the next pulse, resulting in range ambiguity artifact. Higher transducer frequencies with greater attenuation and limited penetration depth allow higher PRFs. The PRF determines the trade-off of image frame rate (temporal resolution) versus image quality (number of lines/frame) and is particularly important in Doppler ultrasound, as there is a direct effect on the sampling rate to accurately determine the velocity of moving objects (see the section below on Doppler ultrasound).

Hardware Components and Data Processing

Acquisition of ultrasound data involves several hardware components: pulser, beam former, transmit/receive switch, receivers, amplifiers, and scan converter, as shown in Fig. 1.13. The *pulser* (also known as the

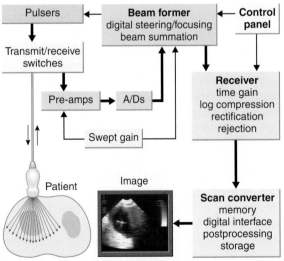

Fig. 1.13 Components of an ultrasound system needed to acquire ultrasound image data is shown. The grayscale image is created from returning echoes detected as a function of time and ultrasound beam direction from A-mode data, converted to B-mode, digitized, and mapped into a 2D digital image matrix.

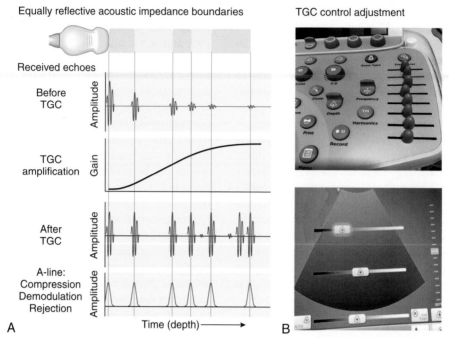

Equally reflective acoustic impedance boundaries

TGC control adjustment

Received echoes

Before TGC — Amplitude

TGC amplification — Gain

After TGC — Amplitude

A-line: Compression Demodulation Rejection — Amplitude

Time (depth) ⟶

A   B

Fig. 1.14 (A) Time gain compensation (*TGC*) is a user adjustment to make equally reflective boundaries appear with the same amplitude, despite attenuation with depth. (B) TGC controls are provided as operator slider bars on the console, electronic sliders on the video monitor, or other methods that allow image gain adjustments at a specific depth.

transmitter) provides the electrical voltage for activating the piezoelectric transducer elements. Transmit power is adjusted by the excitation voltage on the transducer crystal—a higher voltage creates a higher-intensity ultrasound pulse and improves echo detection from weak reflectors but increases power deposition to the patient. Transmit power settings are adjusted for the examination type; for instance, a low power is used for obstetric imaging. *Pulse duration* is the instantaneous "on" time of the ultrasound pulse, on the order of 0.001 ms (one-millionth of a second, or 1 μs). *Duty cycle,* the fraction of the ultrasound beam "on" time, is equal to the pulse duration divided by the PRP and is typically 0.2% to 0.4% for imaging—thus more than 99.5% of ultrasound scan time is spent in the receive mode, listening for returning echoes. The *beam former* provides active beam steering as well as transmit and receive focusing. The *transmit/receive switch* isolates the high voltage (≈150 V) applied to the transducer elements during excitation from extremely low voltages (millivolt to microvolt range) induced by returning echoes. At the initial excitation, a ring-down time, when the PZT

crystals are unable to detect proximal echoes, creates a "dead zone" image region at very shallow depth. For evaluation of surface or near-surface regions of the body, an acoustic stand-off window is often used. The *receiver* accepts data and performs signal processing, including time gain compensation (TGC), dynamic range compression, signal demodulation, and noise rejection. TGC (also described as time-varied gain and depth gain compensation) is a user-adjustable amplification of the returning echo signals as a function of time to compensate for ultrasound attenuation. An ideal adjustment of TGC results in equally reflective boundaries with the same signal amplitude, independent of depth, as shown in Fig. 1.14A. Depending on equipment, user adjustment occurs with multiple slider potentiometers designated for a certain image depth (Fig. 1.14B) or by TGC controllers to manipulate initial gain, slope, and far gain of the echo signals. Subsequent processing steps include signal compression, rectification, demodulation, and noise rejection. The output is an amplitude-modulated (A-mode) line of data representing a time sequence of detected echoes.

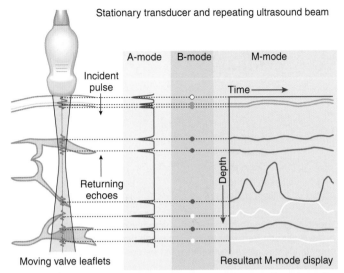

Stationary transducer and repeating ultrasound beam

Fig. 1.15 Time–motion mode ultrasound operation is used for the evaluation of moving anatomy, such as valve leaflets. A stationary transducer and repeating pulse-echo beam that insonates the same area is used to create the M-mode trace of motion that provides analysis of periodic and aperiodic motion.

The scan converter, image memory, and display monitor are required to process A-mode line data into a brightness (B-mode) signal to create time–motion (T-M or M-mode) and grayscale image (B-scan) outputs. B-mode represents the echo amplitudes converted into proportional brightness-modulated dots as a function of depth (time) along the A-line trajectory. M-mode uses a stationary transducer positioned over moving anatomy, such as valve leaflets, where motion in the ultrasound beam is tracked by location of B-mode brightness dots, recorded as a function of depth (vertical position) and time (horizontal deflection) of the traces to enable diagnosis of periodic or aperiodic motion, as illustrated in Fig. 1.15.

Two-dimensional grayscale images are constructed by identifying beam directions relative to the transducer position with the scan converter and mapping B-mode data to build an image in computer memory for display on the device monitor. Digital processing is subsequently applied, with application of a variety of electronic and mathematical functions, including gain, window width and window level adjustment, edge enhancement, noise reduction, and data interpolation for diverging beams, among other schemes. Each image is typically rendered into a 512 × 512 × 8 bit (1 byte) per pixel matrix, equal to ¼ megabyte (MB). For color encoding, the bit depth

is usually 24 bits (3 bytes), with each byte encoding for red, green, and blue color combinations, and an uncompressed size of ¾ MB. Image compression schemes such as JPEG and MPEG are often used in the final output image or image stream to substantially reduce the overall size of the image data.

Time for a single ultrasound image is determined by the number (N) of A-lines acquired across the FOV (the line density) and the PRF/PRP (governed by the needed depth of penetration). These parameters are part of acquisition protocols and can be directly or indirectly changed by operator adjustments. Protocols represent a decision of diagnostic need in terms of temporal resolution versus image quality. For instance, if high frame rates are needed, the number of A-lines, FOV, or penetration depth (with high-frequency operation to allow a higher PRF) can be reduced. When image quality is more important, line density (number of A-lines sampled across the FOV) is increased, with a loss of frame rate. Insufficient line density can cause the image to appear pixelated, which is caused by interpolation of several pixels to fill unscanned image regions. For sector and trapezoidal scans, increased line spacing with depth also results in decreased image quality. Increasing the number of A-lines sampled over a specified FOV or reducing the FOV for the same

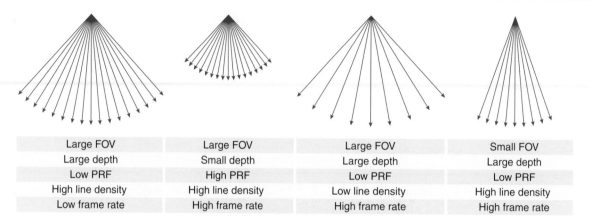

Large FOV	Large FOV	Large FOV	Small FOV
Large depth	Small depth	Large depth	Large depth
Low PRF	High PRF	Low PRF	Low PRF
High line density	High line density	Low line density	High line density
Low frame rate	High frame rate	High frame rate	High frame rate

Fig. 1.16 Factors determining the trade-off between image quality and temporal resolution are field of view, penetration depth, pulse repetition frequency/pulse repetition period, and ultrasound line density, as shown. Examination requirements identify parameters that must be considered when designing an acquisition protocol.

number of lines can achieve adequate line density. These trade-offs are illustrated in Fig. 1.16 for a sector scan. On advanced systems, multiple lateral focal zones that can be set by the operator provide better lateral depth resolution, but at the loss of frame rate and temporal resolution. Ultrasound image rates from 10 to up to 60 frames per second (and higher for specialized ultrasound equipment) are typically achieved, with trade-offs of image quality versus temporal resolution that must be considered, given the requirements of the examination.

Specialized Acquisition Modes

Spatial compounding is an option on many PoC ultrasound systems to obtain ultrasound data from several different angles of insonation (typically from 3 to 5), which are subsequently combined to produce a single image, as shown in Fig. 1.17. As each image is produced from data derived from multiple beam angles, the probability of perpendicular incidence to a boundary reflector is increased, providing better boundary definition, more continuity with curved structures, and improved signal-to-noise ratio due to data averaging. A downside to spatial compounding is the loss of temporal resolution frame rate by a factor equal to the number of insonation angles and the loss of spatial resolution when moving anatomy is present in the scan. Spatial compounding is less useful for imaging situations that have substantial voluntary or involuntary patient motion.

Harmonic imaging is a method that uses higher frequencies generated by nonlinear propagation of ultrasound in tissues to introduce harmonics, which are integer multiples (e.g., 2×, 3×) of the incident frequency. A distortion of the wave occurs as the high-pressure compression part of the wave travels faster than the low-pressure rarefaction, introducing higher-order frequency harmonics that localize in the central area of the low frequency beam, as shown in Fig. 1.18. Reflected echoes of the harmonic frequencies (typically the second harmonic) are detected by use of a multifrequency transducer set to the higher frequency. For instance, a transmit frequency of 2 MHz (3 MHz) has the receive frequency tuned to 4 MHz (6 MHz). This reduces low-frequency echo clutter occurring in the shallow regions of the image and benefits from improved axial resolution due to higher-frequency returning echoes. As the harmonic frequencies are concentrated in the central area of the beam, lateral resolution is also improved by the smaller effective beam diameter. Although not always advantageous, native tissue harmonic imaging is best applied in exams requiring a lower transmit transducer frequency for depth penetration, allowing for the harmonics to build and return as a higher-frequency harmonic echo, but without too much attenuation returning to the transducer. With the receiver frequency switched to the higher-frequency harmonic, the outcome is improved spatial resolution and substantially less clutter from proximal low-frequency echoes (Fig. 1.19).

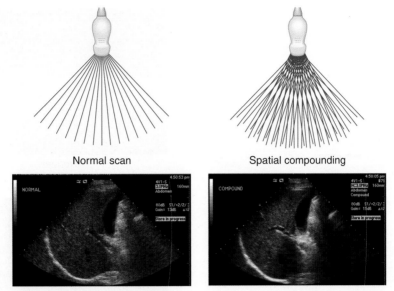

Fig. 1.17 Spatial compounding is applied to linear, curvilinear, and phased array transducer acquisitions by transmitting ultrasound into the tissues at slightly different angles to increase reception of returning echoes from otherwise nonperpendicular boundaries and decreasing image noise by averaging the results.

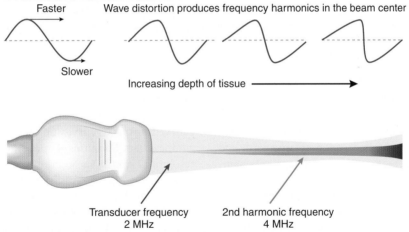

Fig. 1.18 Harmonic ultrasound frequencies are introduced into tissue, with the distortion of the ultrasound wave resulting from the compression traveling faster than the rarefaction. Harmonic frequencies build up in the center of the beam with travel distance, shown in the lower illustration.

Ultrasound Image Modifications

Grayscale ultrasound images can be modified by window width and window level adjustments at the control panel to nondestructively modify the brightness and contrast of the displayed image, implemented with look-up-table (LUT) transformations. The pixel density can limit the quality and resolution of the displayed image. A "zoom" feature on many ultrasound instruments can

enhance the image to delineate details within the image that are otherwise blurred. Two methods, "read" zoom and "write" zoom, are usually available. "Read" zoom enlarges a user-defined region of the stored image and expands the information over a larger number of pixels in the displayed image with replication and interpolation. Even though the displayed region becomes larger, the resolution of the image itself does not change. Using

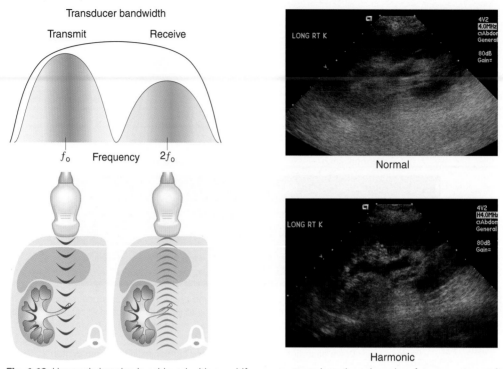

Fig. 1.19 Harmonic imaging is achieved with a multifrequency transducer by using a low-frequency transmit pulse (e.g., 2 MHz) and a higher-order harmonic receive frequency (e.g., 4 MHz). Normal and harmonic images depict the noticeable improvement in image contrast and resolution.

"write" zoom requires the operator to rescan the area of the patient that corresponds to the user-selectable area. When enabled, the transducer scans the selected area; echo data within the limited region are acquired; and line density is increased to improve image data sampling, spatial resolution, and contrast.

Besides the B-mode data used for the 2D image, other information from M-mode and Doppler signal processing (to be discussed) can also be displayed. During operation of the ultrasound scanner, information in the memory is continuously updated in real time. When ultrasound scanning is stopped, the last image acquired is displayed on the screen until ultrasound scanning resumes.

Image Quality

Image quality is dependent on the ultrasound equipment, transducers, frequency, modes of imaging selected, positioning skills of the operator, and acquisition protocols, which should be set with examination-specific needs in mind. The operator has control over equipment parameters such as selection of transducer frequency, ultrasound intensity through transmit gain settings, TGC curves, and noise threshold settings, among others. Measures of image quality include spatial resolution, contrast resolution, image uniformity, and noise characteristics. Additionally, image artifacts can enhance or degrade the diagnostic value of the ultrasound image, as covered in Chapter 2, on ultrasound artifacts. Ultrasound spatial resolution, as previously described, includes axial, lateral, and elevational resolutions. Axial and lateral resolutions are in the plane of the image. Elevational (slice-thickness) resolution, perpendicular to the plane of the image, is not directly discernable. It varies as a function of depth, like lateral resolution, but is typically fixed and not adjustable. Contrast resolution is the ability to discern differences in acoustic impedance that are assigned certain grayscale values as rendered on the display monitor. Degradations can limit contrast, including insufficient signal strength with transmit gain set too low, very large patients, inappropriate TGC adjustments, anatomic

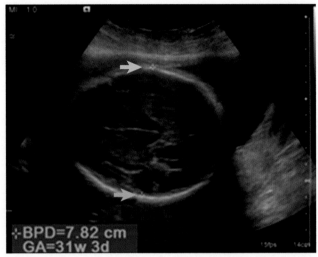

Fig. 1.20 Measurement of the biparietal diameter of a developing fetus, indicating 7.82 cm measurement and gestational age of 31 weeks and 3 days. Notice the caliper markers along the axial direction of the beam. Also note the dropout of the curved surface of the skull due to echoes reflecting away from the transducer.

clutter, excessive electronic noise, transducer element malfunction, image artifacts, display monitor quality/calibration, and room viewing conditions, many of which the operator has no control over. Image noise is chiefly generated by electronic amplification of weaker signals with depth, so deeper anatomic regions have diminished contrast-to-noise ratios. Image processing that specifically reduces noise, such as temporal or spatial averaging, can increase the contrast-to-noise ratio; however, trade-offs include lower frame rates and/or poorer spatial resolution. Spatial compounding better depicts tissue boundaries with multiple-angle incidence of the ultrasound beam and reduces stochastic speckle and electronic noise through averaging. Harmonic imaging improves image contrast by reducing clutter due to low-frequency echoes. Although these and other tools and acquisition modes can assist in delivering the best image quality possible, it is also very important to recognize the limitations that can only be partially mitigated.

Quantitative Ultrasound Measurements

Distance, area, and volume measurements are routinely and accurately performed on calibrated diagnostic ultrasound systems, based on the relationship of ultrasound speed to the round-trip time of the pulse and the echo. From the physics perspective, measurements between points along the direction of the ultrasound beam are usually more reliable because of better axial spatial resolution. Measurement accuracy is improved by careful selection of reference positions, such as the leading edge of the first boundary to the leading edge of the second boundary along the axis of the beam. Along the lateral direction, the echoes are smeared out due to poorer lateral resolution, dependent on the beam diameter at a given depth, with less reproducibility and accuracy. Distance measurements can be extended in a straightforward way to area measurements by assuming a specific geometric shape in the plane of the image. With multiple planar images, area measurements can likewise extend to three-dimensional (3D) volumes by estimating the slice thickness as a function of depth. An example is illustrated in Fig. 1.20 of an obstetric examination and the measurement of biparietal diameter to estimate gestational age based on the age-related values. Ultrasound assumes a speed of 1540 m/s to determine distances and is very accurate in these types of examinations. When the speed of sound is largely different (e.g., in fat and bone) the accuracy of measurements can be compromised, so acknowledgment of these issues is important.

DOPPLER ULTRASOUND

Doppler ultrasound assesses the velocity of moving reflectors, typically blood cells in the vasculature, based on frequency shifts occurring with the incident pulse and returning echo. A familiar analogy is an observer encounter with a train and its whistle that has a high pitch as the train moves toward the person and changes to a low pitch as the train passes and moves away. The approaching sound waves are compressed with motion, resulting in decreased distance between the source and observer, causing a shorter wavelength and higher frequency. The opposite, longer wavelength and lower frequency occur as the sound waves recede from the observer. The magnitude of the frequency shift is dependent on the velocity of the train relative to the observer, and also the angle with respect to the direction of motion.

The Doppler Shift

When an ultrasound wave of known frequency reflects from blood cells in a vessel moving toward the transducer, the echoes have a higher frequency; if moving away from the transducer, they will have a lower frequency, as shown in Fig. 1.21. The frequency shift generated is a fraction of the initial ultrasound (transducer) frequency, proportional to the ratio of the velocity of the blood cells relative to the velocity of the speed of sound. The *Doppler shift*, f_d, is the difference between the incident frequency f_i and reflected frequency f_r from the blood cells for parallel incidence of the blood vessel with the ultrasound beam:

$$f_d = f_i - f_r = \frac{v}{c} \times f_i \times 2$$

where v is the velocity of the blood cells and c is the velocity of ultrasound. The factor of 2 arises to compensate for transmitting the ultrasound and receiving a reflection. As an example, blood cell velocity of 30 cm/s is a tiny fraction of the speed of sound, equal to 154,000 cm/s. For an incident frequency of 4 MHz, the Doppler shift at this specific measurement point in time is calculated as

$$\frac{30}{154,000} \times \left(4 \times 10^6 Hz\right) \times 2 \cong 1558 hz \cong 1.5 kHz.$$

One can hear the frequency shift on an audio speaker, as this is within the audible frequency range. With a periodic heartbeat and pulsatile blood motion, velocity changes can be heard as changes in pitch of the Doppler frequency. If the observation and returning echoes are at an angle relative to the direction of motion, there will be

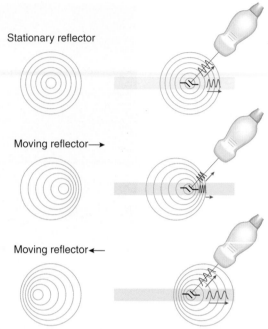

Fig. 1.21 A moving reflector such as a blood cell in a vessel changes the wavelength of the returning echo and thus the frequency, the degree to which is proportional to the velocity of motion and angle of the echo trajectory. For the reflector moving toward the transducer, the wavelength is shortened, and the frequency is increased (*middle*), whereas the opposite occurs for the reflector moving away from the transducer (*bottom*). When at an angle to the reflector motion direction, the measured wavelength (frequency) is not equal to that along the direction of the reflector, except in the case of a stationary reflector, where there is no change in wavelength or frequency (*top*).

a difference in the observed changes in wavelength and therefore frequency, which must be corrected for accurate evaluation of the true blood velocity.

To quantitatively measure blood velocity, a "duplex" mode of operation allows the user to simultaneously perform grayscale B-mode imaging and pulsed Doppler evaluation, the latter with a separate transducer element group within the transducer array. Over a vessel of interest visualized in the image, a user-positioned gate region is located and a Doppler angle, θ, relative to the vessel is determined, as shown in Fig. 1.22. For blood moving toward the transducer, the frequency that is proportional to the velocity vector along the blood vessel axis is greater than the frequency measured along the direction of the Doppler transducer, causing the measured Doppler shift, f_d, to be less by a fraction equal to the cosine of the Doppler angle as

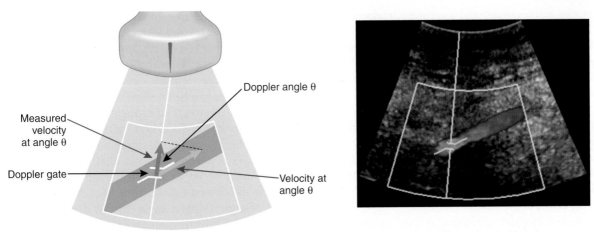

Fig. 1.22 (*Left*) Doppler evaluation of frequency shift associated with blood velocity, illustrating the Doppler gate, the Doppler angle, and the calculated velocity vectors in the direction of blood flow and in the direction of the transducer. (*Right*) Image acquired with duplex acquisition and color flow active area (trapezoidal white boundary, see the text for an explanation) shows the vessel location that aids in placing the Doppler gate.

determined by trigonometry. Thus cos(θ) is the correction to the calculated Doppler shift at an angle other than 0 degrees, resulting in the generalized Doppler shift equation:

$$f_d = \frac{2f_i v \cos(\theta)}{c}$$

Blood velocity is determined by rearranging the equation and solving for v:

$$v = \frac{f_d c}{2f_i \cos(\theta)}$$

where the measured Doppler shift is adjusted by 1/cos(θ). As the Doppler angle increases, the measured Doppler shift decreases, necessitating correction to determine the actual blood velocity. Typical Doppler angles range from 30 to 60 degrees for two major reasons: (1) the vessel should be displayed in profile, which needs a minimum of about 30 degrees relative to the vessel axis for recognition in the image, and (2) at angles greater than 60 degrees, small errors in the angle estimate cause increasingly larger errors in the velocity correction factor 1 / cos(θ) as the Doppler angle approaches 90 degrees, and thus large errors in the actual velocity. For example, making a +5% error in the Doppler angle at 60 degrees is 63 degrees and at 80 degrees is 84 degrees. Corresponding cosine values are cos 60° = 0.5,

cos 63° = 0.454, cos 80° = 0.174, and cos 84° = 0.105. Plugging these values into the equation results in a velocity estimate error of ≈10% for a 63-degree Doppler angle (actual 60 degrees) and ≈66% for an 84-degree Doppler angle (actual 80 degrees). Doppler angles less than 20 degrees are also problematic because of the difficulty in clearly identifying the vessel in profile, and with pulsed Doppler methods (discussed later), the measurements are prone to insufficient sampling rates to identify the maximum Doppler shift. High-velocity blood flow can exhibit an artifact known as *aliasing*, which is represented as reverse velocity (flow) in the quantitative estimate.

Continuous and Pulsed Doppler Modes

Two distinct methods using continuous wave or pulsed ultrasound transducer operation are used to measure blood velocity. The continuous wave Doppler system is the simplest and least expensive, with two transducers—a transmitter for the incident ultrasound generating continuous, narrow-bandwidth ultrasound and a receiver detecting the returning continuous echoes from the vasculature. Positional adjustment of the transmit and receive transducers identifies an overlap area that includes the vessel of interest. In operation, a demodulator compares the transmit and receive frequencies from which the Doppler shift frequency is extracted. An amplifier converts the Doppler shift signal into an audio output, and a recorder tracks spectrum changes as a function of time for analysis of pulsatile flow. The advantages of continuous mode include high accuracy of the Doppler shift measurement due to a narrow operational frequency bandwidth and no signal aliasing of high-velocity motion because of continuous transmit and receive operation. The disadvantages include difficulty in determining depth and overlap area from which to evaluate a vessel, multiple overlying vessels making it difficult to distinguish a specific Doppler signal, and moving objects within either the transmit or receive beams that can disrupt frequency shifts and cause errors in the velocity estimates.

Pulsed Doppler ultrasound is used in conjunction with B-mode and color flow imaging to identify vessels of interest. A separate transducer element array is used for Doppler operation, with a lighter damping block function providing a narrow-frequency bandwidth and longer SPL (see Fig. 1.8). With interactive panel controls, the user positions and adjusts a region and size over the vessel to be interrogated. A Doppler angle is estimated from the direction of the Doppler transmit–receive pulse relative to the vessel axis. Electronic logic and timing algorithms reject all echo signals except those falling within the gate region. Each interrogation pulse and returning echo represent a discrete sample of the frequency shift caused by reflections of moving blood cells within the region, measured as a phase change. The Doppler transducer PRF represents the sampling rate of the returning echo signals and their frequencies. The maximum frequency accurately determined is governed by the Nyquist sampling requirement, where a frequency signal requires at least two samples per cycle, as shown in Fig. 1.23. Thus the maximum frequency shift accurately measured is one-half of the PRF. When Doppler shift frequencies exist beyond this maximum, such as stenotic jets with very high blood velocity, artifactual signals are generated due to insufficient sampling and are represented as reverse flow. In a pulsed Doppler acquisition, the maximum Doppler frequency shift, $f_{d,max}$, is equated to PRF / 2, and the Doppler shift equation becomes

$$\Delta f_{d,\,max} = \frac{PRF}{2} = \frac{2 f_i v_{max} \cos (\theta)}{c}.$$

Rearranging the equation and solving for v_{max} in terms of PRF,

$$v_{max} = \frac{c \times PRF}{4 f_i \cos (\theta)}$$

shows the relationship of the maximum blood velocity to the Doppler PRF, Doppler angle, and transducer frequency. To obtain an accurate measurement of a high velocity, Doppler PRF can be increased, incident transducer frequency can be decreased, or the Doppler angle can be increased. Of these adjustments, the most interactive is adjustment of the Doppler angle by the operator. If a 1.6-kHz maximum Doppler shift is present in the measured signal, a PRF of 2 × 1.6 kHz = 3.2 kHz is needed to avoid aliasing. The Doppler PRF cannot be set to arbitrarily high values because of the ultrasound transit time required during the PRP. A larger Doppler angle (e.g., 60 degrees) reduces the Doppler shift frequencies in the measured signal, which are subsequently adjusted to determine the true blood velocity. At angles larger than 60 degrees, however, small errors in angle estimation cause significant errors in the estimation of blood velocity, as explained previously.

Blood flow (in units of cm^3/s or milliliters/s) is estimated as the product of the vessel's cross-sectional area (cm^2) times the velocity (cm/s). Errors in flow volume may occur due to several circumstances. The vessel axis might not lie totally within the scanned plane, or flow might be altered from the perceived direction. The Doppler gate (sample area) could be mispositioned or of inappropriate size, such that the velocities are an overestimate (gate area too small) or underestimate (gate area too large) of the average velocity. In addition, errors in the cross-sectional area evaluation will cause errors in the flow estimate.

Doppler Spectrum

The Doppler spectrum is a display of the Doppler shift frequencies contained in the Doppler gate region as a function of time, as illustrated in Fig. 1.24. This information is displayed on the ultrasound monitor below the B-mode image as a moving trace, with a range of blood velocities measured from $-V_{max}$ to $+V_{max}$ on the vertical axis and time on the horizontal axis. The spectrum appears as a periodic waveform with a narrow or filled-in trace, depending on the range of frequencies contained in the signals analyzed from the Doppler gate region, and the wall filter settings that remove low-frequency motion not associated with blood flow. As new data arrive, the information is updated and scrolled from left to right. Pulsatile blood takes on the appearance of a choppy repeating wave through the periodic

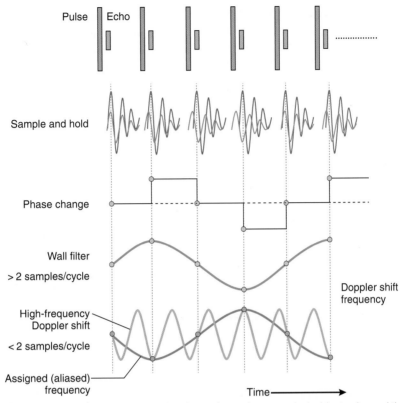

Fig. 1.23 Pulsed Doppler operation evaluates the phase change between the incident pulse and the returning echo that is mapped for each sample and recorded as a phase change. A wall filter smooths the resultant frequencies contained in the evaluation to create the constituent Doppler frequencies. If higher frequencies caused by high blood velocity generate Doppler frequencies greater than one-half the Doppler pulse repetition frequency (two samples/cycle), the assigned frequency values will be misrepresented as lower-frequency signals of opposite phase and will be aliased as slow velocity in the reverse direction (*bottom*).

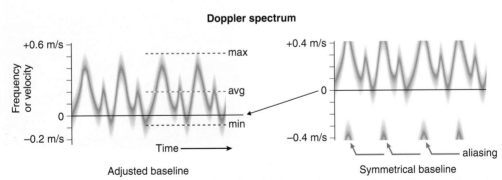

Fig. 1.24 The Doppler spectrum is a plot of the Doppler frequencies present in the Doppler gate region, plotted as a function of time. Scaling of the range of velocities is dependent on the PRF of the Doppler transducer elements; in this example, symmetrical allocation is shown on the spectrum, but aliasing is evident (*right*). To avoid aliasing, the operator can adjust the baseline to reallocate sampling (*left*). Maximum, average, and minimum velocities are extracted to calculate pertinent clinical measures, including pulsatility index and resistive index.

cycle of the heartbeat. Depending on the Doppler gate positioning, vessel size, and shape, blood movement exhibits laminar, blunt, or turbulent flow patterns. In the center of large vessels, fast and laminar flow occurs; near vessel walls, frictional forces slow blood velocity. Plaque buildup on vessel walls and narrowing (stenosis) of the vessel result in turbulent flow. When a Doppler gate area is positioned to encompass the entire vessel lumen, there exists a large range of blood velocities and corresponding large range of Doppler frequencies in the spectrum. Conversely, a centrally positioned small gate contains a narrow range of faster velocities and narrow-frequency content. A Doppler gate positioned over a stenosis results in the largest range of velocities and the greatest likelihood of aliasing. The spectral Doppler display demonstrates the presence, direction, and velocity characteristics of blood movement. The direction of flow is best determined with a small Doppler angle of about 30 degrees. Normal versus diseased vessels can be characterized by the respective spectral Doppler display waveforms and shapes due to their hemodynamic features. Quantitative vascular measures such as pulsatility index (PI) and resistive index (RI) are extracted from the Doppler spectrum waveform using the maximum, minimum, and average velocity values. PI = (max − min) / average, and RI = (max − min) / max, which can be very useful in many clinical situations.

In a spectral Doppler display, aliased signals demonstrate reversed flow with negative amplitudes. Reducing or eliminating aliasing errors requires the user to adjust the spectral Doppler velocity scale to a wider range, as the PRF of the Doppler element is linked to the scale setting. When the maximum PRF has been reached, the *spectral baseline,* which represents 0 velocity, can be adjusted to allocate a greater frequency sampling for high-velocity reflectors in arterial vessels moving toward or away from the transducer, as there is much lower velocity of blood cells in the venous vessels. For instance, instead of allocating the sampling equally in negative and positive directions, as shown in Fig. 1.24 (*right*) of +0.4 m/s to −0.4 m/s, the baseline is adjusted to scale the velocity from +0.6 m/s to −0.2 m/s in the case of arterial flow moving toward the transducer, which allows a greater fraction of the frequency sampling to be assigned to positive frequency shifts resulting from higher blood velocity moving toward the transducer.

Color Flow Imaging

Color flow imaging (also known as *color Doppler*) is a 2D visual display of moving blood superimposed on the conventional grayscale image, as shown in Fig. 1.25. In this mode, a subarea of the image is activated, with multiple small subregions individually evaluated to identify areas of motion using phase-shift or time-domain autocorrelation techniques. These calculation methods are very fast to enable color-encoded, real-time updates of blood vessel velocity that are

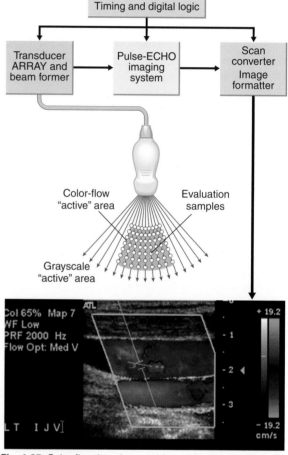

Fig. 1.25 Color flow imaging provides a 2D analysis of moving blood by sampling coarse areas within an operator-designated area on the B-mode grayscale active area. Assignments of color represent direction of blood velocity. In the image, both arterial and venous flow are present. A Doppler gate for evaluating Doppler spectra is placed for further evaluation of velocity and flow.

superimposed on the real-time grayscale image. Vasculature representing arterial and venous flow is usually within the active area, and color encoding, with shades of red for blood moving toward the transducer and blue for blood moving away from the transducer, is typically applied. Color flow systems do not calculate the full Doppler shift but estimate the shift based on the similarity of one scan line measurement to another using an autocorrelation processor to compare the entire echo pulse of one A-line with that of a previous echo. The output correlation varies proportionately with the phase change, which in turn varies proportionately with the velocity at the point along the echo trace. Four to eight traces are used to determine the presence of motion. Direction is preserved through phase detection of the echoes. For visualization, the grayscale B-mode image and the color flow information must be interleaved. A trade-off of color flow active image area and frame rate must be considered, as a larger area requires more computation time, which leads to slower updates. The color flow image depicts flow direction and vessel boundaries and provides a nice locator for placing a Doppler gate for more precise evaluation of blood velocity, as shown in Fig. 1.25.

There are several limitations with color flow imaging. Noise and clutter of slowly moving, solid structures can overwhelm smaller echoes returning from moving blood cells in color flow images. The spatial resolution of the color display is much coarser than the grayscale image because regions are used to identify areas of motion. Estimates of velocity can be limited, and velocity variations are not as well resolved as with pulsed Doppler. Aliasing artifacts affect the color flow image due to insufficient sampling, so areas of high velocity are represented as reverse flow with a different color assignment.

Power Doppler

Power Doppler mode is a signal processing method used with color flow acquisition that gives up direction and quantitative flow estimates but dramatically increases the sensitivity to any motion by relying on the total strength and amplitude of all Doppler signals, regardless of the frequency shift. A color scale presented with power Doppler reflects the magnitude (but not direction) of motion, and by eliminating directionality, the greater sensitivity allows detection and interpretation of very subtle and slow blood flow. Acquisition frame rates are typically slower than with color flow acquisition, and "flash artifacts" are common with power Doppler imaging mode, arising from moving tissues, patient motion, or transducer motion in conjunction with very high sensitivity. Aliasing is not a problem, as only the strength of the frequency-shifted signals are analyzed, and not the phase. The name *power Doppler* can be mistaken for higher deposition of energy to the patient, but this is not the case, as the technique involves computational processing. Images acquired with color flow and power Doppler are illustrated in Fig. 1.26.

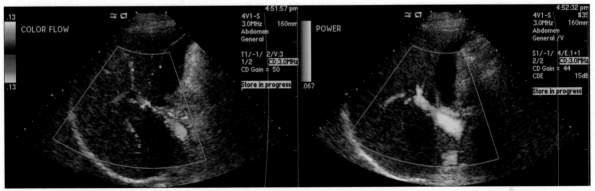

Fig. 1.26 (*Left*) Abdominal color flow image demonstrating vasculature and directionality of blood velocity; note color flow scale. (*Right*) Power Doppler acquisition of the same region, demonstrating increased sensitivity but no directionality of motion.

ULTRASOUND SYSTEM PERFORMANCE

The system performance of a diagnostic ultrasound unit is described by several parameters, including sensitivity and dynamic range, spatial resolution, contrast sensitivity, range/distance accuracy, dead zone thickness, and TGC operation. For Doppler studies, PRF, transducer angle estimates, and range gate stability are key issues. To ensure the performance, accuracy, and safety of ultrasound equipment, periodic quality control (QC) evaluations are recommended, preferably performed by trained sonographers and/or service engineers. The periodic QC testing frequency of ultrasound components should be adjusted to the probability of finding instabilities or maladjustment. This can be assessed by initially performing tests frequently, reviewing logbooks over an extended period, and, with documented stability, reducing the testing rate.

Quality Control

Simple equipment QC should be performed every day during routine scanning by the sonographer to recognize major problems with the images and the equipment. Ensuring ultrasound image quality, however, requires implementation of a QC program with periodic measurement of system performance to identify problems before serious malfunctions occur. Tissue-mimicking phantoms with acoustic targets of various sizes and echogenic features embedded in a medium of uniform attenuation and speed of sound characteristic of soft tissues are used. Various multipurpose phantoms are available to evaluate the clinical capabilities of the ultrasound system. The same tests must be performed during each testing period so that changes can be monitored over time and effective corrective action can be taken. Testing results, corrective action, and the effects of corrective action should be documented and maintained on-site. Other equipment-related issues involve cleaning air filters; checking for loose or frayed cables; and checking handles, wheels, and wheel locks as part of the QC tests. These tasks are usually handled by clinical engineering specialists or by service engineers of the manufacturer's equipment.

The most frequently reported source of performance instability of an ultrasound system is related to the display on maladjusted video monitors. Drift of the ultrasound instrument settings and/or poor viewing conditions (for instance, portable ultrasound performed in a very bright patient room, potentially causing inappropriately gain-adjusted images) can lead to suboptimal images on the softcopy monitor. The analog contrast and brightness settings for the monitor should be properly established during installation.

Doppler techniques are becoming more common in the day-to-day use of medical ultrasound equipment. Reliance on flow measurements to make diagnoses requires demonstration of accurate data acquisition and processing. QC phantoms to assess velocity and flow contain one or more tubes in tissue-mimicking materials at various depths. A blood-mimicking fluid is pushed through the tubes with carefully calibrated pumps to provide a known velocity for assessing the accuracy of the Doppler velocity measurement. Several tests can be performed, including maximum penetration depth at which flow waveforms can be detected, alignment of the sample volume with the duplex B-mode image, accuracy of velocity measurements, and volume flow. For color flow systems, sensitivity and alignment of the color flow image with the B-scan grayscale image are assessed.

ACOUSTIC POWER AND BIOEFFECTS

Acoustic power is the rate of energy production, absorption, or flow. The SI unit of power is the watt (W), defined as one joule of energy per second. Acoustic intensity is the rate at which sound energy flows through a unit area, and is usually expressed in units of watts per square centimeter (W/cm^2) or milliwatts per square centimeter (mW/cm^2).

Ultrasound acoustic power levels are strongly dependent on the operational characteristics of the system, including the transmit power, PRF, transducer frequency, and operation mode. Biological effects (bioeffects) are predominately related to the heating of tissues caused by high-intensity levels of ultrasound used to enhance image quality and functionality. For diagnostic imaging, the intensity levels are below the threshold for documented bioeffects. In the pulsed mode of ultrasound operation, the instantaneous intensity varies greatly with time and position. At a specific location in tissue, the instantaneous intensity is quite large while the ultrasound pulse passes through the tissue, but the pulse duration is short (only about a microsecond), and for the remainder of the PRP the intensity is nearly zero. The temporal peak intensity, I_{TP}, is the highest instantaneous intensity in the beam; the temporal average, I_{TA}, is the time-averaged intensity over the PRP; and the pulse average, I_{PA}, is the average intensity of the ultrasound pulse. The spatial peak, I_{SP}, is the highest intensity spatially in the beam, and the spatial average, I_{SA}, is the average intensity over the beam area, usually taken to be the area of the transducer.

Thermal and mechanical indices of ultrasound operation are now the accepted method of identifying power levels for real-time instruments that provide the operator with quantitative estimates of power deposition in the patient. These indices are selected for their relevance to risks from bioeffects and are constantly updated on the monitor during real-time scanning. The sonographer can use these indices to minimize power deposition to the patient and fetus consistent with obtaining useful clinical images in the spirit of the ALARA (as low as reasonably achievable) concept.

Thermal Index

The *thermal index*, TI, is the ratio of the acoustic power produced by the transducer to the power required to raise tissue in the beam area by 1°C. This is estimated by the ultrasound system using algorithms that consider the ultrasonic frequency, beam area, and acoustic output power of the transducer. Assumptions are made for attenuation and thermal properties of the tissues with long, steady exposure times. An indicated TI value of 2 signifies a possible 2°C increase in the temperature of the tissues when the transducer is stationary over a given volume of tissue. On some scanners, other thermal indices that might be encountered are TIS (S for soft tissue), TIB (B for bone), and TIC (C for cranial bone). These quantities are useful because of the increased heat buildup that can occur at a bone–soft tissue interface when present in the beam, particularly for obstetric scanning of late-term pregnancies, and with the use of Doppler ultrasound (where power levels can be substantially higher). TI values are usually less than 1 for most ultrasound imaging applications. The limit of TI varies with scanning time; as TI increases, the acceptable scanning time decreases. It is prudent to keep TI values less than 0.7.

Mechanical Index

The *mechanical index*, MI, is a value that estimates the likelihood of cavitation by the ultrasound beam.

Cavitation is a consequence of the negative pressures (rarefaction of the mechanical wave) that induce bubble formation from the extraction of dissolved gases in the medium. The MI is directly proportional to the peak rarefactional (negative) pressure and inversely proportional to the square root of the ultrasound frequency (in MHz). Cavitation can cause disruption of tissue structures by gas bubble implosion and is associated with the formation of free radicals. For ultrasound imaging applications, the MI is typically maintained at low, safe levels, with values substantially less than 1. The United States Food and Drug Administration (FDA) has established a maximum MI of 1.9 for diagnostic imaging and 1.0 for obstetric imaging.

Biological Mechanisms and Effects

Diagnostic ultrasound has a remarkable safety record. Despite the lack of evidence that any harm has been the result of ultrasound diagnostic intensities, it is prudent and indeed an obligation of physicians and sonographers to consider issues of benefit versus risk when performing an ultrasound examination and to take all precautions to ensure maximal benefit with minimal risk. The American Institute of Ultrasound in Medicine recommends adherence to the ALARA principles. The FDA, which oversees requirements for new ultrasound equipment, requires the inclusion of MI and TI output indices to give the user feedback regarding power deposition to the patient. At very high intensities, ultrasound causes consequential bioeffects by thermal and mechanical mechanisms. The levels and durations for typical imaging and Doppler studies are substantially below the threshold for known undesirable effects. Even though ultrasound is considered safe when used properly, prudence dictates that ultrasound exposure be limited to only those patients for whom a definite benefit will be obtained.

BIBLIOGRAPHY

Abu-Zidan FM, Hefny AF, Corr P. Clinical ultrasound physics. *J Emerg Trauma Shock.* 2011;4(4):501–503. https://doi.org/10.4103/0974-2700.86646.

Anvari A, Forsberg F, Samir AE. A primer on the physical principles of tissue harmonic imaging. *Radiographics.* 2015;35:1955–1964.

Baad M, Liu ZF, Reiser I, Paushter D. Clinical significance of US artifacts. *Radiographics.* 2017;37:1408–1423.

Bakhru RN, Schweickert WD. Intensive care ultrasound: physics, equipment, and image quality. *Ann Am Thorac Soc.* 2013;10(5):540–548. https://doi.org/10.1513/Annals ATS.201306-191OT.

Bushberg JT, Seibert JA, Leidholdt EM, Boone JM. *The Essential Physics of Medical Imaging.* 3rd ed. Baltimore: Wolters Kluwer, Lippincott Williams and Wilkens; 2012:500–576. Chapter 14-Ultrasound.

Hangiandreou NJ. AAPM/RSNA physics tutorial for residents. Topics in US: B-mode US: basic concepts and new technology. *Radiographics.* 2003;23:1019–1033. https://doi.org/10.1148/rg.234035034.

Hedrick WR, Hykes DL, Starchman DE. *Ultrasound Physics and Instrumentation.* 4th ed. St. Louis: Elsevier Mosby; 2005.

Zagzebski JA. *Essentials of Ultrasound Physics.* St. Louis: Mosby; 1996.

2

Ultrasound Artifacts

J. Anthony Seibert, Ghaneh Fananapazir

INTRODUCTION

Ultrasound artifacts represent a false portrayal of image anatomy or image degradations related to false assumptions regarding the propagation and interaction of ultrasound with tissues, as well as malfunctioning or maladjusted equipment. Understanding how artifacts are generated and how they can be recognized is crucial, which places high demands on the knowledge of the sonographer and the interpreting physician. Most artifacts arise from violations of assumptions for creating the ultrasound image, including but not limited to (1) ultrasound travels at a constant speed in all tissues (1540 m/s); (2) ultrasound travels in a straight path; (3) reflections occur from the initial ultrasound beam with one interaction at a perpendicular incidence for each boundary; (4) attenuation of ultrasound echoes is uniform; (5) all of the energy emitted by the ultrasound transducer exists in the main beam; (6) the operator has transmit, receive gain, and other settings properly adjusted; and (7) all of the elements in the transducer array, as well as the remainder of the imaging system, are operating optimally.

Artifacts are caused by a variety of mechanisms that contradict the assumptions listed above. In respective order are responses to these assumptions: (1) Sound travels at different speeds in different media based on compressibility and density characteristics. The ultrasound system uses the average speed in soft tissue of 1540 m/s to map echo amplitude depths as a function of time in the image matrix. Most notably, for fat with a speed of 1450 m/s (about a 6% difference), echoes along the trajectory, including fat structures,

are displaced farther in terms of depth from the actual location. (2) Even minor differences in ultrasound speed between tissues alter the transmitted beam direction from a straight-line trajectory when the incident ultrasound beam is nonperpendicular to the boundary, causing a change in wavelength (the ultrasound frequency remains constant in stationary tissues). The transmitted ultrasound beam is redirected at an angle of transmission different from the angle of incidence (known as *refraction*), potentially causing mismapped anatomic locations. (3) Multiple reflections of ultrasound occur from all directions within the complex environment of the human body, complicating the mapping of anatomic boundaries in the ultrasound image. (4) Ultrasound attenuation varies greatly from high to low in typical tissues and structures encountered, with resultant artifactual shadowing or enhancement of tissues at greater depths in the image. (5) Transducer crystal expansion and contraction in the thickness mode produces the main ultrasound beam, but at the same time radial contraction and expansion also occur. This results in ultrasound energy emitted outside of the main beam producing echoes that can appear as if in the beam and creating false information in the image. (6) Improper use of user-adjusted overall receive-gain or time gain compensation (TGC) results in images that may not be representative of the acoustic properties at a given depth in the image. Pulse repetition frequency (PRF) settings must ensure adequate time for listening for echoes before the next pulse. Additionally, proper transducer frequencies must be selected to achieve the desired depth of penetration in the image.

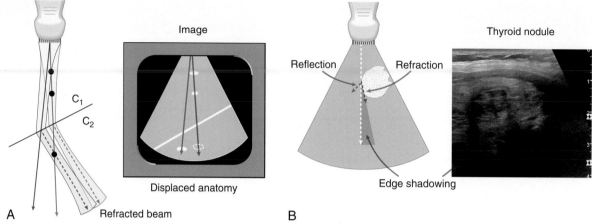

Fig. 2.1 (A) Refraction artifacts arise from a change of direction of the ultrasound beam at a tissue boundary, with nonperpendicular incidence caused by a speed of sound difference and a change in wavelength. The illustration on the left demonstrates how anatomy can be displaced as the ultrasound beam sweeps over the field of view, where the actual colinear structures are incorrectly mapped. (B) Edge shadowing occurs at the edges of rounded tissue structures caused by reflection away from the beam at the boundary edge and refraction of the beam within the structure. These interactions result in an edge shadow, an example of which is shown for a thyroid nodule on the right.

(7) The ultrasound system is dependent on all components of the imaging chain, including the transducer array, gain and filter settings, and image display, to be functioning normally. When there are component failures, the ultrasound images may not be accurately portrayed.

Fortunately, most ultrasound artifacts can be identified by the experienced sonographer because of obvious effects on the image or the transient nature of mismapped anatomy that appears and disappears during the scan. Some artifacts can be used to advantage as diagnostic aids in the characterization of tissue structures and composition. The following descriptions represent some typical artifacts encountered in diagnostic ultrasound.

Refraction

Refraction represents a change in the transmitted ultrasound pulse direction at a boundary with nonperpendicular incidence when the two adjacent tissues support a different speed of sound. Misplaced anatomy can occur in the image from the beam redirection as the echoes propagate back to the transducer over a similar return path (Fig. 2.1A). The sonographer must be aware of objects appearing and disappearing with slight differences in orientation of the transducer array. At the edges

of smooth-rounded organs, refraction of the beam at nonnormal incidence can redirect the beam away from the edge, creating a shadow of reduced intensity beyond the edge and resulting in an edge artifact (Fig. 2.1B). In many situations, the cause of the refraction artifact can be traced back to anatomic structures.

Speed Displacement

The speed displacement artifact results from the substantial variability of sound speed in fat (1450 m/s) relative to soft tissues (1540 m/s)—about a 6% slower propagation speed. Anatomic borders are displaced distally when ultrasound interacts with structures containing fat compared with the nondisplaced borders through the soft tissues (Fig. 2.2A). In the situation of a soft tissue structure surrounded by a fatty liver, the border is proximally displaced behind the soft tissue structure (Fig. 2.2B). An image of a liver with a fatty region demonstrates a displacement and disruption of the distal border (Fig. 2.3). The differences in speed also affect the accuracy of distance measurements along the direction of ultrasound travel when fat is present in the beam.

Shadowing and Enhancement

Acoustic shadowing is the result of several physical mechanisms. Objects with high attenuation, such as

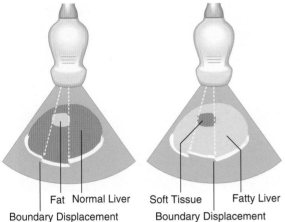

Fat   Normal Liver   Soft Tissue   Fatty Liver
Boundary Displacement   Boundary Displacement

Fig. 2.2 Speed displacement is caused by the substantial speed of sound differences in most soft tissues (1540 m/s) to that of fat (1450 m/s), which causes artifactual displacement of boundaries and errors in distance measurements along the direction of ultrasound beam travel. (A) Fatty structure surrounded by soft tissue. (B) Soft tissue structure surrounded by fatty replaced tissues (*right*).

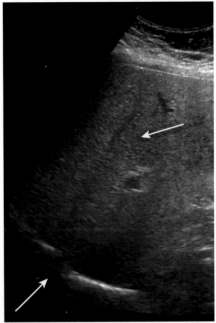

Fig. 2.3 Ultrasound of the liver with irregular fatty deposits (*upper arrow*) and resultant distal displacement of the diaphragm due to the slower speed of sound in fat (*lower arrow*).

kidney stones and gallstones, can assist in diagnosis by producing shadowing or streaks (Fig. 2.4), but they can also be a hindrance if a large attenuator, such as a rib, produces shadows that precludes optimal imaging of distal anatomy. Shadowing is also the result of reflection and refraction, as shown in the edge shadowing artifact in Fig. 2.1. Acoustic enhancement occurs distal to low-attenuation, fluid-filled structures such as cysts and the bladder where increased transmission of sound occurs, resulting in distal hyperintense signals. "Through transmission" is commonly described for this occurrence.

Reverberation, Comet Tail, and Ring-Down

Reverberation artifacts arise from multiple echoes generated between highly reflective and parallel structures that interact at a perpendicular angle to the ultrasound beam. These artifacts are often caused by reflections between a reflective interface and the transducer or between reflective interfaces, such as metallic objects (e.g., bullet fragments), calcified tissues, or air pocket/partial liquid areas of the anatomy, and are typically manifested as multiple equally spaced parallel lines at progressive depth with decreasing amplitude (Fig. 2.5). Comet tail artifact is a form of reverberation between two closely spaced reflectors and appears as bright lines along the

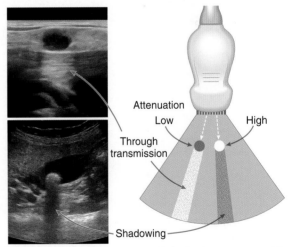

Attenuation
Low   High

Through
transmission

Shadowing

Fig. 2.4 Image enhancement and shadowing are created by anatomy with low attenuation, such as fluid-filled cysts, and high attenuation, such as calcifications. Anatomic examples illustrate through transmission (enhancement) distal to a cyst and shadowing distal to a gallstone.

direction of ultrasound propagation. It is manifested as a tapering shape and decreasing width with depth

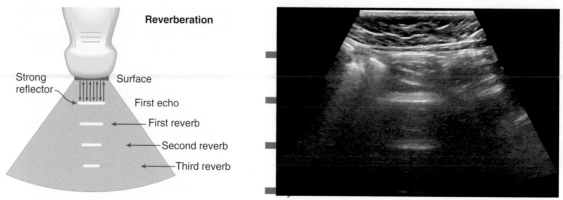

Fig. 2.5 (*Left*) Reverberation artifacts arise from a highly reflective boundary close to the transducer surface that then reflects echoes from the transducer back to the boundary several times. The consequence is a number of equally spaced structures that diminish in intensity with depth. (*Right*) Ultrasound image shows ring-down artifacts from the anterior abdominal wall, which are equally spaced and decrease in intensity with distance from the ultrasound probe.

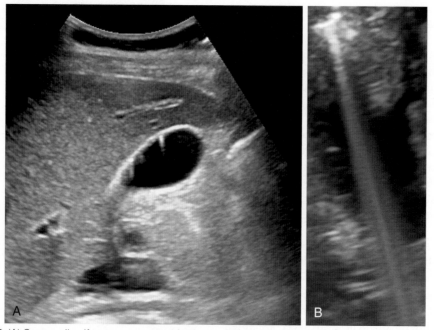

Fig. 2.6 (A) Comet tail artifacts are generated from closely spaced, highly reflective interfaces. Ultrasound of the gallbladder with adenomyomatosis demonstrating comet tail artifacts from the anterior gallbladder wall, probably due to cholesterol crystals within Rokitansky–Aschoff sinuses. (B) Ring-down artifacts are generated by resonant vibrations in air bubbles contained in abscesses, emphysematous infections, and other processes that contain air, often resulting in long reverberations at depth in the image.

of travel (Fig. 2.6A). Reverberation artifacts are useful in assessing the characteristic structures of tissues but can also hinder visualization of deeper anatomy.

Effects of reverberation can be reduced by adjusting the transducer angle of incidence or by decreasing the distance between the reflective structure and the transducer. Harmonic imaging reduces these artifacts by receiving the first harmonic frequency and filtering out the fundamental frequency.

Ring-down artifacts arise from resonant vibrations within fluid trapped between a tetrahedron of air bubbles, which creates a continuous sound wave that is transmitted back to the transducer and displayed as a series of parallel bands extending posterior to a collection of gas (Fig. 2.6B).

Mirror Image and Multipath Reflection

Mirror image artifacts occur when the ultrasound beam encounters a highly reflective nonperpendicular or curved boundary such as the diaphragm. The redirected beam encounters a specular reflector, producing a series of echoes that are reflected along the same path back to the transducer. As the field of view is scanned, the beam interacts with the same specular reflector to record its true position. Later echoes of the specular reflector from the redirected beam arrive and are mapped as distal objects on the opposite side of the strong reflector, appearing as a mirror image because of the double reflection. A common mirror image artifact occurs at the interface of the liver and the diaphragm in abdominal imaging. In one direction, the ultrasound beam correctly positions the echoes emanating from a lesion in the liver. As the ultrasound beam moves through the liver, echoes are strongly reflected from the curved diaphragm away from the main beam to interact with the lesion, generating echoes that travel back to the diaphragm and ultimately back to the transducer. The back-and-forth travel distance of these echoes creates artifactual anatomy that resembles a mirror image of the mass, placed beyond the diaphragm that would otherwise not have anatomy present in the image (Fig. 2.7). Other strong reflectors that generate mirror image artifacts include the pericardium and bowel, which might be more difficult to detect due to the presence of other anatomic structures in the same area.

Side Lobes and Grating Lobes

Ultrasound energy produced outside of the main longitudinal wave arises from the height and width expansion and contraction of the piezoelectric element that occurs when the crystal thickness mode undergoes contraction and expansion. The resultant ultrasound energy is slightly off axis from the main

beam and creates side lobe emissions (Fig. 2.8). Tissues along the trajectory of the side lobes can create echoes that are positioned in the image as if they occurred along the main beam, generating artifactual signals. This is quite noticeable when side lobes redirect diffuse echoes from adjacent soft tissues into an organ that is normally hypoechoic or anechoic. For instance, in imaging of the gallbladder, the side lobes can produce artifactual "pseudo-sludge" in an otherwise echo-free organ (Fig. 2.9). Side lobe artifacts are reduced with lower transmit gain (at the loss of penetration depth), with a process called *apodization* (excitations from the center of the transducer array are modified to reduce the amplitude of the side lobes), or with the use of harmonic imaging (higher-order frequency harmonics are generated in the center of the main ultrasound beam). Most often, if artifacts from side lobes are suspected, the sonographer should scan the anatomy from a different direction to determine whether the signals persist.

Grating lobes are caused by the division of the multielement transducer surface into small discrete emitters, each creating a diverging radial wave pattern. The individual waves interact with constructive and destructive interference (in-phase and out-of-phase frequencies) to produce the forward directed main beam; however, a small fraction of the emitted energy escapes at large angles relative to the main beam direction, resulting in the presence of grating lobe energy (Fig. 2.10). Although weak in intensity, grating lobes generate signals in the main beam from off-axis, highly reflective objects that can be recognized in hypoechoic structures. Designing transducer arrays with elements less than one-half wavelength spacing can somewhat mitigate grating lobe energy emission. These artifacts are more likely present when using phased array transducers, as the leakage occurs most at the edges of the array.

Ambiguity

Range ambiguity artifacts are caused by a high PRF acquisition that decreases the time allocated to listening for echoes during the pulse repetition period (PRP). Returning echoes arriving from depth at a time longer than the PRP will be detected after the next pulse excitation and mismapped to shallow positions in the image. These artifacts are most easily identified in regions of low attenuation and echogenicity, such as a fluid-filled

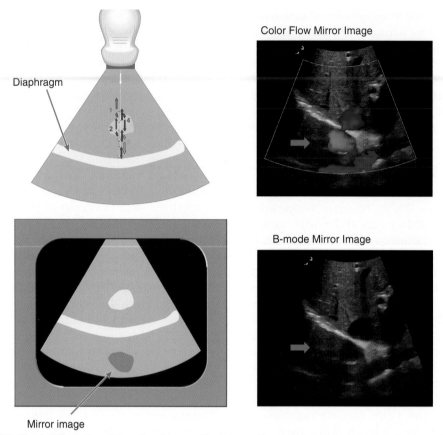

Color Flow Mirror Image

B-mode Mirror Image

Diaphragm

Mirror image

Fig. 2.7 (*Top left*) Evolution of the mirror image artifact shows the multiple echoes generated at tissue boundaries early and then later in time caused by a strong reflector such as the diaphragm. The white arrows depict the initial ultrasound pulse and first and second echoes generating the acoustic anatomy in the normal mode. At the diaphragm, most of the transmitted ultrasound pulse is reflected (*red arrow*). On the return trip, echoes are generated from the distal (third echo) and proximal (fourth echo) boundaries of the same anatomy. These echoes travel to the diaphragm and then back to the transducer later in time, generating signals at greater depth, with boundaries flipped along each ultrasound A-line during the scan. (*Bottom left*) An artifactual mirror image is generated beyond the strong reflector where there should be no signal. (*Top right*) Color flow image shows the mirror image artifact and a reversal of flow, as demonstrated by the red color of the vessel beyond the diaphragm. (*Bottom right*) B-mode image of the mirror image artifact.

cyst in the proximal field of the transducer. Ambiguity artifacts can be eliminated by decreasing the PRF, but lower acquisition frame rate and/or reduced image quality will occur as a trade-off. When possible, selecting a higher operational transducer frequency will reduce penetration depth so that echoes from depth are insignificant in amplitude.

Twinkling Artifact

Two-dimensional color flow imaging detects blood flow in a selected subregion in the image and displays moving blood as red or blue (or any selectable color) on the monitor, depending on direction and velocity. In the presence of a small, strong reflector such as a calculus, a rapidly changing mixture of colors often appears and can be mistaken for an aneurysm. This artifactual appearance is caused by echoes undergoing frequency changes of narrow-band "ringing" from the small reflectors. Twinkling artifact may be used to identify small renal stones (Fig. 2.11) and differentiate echogenic foci from calcifications within the kidney, gallbladder, and liver. Turning off color flow acquisition allows the differentiation of calcific from other anatomic structures.

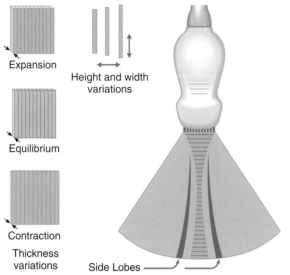

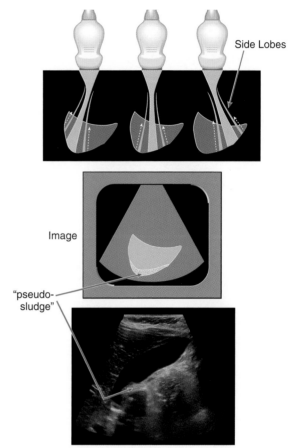

Fig. 2.8 Side lobes represent ultrasound energy produced outside of the main ultrasound beam along the same direction and are caused by nonthickness modes of vibration by the transducer elements (*upper left*). The act of compression and expansion of the thickness causes a corresponding expansion and compression of the height and width of each crystal element from which the side lobe energy is generated.

Doppler Artifacts

Aliasing is an error caused by insufficient Doppler transducer PRF relative to the Doppler shift frequency signals generated by fast-moving blood. A minimum of two samples per cycle of Doppler shift frequency is required to unambiguously determine the corresponding velocity, as defined by the Nyquist sampling theorem. In measurements containing frequencies beyond this minimum sampling rate, a Doppler signal of lower frequency and of opposite phase is generated (Fig. 2.12), as if the blood is flowing in the opposite direction in the vessel. In some situations, aliasing may be a useful indicator of higher-velocity flow (e.g., the presence of a stenosis). In the spectral Doppler display, the aliased signals wrap around to negative amplitude and reversed flow (Fig. 2.13). A straightforward adjustment to reduce or eliminate the aliasing error is to increase the PRF to enable a wider-range Doppler spectrum velocity scale. If the maximum PRF is set, then the spectral baseline can be readjusted to allocate a greater frequency range in the direction with the highest frequency shift. (This is shown in Fig. 2.13, with greater allocation of the sampling applied to the positive velocity scale.) Another

Fig. 2.9 Common side lobe artifacts are manifested when imaging curved structures of hypoechogenicity, such as the gallbladder, where the side lobe energy echoes adjacent to the beam are integrated within the beam. The example in the illustration demonstrates artifactual "pseudo-sludge" in the gallbladder that can be ameliorated by scanning at a different angle. (*Left*, adapted from Bushberg JT, Seibert JA, Leidholdt EM Jr, Boone JM. Ultrasound. In *The Essential Physics of Medical Imaging*. 3rd ed. Philadelphia, PA: Lippincott Williams & Wilkins; 2012:500–576.)

adjustment is for the sonographer to adjust the transducer for a larger Doppler angle, which lowers the measured Doppler shift and enables use of a lower PRF to meet the Nyquist criterion. Subsequent correction by $1/\cos(\theta)$ is used to calculate the actual blood velocity. At angles larger than 60 degrees, however, small errors in angle measurement can cause large errors in estimates of blood velocity. Each of these adjustments is described in Chapter 1.

Power Doppler is a way to improve motion sensitivity to slow blood flow by eliminating directionality

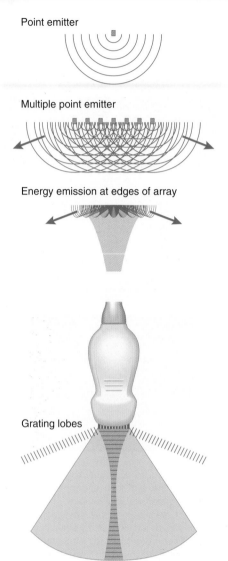

Point emitter

Multiple point emitter

Energy emission at edges of array

Grating lobes

Fig. 2.10 Grating lobes represent emission of energy at large angles relative to the direction of the beam and are caused by the discrete nature of the multielement transducer array. If one models an element as a point irradiator (*top*), the ultrasound beam diverges; for multiple point sources, the diverging waves constructively and destructively interfere, causing the composite (main) beam to converge to a minimum beam diameter and then diverge beyond the focal distance. At the edges there are no interference waves, allowing energy to be emitted away from the transducer array at large angles relative to the main beam (*lower illustration*). This energy represents grating lobes, with much lower intensity than the ultrasound main beam. Grating lobe artifacts manifest in the main beam area and occur when highly reflective objects are situated perpendicular to the grating lobe direction.

and quantitation capabilities of color Doppler. Aliasing is not a problem, as only the strength of the frequency-shifted signals are analyzed, and not the phase, but the greater sensitivity leads to significant *flash artifacts* related to moving tissues, patient motion, or transducer motion.

Beam Width and Slice Thickness

Beam width artifact results from the variable width of the in-plane ultrasound beam as a function of depth, resulting in poor lateral resolution proximal and even poorer lateral resolution distal to the focal zone. The artifact refers to the lateral blurring of objects as a function of beam width. Objects at proximal and deeper depths beyond the focal zone appear to be horizontally stretched (Fig. 2.14). In addition, if two adjacent small objects are separated by less than the beam width, they will appear as one and not be resolved. A solution to the beam width artifact is to implement a lateral focal zone at the depth of interest; on some advanced systems, multiple depths can be selected, but at the cost of temporal resolution. Use of higher-frequency transducer operation results in a narrower beam width, which can improve lateral resolution, as can the use of harmonic imaging with the generation of harmonic frequencies in the center of the beam (see Chapter 1).

The slice thickness profile, which is perpendicular to the displayed ultrasound image, varies with depth, similar to the in-plane lateral beam width. Proximal to the transducer array, the slice thickness is broad, becomes narrower at the mid-depth zone, and widens with greater depth. Consequences are loss of signal from objects smaller than the slice thickness due to partial volume averaging and inclusion of signals from highly reflective objects adjacent to the imaging plane. Usually there is no specific solution to slice-thickness artifacts, although 1.5D and 2D array transducers (not used in point-of-care ultrasound) can aid in creating a narrower slice thickness over selected depths.

EQUIPMENT SETTINGS AND EQUIPMENT FAILURES

Artifacts can be caused by inappropriate equipment settings and protocols. Variations in image echogenicity and uniformity are affected by TGC settings inappropriately adjusted by the user (Fig. 2.15). High wall filter

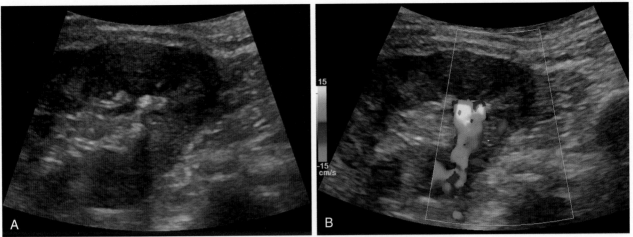

Fig. 2.11 (A) B-mode longitudinal image of the left kidney with a high-attenuation object and distal shadowing. (B) Color flow image with an obvious multicolor "twinkle" related to the object, due to ultrasound beam interactions with the calcified structure and associated narrow-band ringing.

settings can significantly affect the Doppler spectrum by overcompensating the low-frequency cut-off, which can have significant repercussions on the determination of quantitative values such as resistive index (Fig. 2.16).

Loss of transducer element function in a multielement array can be difficult to detect, as adjacent transducers and image processing can compensate for malfunctions. Specialized electronic equipment is often needed to evaluate and detect functionality of individual transducer elements. When two or more adjacent elements are malfunctioning, a uniformity phantom can assist in indicating the location and effects on the image in the form of vertical dark streaks (Fig. 2.17). Horizontal banding in the ultrasound image is attributed to the use of multiple focal zones that can be set on advanced ultrasound equipment. This artifact is the result of errors in creating a single image from the multiple partial images acquired for each focal zone depth. The banding artifact occurs at depths coincident with the location of the focal zones (Fig. 2.18). Service adjustment with calibration is necessary to correct this artifact.

CONCLUSIONS

Artifacts—whether resulting from violations of the underlying assumptions used for acquiring and creating an ultrasound image or from improper equipment settings or malfunctioning equipment—are common and widespread, so understanding the physical principles and underlying causes is important in recognizing and diminishing those that interfere with image interpretation. At the same time, some artifacts can reveal important information regarding tissue structure and composition that can assist in diagnosis. Periodic quality control is an important and useful activity to identify component failure effects on the ultrasound images and to direct repair and replacement by service engineers to maintain optimal image quality.

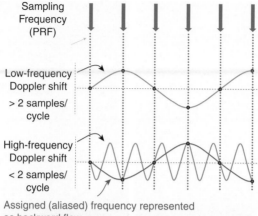

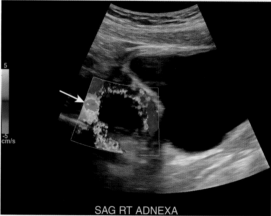

Fig. 2.12 In pulsed-Doppler acquisitions, the maximum Doppler shift frequency accurately measured is equal to one-half PRF described by the Nyquist sampling theorem. (*Top*) A low-frequency Doppler shift signal (*in red*) is properly identified when there are more than two samples/cycle; however, for a higher-frequency Doppler shift (*also red*), the criterion is not met. The insufficient sampling assigns a low-frequency signal (*in blue*) that is out of phase and moving in the opposite direction as the artifactual aliased signal. (*Bottom*) A sagittal B-mode acquisition through the bladder with color flow shows a corpus luteal cyst in the right adnexa with a "ring of fire" and color aliasing (*arrow*). Note the color scale is set to 5 cm/s. Any velocities above that will appear as a mosaic pattern of color due to aliasing. By increasing the PRF, the range of velocities also increases, which can eliminate the aliasing artifact. ((*Top*) from Bushberg JT, Seibert JA, Leidholdt EM Jr, Boone JM. Ultrasound. In *The Essential Physics of Medical Imaging*. 3rd ed. Philadelphia, PA: Lippincott Williams & Wilkins; 2012:500–576.)

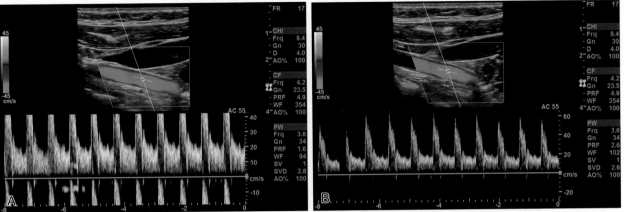

Fig. 2.13 (A) Aliasing in the Doppler spectrum is demonstrated by wrap around of the high-velocity signals (lower traces in the image below the baseline). The PRF of 1.6 kHz was insufficient to provide adequate sampling of the higher Doppler shift frequencies. (B) The PRF is increased to 2.6 kHz, expanding the velocity range of the Doppler spectrum from +40 cm/s and −20 cm/s to +60 cm/s and −30 cm/s to avoid the aliasing, but at the cost of finer spectral detail.

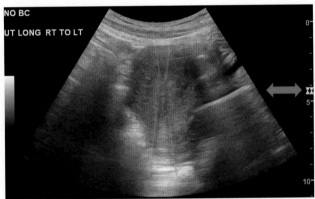

Fig. 2.14 Beam width variations occur with depth in the ultrasound image, causing horizontal lateral spread of anatomy and loss of lateral resolution proximal and distal (*red arrows*) to the focal zone depth (*blue arrow*).

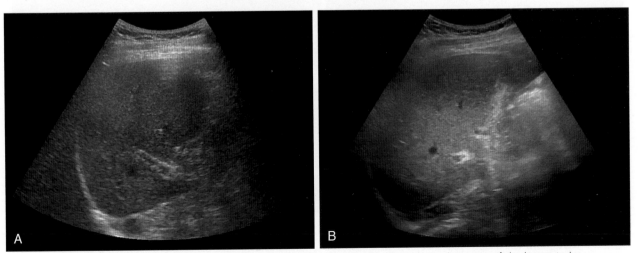

Fig. 2.15 Time gain compensation (TGC) settings can be improperly adjusted, causing areas of the image to be underemphasized or overemphasized, potentially leading to misdiagnosis or other untoward outcomes. (A) Liver image with proper TGC. (B) Liver image with too much gain in the mid-depths and insufficient gain in the proximal and distal areas of the image.

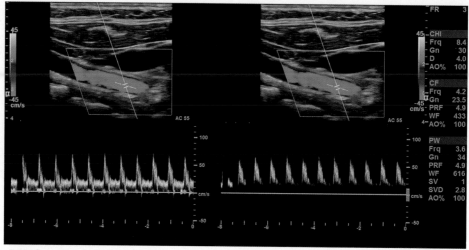

Fig. 2.16 Color flow image demonstrating effect of wall filter on the Doppler spectrum when the wall filter settings are too high (*right*), resulting in loss of spectral information and inability to make quantitative measurements.

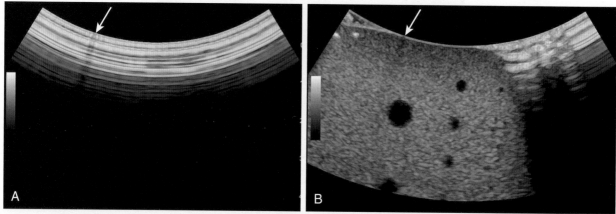

Fig. 2.17 (A) Curvilinear transducer array shows element dropout (*arrow*). (B) The same transducer array shows the effect on the image of an ultrasound quality-control phantom with no acquisition processing (*arrow*). Phased array transducer operation and compound scanning mode reduce the effects and impact of small numbers of malfunctioning elements.

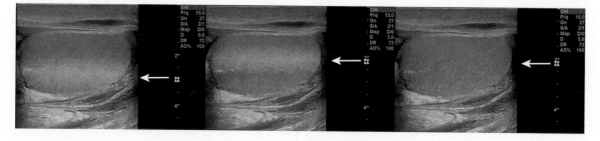

Focal zone banding   After calibration

Fig. 2.18 Lateral focal zones are user-identified depths within the image that benefit from improved resolution. Focal zone banding occurs at the location of a user-placed lateral focal zone, which requires the joining of two or more separate acquisitions to create the in-focus image. When the subimages are improperly joined due to a lack of system calibration, a nonuniform band occurs at the level of the focal zone.

BIBLIOGRAPHY

Abu-Zidan FM, Hefny AF, Corr P. Clinical ultrasound physics. *J Emerg Trauma Shock*. 2011;4(4):501–503. https://doi.org/10.4103/0974-2700.86646.

Anvari A, Forsberg F, Samir AE. A primer on the physical principles of tissue harmonic imaging. *RadioGraphics*. 2015;35:1955–1964.

Baad M, Liu ZF, Reiser I, Paushter D. Clinical significance of US Artifacts. *RadioGraphics*. 2017;37:1408–1423.

Bakhru RN, Schweickert WD. Intensive care ultrasound: physics, equipment, and image quality. *Ann Am Thorac Soc*. 2013;10(5):540–548. https://doi.org/10.1513/AnnalsATS.201306-191OT.

Bushberg JT, Seibert JA, Leidholdt EM Jr, Boone JM. *The Essential Physics of Medical Imaging*. 3rd ed. Baltimore: Wolters Kluwer, Lippincott Williams and Wilkens; 2012:500–576. Chapter 14-Ultrasound.

Hangiandreou NJ. AAPM/RSNA physics tutorial for residents. Topics in US: B-mode US: basic concepts and new technology. *Radiographics*. 2003;23:1019–1033. https://doi.org/10.1148/rg.234035034.

Hedrick WR, Hykes DL, Starchman DE. *Ultrasound Physics and Instrumentation*. 4th ed. St. Louis: Elsevier Mosby; 2005.

Zagzebski JA. *Essentials of Ultrasound Physics*. St. Louis: Mosby; 1996.

SECTION 2

Head and Neck Ultrasound

3

Peritonsillar Abscess

Leigha J. Winters, Christine N. McBeth, Michael A. Schick

CLINICAL CONSIDERATIONS

Patients with soft tissue infections of the oropharynx and neck commonly present to the emergency department and other frontline medical providers. Peritonsillar abscess (PTA) is the most common deep infection of the neck and face. PTAs develop from tonsillitis, which progress to peritonsillar cellulitis and then onto abscesses. Although peritonsillar cellulitis and PTAs may be considered a spectrum of disease, they are important to differentiate as their definitive management differs. Peritonsillar cellulitis is treated with antibiotics, analgesics, and at times steroids for symptom management, whereas PTAs may require aspiration or incision and drainage (I&D).

It can be difficult to differentiate between cellulitis and abscess by history and physical alone, as signs and symptoms may be nonspecific and unreliable. One distinguishing feature for PTAs is that they often develop unilaterally, whereas tonsillitis usually develops bilaterally. However, studies have shown that clinical evaluation by otolaryngologists is only 78% sensitive and 50% specific for identification of PTA. Historically, patients presenting with sore throat, fever, chills, and/or peritonsillar erythema and edema were managed with a diagnostic needle aspiration of the peritonsillar swelling to search for pocket(s) of purulence. This blind aspiration poses significant risks, including carotid artery injury (as the carotid artery is frequently within millimeters of the area of swelling), hemorrhage, insufficient aspiration leading to recurrence of the PTA, and false-negative aspirations in 10% to 24% of cases. Today, the gold standard for identifying a PTA is computed tomography (CT) of the neck with intravenous (IV) contrast.

Although CT is the gold standard, there is growing concern for radiation exposure, especially in adolescents and young adults (who have the highest incidence of PTAs). CT is also costly and time consuming. For these reasons, medical specialists are turning to ultrasound to help identify PTAs.

The use of intraoral ultrasound for the diagnosis of PTA was first described in 1993. This imaging modality has the advantage of being rapid (done at the bedside), noninvasive, lacking in radiation exposure, and usually well tolerated. It may be used to detect occult abscesses and localize the optimal site for aspiration or I&D. Studies report a sensitivity of 89% to 100% and specificity of 83% to 100% in detecting abscess compared with CT, magnetic resonance imaging (MRI), or surgical follow-up.

ANATOMY

Posterior oropharyngeal anatomy is complex and potentially hazardous during PTA management, so it is important to have a clear understanding of regional anatomy.

The palatine tonsils are ovoid masses composed of lymphoid tissue that reside in the lateral walls of the oropharynx between the anterior and posterior tonsillar pillars. The tonsils lie in the depression between the palatoglossal arch anteriorly and the palatopharyngeal arch posteriorly. Each tonsil is surrounded by a capsule (Fig. 3.1). Each tonsil is composed of a medial and lateral surface and an upper, middle, and lower pole. A PTA forms between the palatine tonsil and its capsule, rather than within the tonsil itself. As an abscess progresses, it may involve the surrounding anatomy and even penetrate the carotid sheath, which is situated posterolateral to each

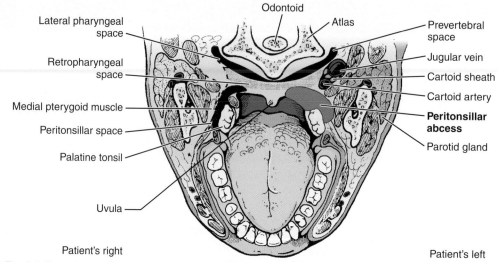

Fig. 3.1 Posterior oropharynx anatomy. (From Roberts J, Custalow CB, Thomsen TW. *Roberts and Hedges' Clinical Procedures in Emergency Medicine and Acute Care*, 7th ed. Philadelphia, PA: Saunders; 2019: 1338-1383.e2.)

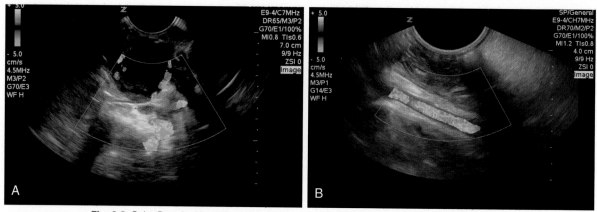

Fig. 3.2 Color Doppler identifying the carotid artery in (A) short access and (B) long access.

tonsil. Another complication of pharyngitis is Lemierre's syndrome, a suppurative thrombophlebitis of the internal jugular vein. This complication can be accompanied by bacteremia or septic emboli and is most commonly caused by the gram-negative anaerobe *Fusobacterium necrophorum*. This condition should be treated with penicillin, clindamycin, or a third-generation cephalosporin, as macrolide resistance is high in *F. necrophorum*.

When utilizing bedside ultrasound in the posterior oropharynx, one can visualize several structures, including the palatine tonsil, margin of the bony hard palate, styloid process of the temporal bone, medial pterygoid muscle, various fascial planes, internal jugular vein, and internal carotid artery. When evaluating a possible PTA with ultrasound, it is imperative to identify the location of the carotid artery. The carotid artery courses anterior to the jugular vein within the carotid sheath (Fig. 3.2). It is normally located posterolateral to the tonsil and within 5 to 25 mm of the PTA.

PREPARATION AND TECHNIQUE FOR INTRAORAL ULTRASOUND EVALUATION

Probe

When evaluating for a PTA, it is best to use a high-frequency probe. We recommend the 5- to 13-MHz curved array endocavitary probe. Other probe options include the 5.0- to 7.5-MHz linear array or dedicated flexible endoscopic transducer. Prepare the probe as follows:

1. Choose the appropriate probe. Ensure it has been sterilized since its most recent use.
2. Apply ultrasound gel to the tip of the probe.
3. Sheath the probe in a probe cover (nonlatex glove if patient has a latex allergy).
4. Securely fasten the probe cover with an elastic band or by the built-in retaining bar.
5. Gently remove any air bubbles in the gel at the tip of the probe.
6. On the ultrasound machine, set the initial depth to 5 cm and the probe to the highest frequency available.

After use, sterilize the probe according to institutional policy.

Premedication

Although evaluation for PTA by ultrasound is non-invasive, the pressure of the probe on the swollen tissue can cause pain and anxiety, as well as trigger the patient's gag reflex. Hence, these procedures often proceed more smoothly with premedications. Consider an IV anxiolytic or light analgesic if the patient is anxious or trismus is present. Also consider an IV steroid (e.g., dexamethasone) to help with inflammation and symptom control before the procedure. Finally, consider nebulized, atomized, viscous, or topical lidocaine for local anesthesia. If you are concerned the patient may not be sufficiently cooperative, consider a bite block for protection.

Technique

1. Position the patient in a seated or upright position. Place a pillow or stacked towels behind the patient's head for comfort.
2. Carefully place the probe on the tonsil in the transverse plane, with the indicator to the patient's right. The probe should contact the glossopalatine arch (anterior pillar) to visualize the lateral tonsil.

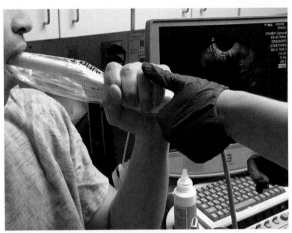

Fig. 3.3 Endocavitary probe in dual hold by practitioner and patient to avoid gag reflex. Probe indicator is to the patient's right.

3. Operators often need to hold the probe with both hands for stability. Place your dominant hand on the probe handle and your nondominant hand on the probe shaft abutting the perioral area. Alternatively, consider allowing the patient to place their hand on top of the operator's dominant hand. This allows the patient to help control insertion and pressure, as well as to remove the probe if their gag reflex may trigger emesis (Fig. 3.3).
4. Identify the tonsil. When not inflamed, the tonsil is an ovoid structure approximately 2 cm in diameter. As the tonsil is a solid organ, it will appear as a homogeneous, hypoechoic structure distinct from surrounding tissue on ultrasound (Fig. 3.4).
5. Center the tonsil on the screen, then magnify the tonsil by decreasing the depth as needed. Do not decrease the depth so much that the location of the carotid artery is lost.
6. Systematically sweep through the tonsil in two perpendicular planes (sagittal/longitudinal and transverse) to evaluate for an abscess. With trismus, it may be impossible to sweep through the entire tonsil. Usually when this occurs, the inferior pole is difficult to scan. The solution to this problem is to scan through the tonsil in the longitudinal plane to ensure visualization of the superior and inferior poles. However, only scanning in the longitudinal plane makes the position of the carotid artery more difficult to determine.

7. Once centered upon the largest area of fluid collection, note the location of the probe contact with the tonsil and the angle of the probe. Needle aspiration will need to be done at this location and angle.

8. Measure the depth of the anterior and posterior edges of the abscess to determine the depth required during needle aspiration.

9. Identify the carotid artery, which will be posterolateral to the tonsil. Use color flow Doppler to ensure this is a vessel and not another fluid collection. Note the total depth of the artery, as well as the distance from the most posterior aspect of the abscess.

10. Note the depth of the most posterior aspect of the tonsil so you know the maximum depth to inject the needle during aspiration (Fig. 3.5). This will prevent you from accidentally injuring the carotid artery.

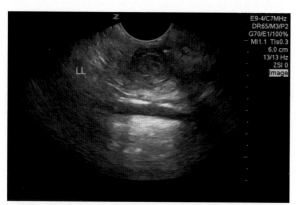

Fig. 3.4 Normal tonsil identified by endocavitary probe in long axis.

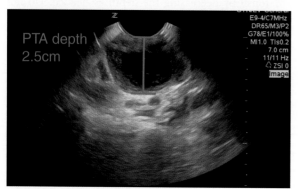

Fig. 3.5 Posterior aspect of PTA measures 2.5 cm deep to the tip of the endocavitary probe.

ULTRASOUND FINDINGS

To differentiate peritonsillar cellulitis from abscess, it is important to be able to recognize normal tissue and identify surrounding anatomy. Normal subcutaneous tissue is composed primarily of fat. Under ultrasound, this appears as hypoechoic tissue that may be interspersed with echogenic linear streaks of connective tissue.

When cellulitis arises, the edema found within the subcutaneous tissues is seen under ultrasound as diffusely increased echogenicity (hyperechoic) with traversing hypoechoic strands. This is often described as a "cobblestone" or reticular pattern (Fig. 3.6). Findings may be subtle; consider comparing the unaffected side to help identify pathology.

In comparison, an abscess most often appears as a hypoechoic, anechoic, or complex round cystic mass on ultrasound. Most PTAs contain purulent material, so compression of the abscess by the ultrasound probe may induce motion (swirling). Recall that PTAs develop between the tonsil and its capsule and the tonsillar tissue will be behind the well-demarcated, hypoechoic abscess. However, the tonsil may be obscured by posterior acoustic enhancement and/or displaced medially and caudally by the abscess. Color flow Doppler is helpful to identify a PTA, as it can show hyperemia adjacent to the abscess cavity and absent flow within it (Fig. 3.7). Central tonsillar necrosis may be seen in severe PTA infections (Fig. 3.8).

Once a PTA is identified, note its size, shape, and depth. It is important to identify the internal carotid artery and note its relationship to the abscess. The carotid artery will appear anechoic and tubular on ultrasound. It is pulsatile and relatively noncompressible (especially compared with the internal jugular vein). Color flow Doppler is helpful in identifying the pertinent vascular structures of the posterior oropharynx (see Fig. 3.2).

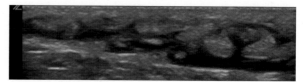

Fig. 3.6 In late cellulitis, the accumulation of fluid in the subcutaneous tissue appears as "cobblestoning" under ultrasound.

ULTRASOUND-GUIDED DRAINAGE OF PTA

Intraoral ultrasound can be helpful in identifying PTAs, as well as identifying the ideal location for aspiration of purulent material. However, ultrasound-guided PTA drainage is usually a static technique, as keeping the endocavitary probe and the needle and syringe in the patient's mouth at the same time is difficult and awkward.

Once a PTA is identified, always consider contraindications to aspiration or I&D before proceeding. Absolute contraindications to attempted drainage are malignancy and vascular malformations. Relative contraindications are pediatric patients, severe trismus, and the uncooperative patient.

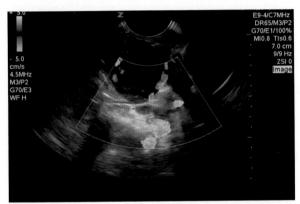

Fig. 3.7 Color flow Doppler identifies hyperechoic PTA without flow within the abscess surrounded by hyperemic tissue with significant flow.

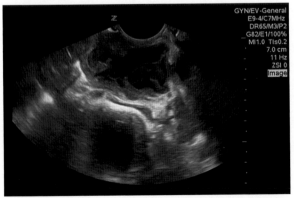

Fig. 3.8 Severe PTA infection with central tonsillar necrosis.

Procedure: PTA Aspiration

1. Identify the ideal location and angle for aspiration following the steps listed in the "Preparation and Technique for Intraoral Ultrasound Evaluation" section above. The most fluctuant area is usually located in the upper pole of the tonsil.
2. Consider additional analgesic administration with atomized, nebulized, viscous, and/or local infiltration of lidocaine.
3. Prepare an 18- or 20-gauge, 1.5-inch needle on a 10- or 20-mL syringe. Conversely, you may use an 18- or 20-gauge, 3.5-inch spinal needle on a syringe to provide additional length to reach the posterior oropharynx (Fig. 3.9).
4. Fix a needle guard at the base of the 18- or 20-gauge needle to prevent it from advancing past the depth of the posterior aspect of the tonsil. Cut a needle cap to the appropriate length and fit it back on the needle, or use tape directly on the needle (Fig. 3.10).
5. A light source is needed to properly visualize the posterior oropharynx to facilitate drainage. Consider using the lower half of a disposable lighted speculum (Fig. 3.11).

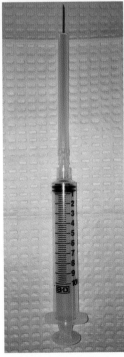

Fig. 3.9 Spinal needle attached to 10-mL syringe with needle guard in place to prevent penetration of deep vascular structures.

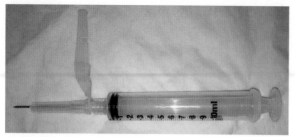

Fig. 3.10 Eighteen-gauge needle with guard to prevent penetration of vascular structures.

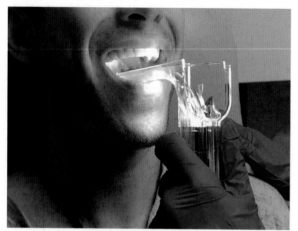

Fig. 3.11 Disassembled disposable plastic speculum with an attached fiber-optic light source to illuminate the posterior oropharynx for PTA drainage.

A headlamp and tongue blade or a Macintosh laryngoscopy blade (size 3 or 4 in adults) may also be used. Some patients prefer to hold the lighted speculum themselves to facilitate a sense of control and decrease gagging. Ask the patient to place the speculum as far back on their tongue as possible while pulling caudally.

6. Ensure suction is readily available, especially when considering I&D for a larger abscess.
7. For aspiration, enter the tonsil at the predetermined location and angle of entry. Aspirate while advancing the needle to the anticipated depth of the abscess.
8. If purulent material is aspirated, remove as much of the drainage as possible. If a large amount of purulence is obtained (>6 mL), I&D may be indicated.
9. If you do not aspirate purulent material on the first attempt, you may attempt aspiration again 1 cm inferiorly to the initial insertion site at the middle pole of the peritonsillar space. If you again do not aspirate purulent material, you may make a final attempt 1 cm inferiorly at the lower pole of the peritonsillar space (Fig. 3.12).

After aspirating as much of the abscess contents as possible, consider sending the fluid for Gram stain and culture. Treat with antibiotics for a presumed polymicrobial infection. Outpatient options include oral clindamycin or amoxicillin–clavulanate for 14 days. If the patient requires admission, consider IV piperacillin–tazobactam or clindamycin. In addition, a single high-dose steroid (e.g., dexamethasone) often improves symptoms.

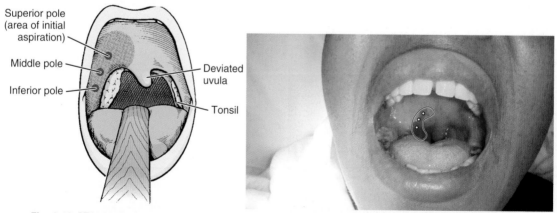

Fig. 3.12 PTA needle insertion locations. (Modified from Roberts J, Custolow CB, Thomsen TW. *Roberts and Hedges' Clinical Procedures in Emergency Medicine and Acute Care,* 7th ed. Philadelphia, PA: Saunders; 2019: 1338-1383.e2.)

PITFALLS/COMMON MISTAKES

Always begin with and prioritize airway, breathing, and circulation when concerned about a head and neck infection. Consider airway protection in large abscesses.

There is a 1% to 15% failure rate for PTA drainage with blind aspiration or drainage, so consider using intraoral ultrasound to identify and optimize PTA management. Remember that intraoral ultrasound will only diagnose a PTA. If the ultrasound is negative for a PTA, consider other head and neck infections (e.g., parapharyngeal space abscess and retropharyngeal abscess).

When attempting aspiration or I&D of a PTA, carotid artery injury is always a risk. Be sure to create a needle (or scalpel) guard with the needle cover (or tape on the scalpel) to prevent inserting the needle too deeply. This also helps prevent inoculating the prevertebral fascia, which is another risk of the procedure. Incision into the tonsil itself may cause excessive bleeding and misdiagnosis if the PTA is missed altogether. When aspirating a PTA, consider I&D if the abscess is large (>6 mL of purulent material is aspirated). After the abscess is drained, continue management with antibiotics and close clinical follow-up. Consider hospital admission for patients who have signs of impending airway compromise, appear toxic, or cannot tolerate oral fluids or oral antibiotics.

BIBLIOGRAPHY

Fernandez MW, Desai BK. Incision and drainage of peritonsillar abscess. In: Latha G, ed. *Atlas of Emergency Medicine Procedures*. New York: Springer; 2016:347–350.

Harris JH, Harris WH. *The Radiology of Emergency Medicine*. 4th ed. Philadelphia: Lippincott Williams & Wilkins; 2000.

Hollinshead WH. *Anatomy for Surgeon*. 3rd ed. Philadelphia: Harper & Row; 1982.

Jones LC, Shafer D. Head, neck, and orofacial infections in pediatric patients. In: Hupp JR, ed. *Head, Neck, and Orofacial Infections: A Multidisciplinary Approach*. St. Louis, MO: Elsevier; 2016:395–405.

Ma OJ, Mateer JR. *Emergency Ultrasound*. New York: McGraw-Hill; 2003.

Mapelli E, Sabhaney V. Stridor and drooling in infants and children. In: Tintinalli JE, ed. *Tintinalli's Emergency Medicine: A Comprehensive Study Guide*. New York: McGraw Hill Education; 2016:800–801.

Socransky S, Wiss R, Hall G. *Point-of-Care Ultrasound for Emergency Physicians: "The EDE Book."* Ontario, Canada: Th EDE 2 Course Inc; 2013.

4

Neck Masses

Alicia A. Gingrich, Michael J. Campbell

INTRODUCTION

In the emergency department setting, the use of head and neck ultrasound has become a valuable tool to expedite the diagnosis of familiar diseases and facilitate common procedures. For head and neck pathology, ultrasound is often favored over computed tomography (CT) because it is readily available at the bedside and does not expose the patient to ionizing radiation. In this chapter we will describe the ultrasound characteristics of common head and neck pathology and outline procedures where ultrasound can facilitate emergent procedures.

Anatomy of the Head and Neck

The neck is historically broken down into two triangles divided by the sternocleidomastoid muscle (SCM). The anterior triangle, which is bordered by the anterior aspect of the SCM, midline of the neck, and inferior mandible, can be further subdivided into the suprahyoid and infrahyoid compartments (Fig. 4.1). The suprahyoid structures include the submandibular glands, the anterior and posterior bellies of the digastric muscle, the mylohyoid, and the stylohyoid muscles. The infrahyoid compartment contains the larynx, trachea, and esophagus, as well as the thyroid and parathyroid glands. Important muscles of the infrahyoid compartment include the sternohyoid, sternothyroid, thyrohyoid, and omohyoid muscles. The posterior triangle is bordered by the SCM anteriorly, the trapezius muscle posteriorly, and the clavicle inferiorly (see Fig. 4.1). In the posterior triangle sits the spinal accessory nerve, brachial plexus, and phrenic nerve. The common carotid artery, internal jugular vein, and vagus nerve sit deep in the SCM and are therefore located on the transition between the anterior and posterior triangles.

Imaging and Technique

Imaging of the neck is performed using a linear transducer with a frequency of 5 to 15 MHz. The choice of frequency will depend on the depth of the pathology, with lower-frequency probes providing better resolution of deep structures. Proper patient positioning is helpful for visualization of anatomic structures, particularly in the obese patient. The patient can be placed in the supine position and a shoulder roll inserted behind the scapulae to aid with extension of the neck. As with all ultrasound imaging techniques, a focused, systematic approach increases the efficiency of the study. Whenever possible, scan the neck in more than one plane to confirm findings.

In the anterior triangle start in the submental region and evaluate the submandibular glands and submental lymph nodes. Move inferiorly in a cranial-to-caudal fashion, noting the trachea as a midline structure with a hyperechoic air–mucosa interface and reverberation artifact. The thyroid gland is located in the midline of the infrahyoid compartment of the anterior triangle. The isthmus of the thyroid will overlie the trachea and connect the right and left lobes (Fig. 4.2). The thyroid will be bound laterally by the common carotid artery and internal jugular vein. The appearance of the thyroid gland is characterized by two homogenous, well-circumscribed lobes connected by a thin isthmus that drapes over the trachea.

When examining the posterior triangle, it helps to have the patient rotate the chin contralateral to the side

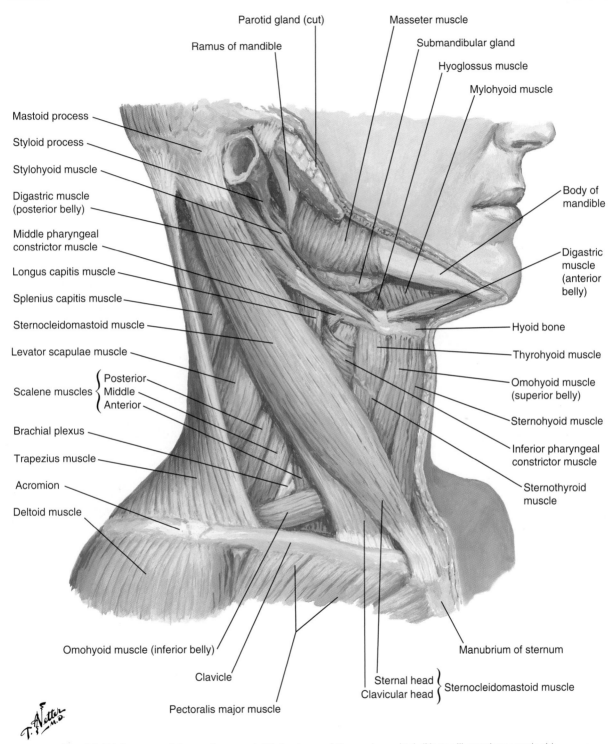

Fig. 4.1 (A) Anatomy of the neck, coronal. (B) Anatomy of the neck, sagittal. (Netter illustrations used with permission of Elsevier, Inc. All rights reserved. www.netterimages.com.)

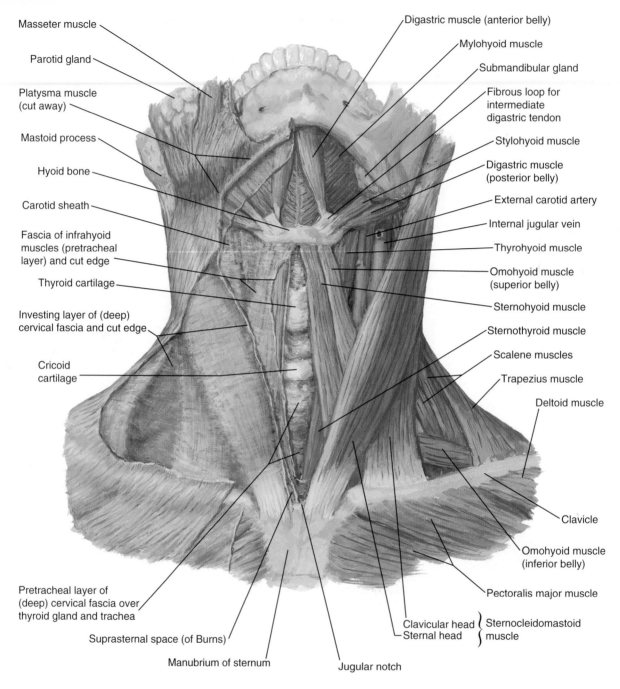

Masseter muscle

Parotid gland

Platysma muscle
(cut away)

Mastoid process

Hyoid bone

Carotid sheath

Fascia of infrahyoid
muscles (pretracheal
layer) and cut edge

Thyroid cartilage

Investing layer of (deep)
cervical fascia and cut edge

Cricoid
cartilage

Digastric muscle (anterior belly)

Mylohyoid muscle

Submandibular gland

Fibrous loop for
intermediate
digastric tendon

Stylohyoid muscle

Digastric muscle
(posterior belly)

External carotid artery

Internal jugular vein

Thyrohyoid muscle

Omohyoid muscle
(superior belly)

Sternohyoid muscle

Sternothyroid muscle

Scalene muscles

Trapezius muscle

Deltoid muscle

Clavicle

Omohyoid muscle
(inferior belly)

Pectoralis major muscle

Clavicular head ⎰ Sternocleidomastoid
Sternal head ⎱ muscle

Pretracheal layer of
(deep) cervical fascia over
thyroid gland and trachea

Suprasternal space (of Burns)

Manubrium of sternum

Jugular notch

Fig. 4.1 Cont'd

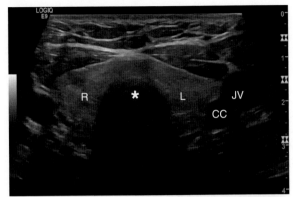

Fig. 4.2 Normal thyroid appearance on ultrasound. *R*, right thyroid. *L*, left thyroid. ***, trachea. *CC*, common carotid artery. *JV*, Internal jugular vein.

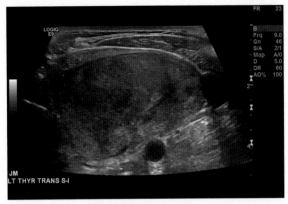

Fig. 4.3 Thyroid nodule.

of examination. Examine the lateral neck in a craniocaudal fashion. The SCM is a bulky, hypoechoic structure overlying the internal jugular vein and common carotid artery. The jugular vein is usually superficial and lateral to the common carotid artery.

PATHOLOGY

Abnormalities of the Anterior Triangle of the Neck and Face

Thyroid Pathology. Thyroid nodules are a common finding on neck ultrasound, occurring in up to 70% of women and 40% of men. A thyroid nodule is seen as a well-circumscribed, hypoechoic, isoechoic, or hyperechoic structure within the thyroid parenchyma. Large thyroid nodules may displace adjacent structures such as the trachea and internal jugular vein (Fig. 4.3). Although the majority of nodules are solid, thyroid cysts are also common. Thyroid cysts appear as anechoic structures without internal vascular flow and with posterior enhancement of the deep margin (Fig. 4.4). Approximately 90% of thyroid nodules are benign; therefore the National Comprehensive Cancer Network and the American Thyroid Association have created guidelines for nodules requiring further workup. Concerning features of malignancy include hypoechoic echotexture (when compared with surrounding thyroid parenchyma); microcalcifications, which appear as small, hyperechoic foci; infiltrative margins and irregular borders; and taller-than-wide orientation in the transverse plane. The decision to perform a fine-needle aspiration for malignancy is done in a nonemergency setting.

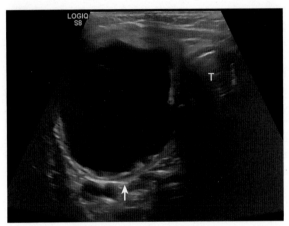

Fig. 4.4 Thyroid cyst. *T*, trachea.

Goiters, or diffuse thyroid enlargement, are fairly common and can present as a large, mobile neck mass. Substernal goiters can extend deep into the mediastinum. Graves' disease is an autoimmune disorder of the thyroid where the gland can become large and hypervascular (Fig. 4.5). Patients often present with signs and symptoms of hyperthyroidism, including anxiety, palpitations, weight loss, and tremor. The ultrasound appearance of goiters will often show a large, heterogeneous thyroid, with or without numerous nodules. Tracheal deviation may be noted, as the tracheal air column can be seen off-center.

Anaplastic thyroid cancer is an uncommon entity that is usually seen in older patients. Unlike goiters, anaplastic cancer is usually rapidly growing and firm and fixed on physical examination. Ultrasound may demonstrate a large, poorly circumscribed neck mass with involvement

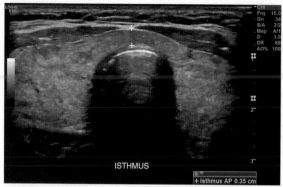

Fig. 4.5 Graves' disease of the thyroid as seen on ultrasound. (+) edges of the thyroid isthmus.

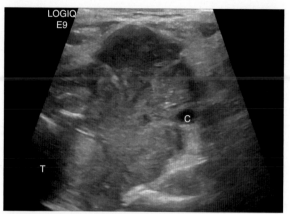

Fig. 4.6 Anaplastic thyroid cancer. *C*, Carotid artery. *T*, trachea.

of the trachea, strap muscles, or lateral neck vessels (Fig. 4.6). The diagnosis of anaplastic thyroid cancer can usually be made on fine-needle aspiration.

Thyroglossal Duct Cyst. Another example of pathology encountered in the anterior triangle is the thyroglossal duct cyst. Although thyroglossal duct cysts can occur at any age, most are detected before age of 20 years. They occur in the midline of the neck, from the base of the tongue to the anatomic position of the thyroid. Eighty percent are found adjacent to the hyoid bone. On physical examination a thyroglossal duct cyst appears as a soft, mobile mass that moves superiorly with swallowing or tongue protrusion.

On ultrasound, a thyroglossal duct cyst appears as a well-circumscribed, anechoic structure with posterior enhancement (Fig. 4.7). Some have a pseudosolid appearance resembling normal thyroid tissue secondary to a proteinaceous component. The wall may appear thickened (3–5 mm) with rim enhancement if the cyst is currently or was previously infected. The presence of a central solid component to the cyst should raise concern for malignancy. Regardless of ultrasound characteristics, patients with thyroglossal duct cysts should be referred to a head and neck surgeon.

Conditions of the Salivary Glands. There are three pairs of major salivary glands: the parotid, the submandibular, and the sublingual glands. The parotid gland is located in the retromandibular fossa, and its size is proportional to body weight. The submandibular gland is located medial to the mandible and is surrounded by the anterior belly of the digastric, the mylohyoid muscle, and the facial vessels. The sublingual gland is located in

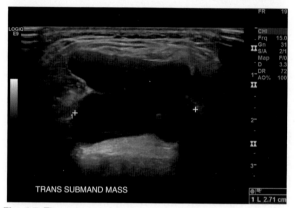

Fig. 4.7 Thyroglossal duct cyst. (+) edges of the thyroglossal duct cyst.

the floor of the mouth, medial to the mandible and lateral to the geniohyoid muscle.

Common conditions of the salivary glands presenting urgently include sialolithiasis, sialadenitis, and salivary tumors (benign and malignant). Sialolithiasis (stones within the salivary glands or ducts) and sialadenitis (inflammation of the gland) usually present with symptoms of pain and swelling that may be exacerbated by eating. Sialadenitis is due to an obstructive process. The most common etiology of obstruction is sialolithiasis, which leads to salivary stasis and ultimately infection. Kinks and strictures within the ductal system can also lead to infection and are usually caused by previous infection, trauma, or instrumentation resulting in inflammation or scarring of the duct. Viral disease, such as the mumps, can also lead to sialadenitis and is more common in unvaccinated children. Sialadenitis may be acute or chronic. The acute infection may result in an abscess and associated swelling of the gland. The peak incidence of acute sialadenitis is between 30 and 60 years and is more common in men. Chronic infections usually result from recurrent indolent inflammation in the setting of sialolithiasis. Over time, remodeling of the parenchyma takes place, and healthy gland tissue can be replaced by fibrosis.

Given the superficial location of the salivary glands, high-resolution ultrasound is the ideal imaging modality for evaluation. This is best performed with a high-frequency, linear array transducer. The first principle of evaluating a salivary pathology is to evaluate the glands in pairs. Comparison between the gland in question and its contralateral counterpart can confirm the presence of abnormal pathology. On ultrasound, salivary stones will have the characteristic appearance of a hyperechoic structure with posterior shadowing (Fig. 4.8). Stones >2 mm in size can be detected by ultrasound. Acute sialadenitis appears as an enlarged, hypoechoic gland with increased vascularity.

Salivary gland tumors comprise a diverse spectrum of neoplasms with a broad range of outcomes. The majority of salivary gland tumors occur in the parotid gland. The risk of malignancy depends on the location of the tumor, with 75% of parotid tumors being benign and 40% of submandibular gland tumors and 80% of sublingual gland tumors being malignant. The most common benign tumor is the pleomorphic adenoma, usually located in the parotid gland. These tumors appear as well-circumscribed, homogenous, hypoechoic lesions with lobulated margins and moderate vascularity (Fig. 4.9). Malignant salivary gland tumors include mucoepidermoid carcinoma, adenoid cystic carcinoma, undifferentiated carcinoma, adenocarcinoma, lymphoma, and squamous cell carcinoma. Ultrasound features concerning for malignancy include irregular borders, hypervascularity, heterogeneity, and necrosis. If there is suspicion for malignancy, follow-up cross-sectional imaging and biopsy are necessary in a nonemergent setting.

Branchial Cleft Abnormalities. Branchial cleft abnormalities are seen primarily in the pediatric population but may present in adults as well. Aberrant development of the branchial arches and clefts results in a variety of anomalies. Such anomalies may present as a cyst (a confined, epithelial-lined structure), a sinus (connection from the pharynx to a blind pouch in the neck), or a fistula (an open tract between the pharynx and skin). Symptoms include neck swelling, pain, and drainage.

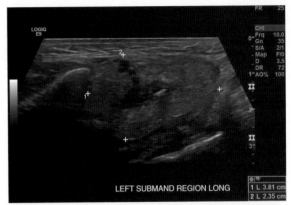

Fig. 4.8 Sialolithiasis. +, edges of the submandibular gland.

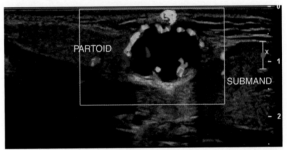

Fig. 4.9 Pleomorphic adenoma.

Branchial cleft abnormalities are classically categorized based on their embryologic origin. First branchial abnormalities are divided into two types. Type 1 abnormalities are located near the external auditory canal and may involve the parotid gland. Type 2 abnormalities start near the angle of the mandible and tract superiorly to join the external auditory canal. Second branchial cleft abnormalities account for 90% of branchial cleft irregularities. Second branchial cleft abnormalities start in the tonsillar fossa and end along the anterior border of the SCM. Abnormalities of the third branchial cleft also present anterior to the SCM, but are usually located on the left side of the neck and are anatomically associated with the thyroid gland. Fourth branchial clefts are very rare and located low in the neck (Fig. 4.10).

On ultrasound a branchial cleft cyst classically appears as a well-defined, cystic mass with uniformly low echogenicity and no internal septations (Fig. 4.11). Branchial cleft cysts in adults may present with more complex ultrasound characteristics, including internal debris or a pseudosolid or heterogeneous appearance.

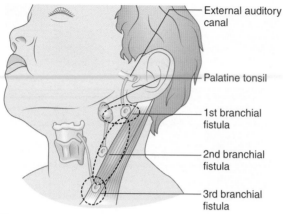

Fig. 4.10 Branchial cleft anomalies. (From Irace A., Adil E. Embryology of congenital neck masses. *Operative Techniques in Otolarnyngology – Head and Neck Surgery.* Elsevier: 2017. 28(3);138-142.)

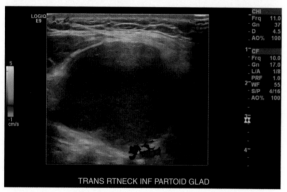

Fig. 4.11 Branchial cleft cyst.

Peritonsillar Infections. In patients presenting with trismus, uvular deviation, and tonsillar asymmetry, a peritonsillar abscess (PTA) and cellulitis must be considered. Intraoral ultrasound has proven to be an effective tool for evaluation of PTAs in the hands of experienced physicians, with studies demonstrating up to 100% sensitivity in the appropriate clinical setting. A high-frequency, cavitary ultrasound transducer is recommended. A PTA can be seen as an organized collection of fluid within the peritonsillar tissues between the palatine tonsils and the pharynx. Cellulitis is characterized as inflammation without an organized fluid collection. The abscess will appear as a hypoechoic or anechoic mass with distinct borders and a hyperechoic rim (Fig. 4.12). Ultrasound is also useful to facilitate drainage of PTAs. Please see Chapter 3 for further information regarding PTAs and Chapter 29 for ultrasound-guided procedures.

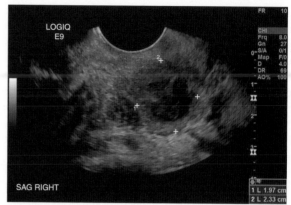

Fig. 4.12 Peritonsillar abscess. +, edges of the peritonsillar abscess.

Abnormalities in the Posterior Triangle of the Neck (Including the Common Carotid Artery and Jugular Adenopathy)

Adenopathy. Cervical adenopathy may be secondary to infectious, inflammatory, or malignant origin. The most common cause of adenopathy in the neck is infectious and can result from viral or bacterial conditions. Malignant adenopathy is less common but has obvious implications to patient management. Ultrasound has a superior sensitivity and specificity for detecting malignant lymph nodes when compared with physical examination.

Cervical adenopathy is a common feature of many carcinomas and lymphomas. Enlargement of cervical lymph nodes can be the presenting symptom for oropharyngeal, nasopharyngeal, thyroid, and even visceral cancers. Cervical lymph nodes are divided into six lymph node levels based on anatomic boundaries (Fig. 4.13). In malignant adenopathy, the pattern and distribution of lymphadenopathy is predictive of the location of the primary tumor (Fig. 4.14). Cervical adenopathy in level I (submental and submandibular nodes) is most commonly associated with malignancy in the floor of the mouth, lower lip, or lower gum. Level II adenopathy (also known as the *jugulodigastric nodes*) may represent metastatic oral cavity, oropharyngeal, and laryngeal cancers. The level III nodes (midjugular chain) drain the pharynx, larynx, and thyroid and thus may represent malignancies from these structures. Level IV nodes (inferior jugular chain) can be the site of metastasis from thyroid, breast, lung, and gastrointestinal cancers. Several diverse sites can drain to the level V (posterior triangle) nodes, with the supraclavicular nodes frequently being the site of metastatic gastrointestinal and thoracic

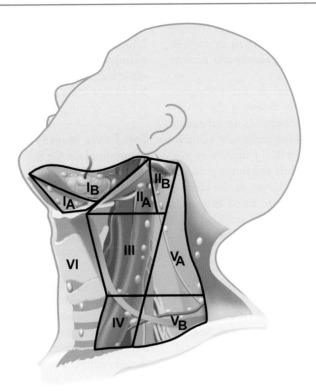

Fig. 4.13 Cervical lymph node levels. (©2019, Memorial Sloan Kettering Cancer Center).

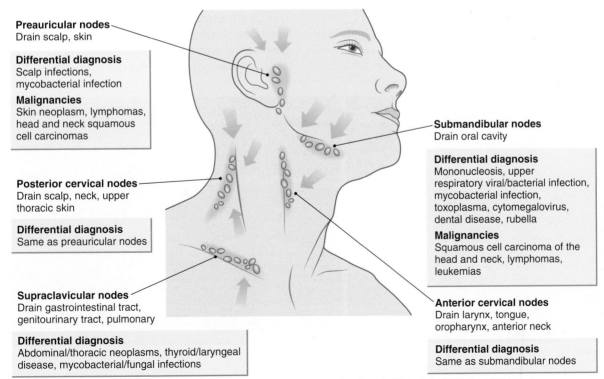

Preauricular nodes
Drain scalp, skin

Differential diagnosis
Scalp infections,
mycobacterial infection

Malignancies
Skin neoplasm, lymphomas,
head and neck squamous
cell carcinomas

Posterior cervical nodes
Drain scalp, neck, upper
thoracic skin

Differential diagnosis
Same as preauricular nodes

Supraclavicular nodes
Drain gastrointestinal tract,
genitourinary tract, pulmonary

Differential diagnosis
Abdominal/thoracic neoplasms, thyroid/laryngeal
disease, mycobacterial/fungal infections

Submandibular nodes
Drain oral cavity

Differential diagnosis
Mononucleosis, upper
respiratory viral/bacterial infection,
mycobacterial infection,
toxoplasma, cytomegalovirus,
dental disease, rubella

Malignancies
Squamous cell carcinoma of the
head and neck, lymphomas,
leukemias

Anterior cervical nodes
Drain larynx, tongue,
oropharynx, anterior neck

Differential diagnosis
Same as submandibular nodes

Fig. 4.14 Patterns of lymph node metastases to the head and neck. (Copyright 2002 David Klemm.)

cancers, and the nodes in the superior posterior triangle being the site of metastatic head and neck squamous cell carcinoma and skin cancers. Lymphomas can present with enlargement of any nodal level.

There is no single sonographic feature pathognomonic for all malignancies, but assessing the node's size, shape, echogenicity, and presence of an echogenic hilum are useful in distinguishing malignant adenopathy from a benign process. Cervical lymph node size may be increased in young patients and in the presence of infection or inflammation. However, in the context of an accurate clinical history, a size cutoff of greater than 7 mm in the short axis had an 85% sensitivity and 79% specificity for predicting malignancy. The shape of the lymph node is also important in determining the malignancy risk. Malignant adenopathy classically has a round shape, whereas oval or flat nodes are usually normal or reactive. The shape can be quantitatively assessed by determining the size ratio of the short-to-long axis (S:L). Round nodes, with an S:L >0.5, are suspicious for malignancy. More oval or elliptical-shaped nodes, S:L <0.5, are more likely to be benign (Fig. 4.15). Metastatic lymph nodes are usually hypoechoic in appearance relative to adjacent musculature. One notable exception is metastatic papillary thyroid cancer, which may appear hyperechoic compared with adjacent musculature. Necrosis can be seen in aggressive or advanced cancer as the tumor exhausts its blood supply and appears as echolucent regions within the node, which correspond to cystic or liquefactive necrosis. Finally, an echogenic hilum is seen in benign lymph nodes. The echogenic hilum is noted as a hyperechoic line contiguous with the perinodal fat that enters the node architecture. Metastatic lymph nodes classically do not show an echogenic hilum, but some studies have suggested that this finding is not as specific as once thought.

Soft Tissue Masses of the Neck. The neck is also a common place for soft tissue tumors, including lipomas, neurofibromas, and schwannomas. Lipomas are benign tumors derived from adipose tissue. Most are located superficially and are soft and mobile on physical examination. On ultrasound, lipomas will have the same echogenicity as adipose tissue, but usually appear as a discreet, well-circumscribed tumor. Neurofibromas and schwannomas are neurogenic tumors located in conjunction with a nerve. The visual difference between the two lies in the relationship to the nerve. Neurofibromas will be centered on the nerve, whereas schwannomas appear adjacent to the nerve but not incorporated in it. Sonographically, these tumors appear as an encapsulated, hypoechoic lesion with a fusiform, oval, or round shape (Fig. 4.16).

The Pulsating Neck Mass. The differential diagnosis of a pulsatile neck mass includes carotid body tumors, tortuosity of carotid arteries, and pseudoaneurysms. Carotid body tumors are paragangliomas that are usually benign, slow growing, and found in the upper cervical region. Importantly, they often present as a pulsatile mass, differentiating

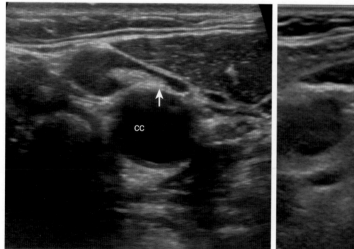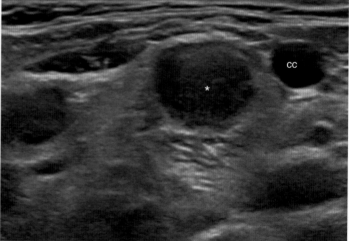

Fig. 4.15 (A) Normal lymph node. (B) Malignant lymph node. Arrows shows a normal fatty hilum in a normal lymph node. *, rounded, abnormal lymph node. *CC*, common carotid artery.

them from an enlarged lymph node or branchial cleft cyst. Ultrasonography classically will show a hypoechoic mass resting near the bifurcation of the common carotid artery. Numerous anechoic, channel-like structures may be seen, which represent the vasculature within the tumor. Color Doppler demonstrates significant vascularity and abundant low-resistance flow (Fig. 4.17). Oftentimes, embolization of these tumors is performed before resection to reduce intraoperative blood loss.

Tortuosity of the internal carotid artery can occur in up to 45% of patients evaluated by high-resolution ultrasound. In the thin patient, tortuosity can be mistaken for a mass. Ultrasound allows the provider to trace the course of the artery and distinguish between a mass and a tortuous course of the carotid. Pseudoaneurysms arise from injury to the carotid artery, typically in the setting of blunt or penetrating neck trauma. They are formed by extravasation of blood into the surrounding tissues. Sonographically, a pseudoaneurysm will appear as a hypoechoic fluid collection located adjacent to the carotid artery with arterial blood flow.

Confirmation of Endotracheal Tube Placement. Endotracheal intubation in the emergency department is a common procedure; however, unrecognized misplacement into the esophagus is a potentially devastating complication. Tracheal ultrasound has been tested to confirm placement of the endotracheal tube (ETT). Studies have shown sensitivities and specificities of up to 100% using tracheal ultrasound for ETT placement.

When assessing ETT placement with ultrasound, the sonographer places the linear probe directly over the trachea just superior to the sternal notch. Once the ETT has been placed using direct laryngoscopy, the image should show one air–mucosa interface with a comet tail artifact and posterior shadowing. This is the trachea with ETT in place. Two air–mucosa interfaces suggest an esophageal intubation. The user can assess ventilation by evaluating for the lung sliding sign. This is done by using the linear transducer probe placed over the second to fourth intercostal space at the midclavicular line. Bilateral sliding confirms ETT placement above the carina.

BIBLIOGRAPHY

Abbasi S, Farsi D, Mohammad AZ, et al. Direct ultrasound methods: a confirmatory technique for proper endotracheal intubation in the emergency department. *Eur J Emerg Med.* 2015;22:1.

Aculate NR, Jones HB, Bansal A, et al. Papillary carcinoma within a thyroglossal duct cyst: significant of a central solid component on ultrasound imaging. *Br J Oral Maxillofac Surg.* 2014;52:277–278.

Ajmal S, Rapoport S, Batlle H, et al. The natural history of the benign thyroid nodule: what is the appropriate follow-up strategy? *J Am Coll Surg.* 2015;200(6):987–992.

Baatenburg de Job RJ, Rongen RJ. Ultrasound of the head and neck. *J Otorhinolaryngol Relat Spec.* 1993;55(5):250–257.

Casarim AL, Tincani AJ, Del Negro A, et al. Carotid body tumor: retrospective analysis on 22 patients. *Sao Paulo Med J.* 2014;132(3):133–139.

Collins B, Stoner JA, Digoy GP. Benefits of ultrasound vs. computed tomography in the diagnosis of pediatric lateral neck masses. *Int J of Ped Otorhinolaryngology.* 2014;(78):423–426.

Costantino TG, Satz WA, Dehnkamp W, et al. Randomized trial comparing intraoral ultrasound to landmark-based needle aspiration in patients with suspected peritonsillar abscess. *Acad Emerg Med.* 2012;19:626–631.

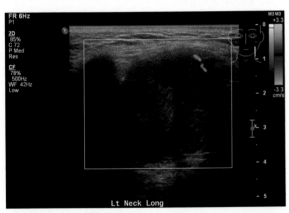

Fig. 4.16 Schwannoma.

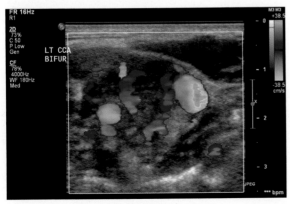

Fig. 4.17 Carotid body tumor.

Giacomini CP, Jeffrey RB, Skin LK. Últrasonographic evaluation of malignant and normal cervical lymph nodes. *Semin Ultrasound CT MR.* 2013;34:236–247.

Gritzmann N, Hollerweger A, Macheiner P, et al. Sonography of soft tissue masses of the neck. *J Clin Ultrasound.* 2002;30(6):356–373.

Kuna SK, Bracic I, Tesic V, et al. Ultrasonographic differentiation of benign from malignant neck lymphadenopathy in thyroid cancer. *J Ultrasound Med.* 2006;25:1531–1537.

Lam EC, Palacios E, Neitzschman H. Carotid pseudoaneurysm of the neck. *Ear Nose Throat J.* 2001;90(11):512–514.

Lyons M, Blaivas M. Intraoral ultrasound in the diagnosis and treatment of suspected peritonsillar abscess in the emergency department. *Acad Emerg Med.* 2005;12(1).

Mallorie CNJ, Jones SD, Drage NA, et al. The reliability of high resolution ultrasound in the identification of pus collections in head and neck swellings. *Int J Oral Maxillofac Surg.* 2012;41:252–255.

NCCN guidelines. https://www.nccn.org/professionals/physician_gls/pdf/thyroid.pdf

Netter FH, Hansen JT, Lambert DR. *Netter's Clinical Anatomy.* Carlstadt, NJ: Icon Learning Systems; 2005.

Niu L, Hao Y, Zhu L, et al. Sonographic diagnosis of carotid body tumor. *Zhonghua Zhong Liu Za Zhi.* 2002;24(5):488–490.

Nogan S, Jandali D, Cipolla M, et al. The use of ultrasound imaging in the evaluation of peritonsillar infections. *Laryngoscope.* 2015;(125):2604–2607.

Prosser JD, Myer CM. Branchial cleft anomalies and thymic cysts. *Otolyarngol Clin N Am.* 2015;48:1–14.

Sanderson RJ. Squamous cell carcinoma of the head and neck. *BMJ.* 2002;325(7368):822–827.

Suh HJ, moon HJ, Kwak JY, et al. Anaplastic thyroid cancer: ultrasonographic findings and the role of ultrasonography-guided fine needle aspiration biopsy. *Yonesi Med J.* 2013;54(6):1400–1406.

Takeuchi Y, Tsutomu N, Konno A, et al. Differential diagnosis of pulsatile neck masses by Doppler color flow imaging. *Ann Otol Rhinol Laryngol.* 1995;104(8):633–638.

Uchida T, Shigihara N, Takeno K, et al. Characteristics of patients with Graves disease and intrathyroid hypervascularity compared to painless thyroiditis. *J Ultrasound Med.* 2014;33(10):1791–1796.

Wadsworth DT, Siegel MJ. Thyroglossal duct cysts: variability of sonographic findings. *AJR Am J Roentgenol.* 1994;163(6):1475–1477.

Ying M, Bbhatia KSS, Lee YP, et al. Review of ultrasonography of malignant neck nodes: greyscale, Doppler, contrast enhancement and elastography. *Cancer Imaging.* 2013;13(4):658–669.

Zander D, Smoker WRK. Imaging of ectopic thyroid tissue and thyroglossal duct cysts. *Radiographics.* 2014;34:37–50.

Zengel P, Schrotzlmair F, Reichel C, et al. Sonography: the leading diagnostic tool for disease of the salivary glands. *Sem in Ultrasound, CT and MRI.* 2013;(11):196–203.

5

Ocular

Gabriel S. Espinoza, Christine N. McBeth, Michael A. Schick

INTRODUCTION

Ocular point-of-care ultrasound (POCUS) can rapidly identify ocular emergencies, including the diagnoses of lens detachment/dislocations, retinal detachment, vitreous detachment, vitreous hemorrhage, ocular infections, the presence of foreign bodies, and secondary signs of elevated intracranial pressure. In a fast-paced clinical practice, a fully dilated ophthalmologic examination may be impractical, and studies have shown that many practitioners lack the clinical skills to perform it effectively. The benefits of performing an ocular ultrasound include ease of use, low cost, sensitivity for identifying pathology, lack of ionizing radiation, and ability to perform imaging at the bedside. POCUS offers few risks, with the exception in the setting of a possible globe rupture, and should not cause significant discomfort to the patient when done correctly. Therefore ultrasound can supplement the acute eye examination, and can accurately detect a range of important eye disorders and attempt to rule out emergent conditions.

ANATOMY

To fully utilize the benefits of the ocular ultrasound, it is imperative to have an accurate understanding of the anatomy of the eye (Fig. 5.1). The white, outermost layer of the eye is the sclera, which surrounds the entire globe and serves as a protective layer. The limbus creates the junction between the sclera and the cornea, which is the transparent part of the eye that covers the colored iris. The pupil allows light to enter the eye. The anterior chamber (AC) is the space between the lens and the cornea. The AC contains aqueous humor produced by the ciliary body, which is continuous with the colored iris, and the choroid, which is the vascular bed for the retina. With ultrasound, this will be the most superficial anechoic chamber. Just deep to the AC is the lens, which is a hyperechoic concave structure. The retina is the innermost layer of the eye, which contains the photoreceptors. It is often not seen unless it is detached from the posterior aspect of the globe. The posterior chamber, which accounts for approximately 80% of the eye, will be the anechoic structure deep to the lens and is filled with vitreous fluid. Finally, the optic nerve is seen as a hypoechoic structure just deep to the retina (Fig. 5.2).

EXAMINATION TECHNIQUE

The structures of the eye are superficial and are best visualized with a high-frequency linear array probe. A transparent dressing can be placed on top of the closed eye for patient comfort and ease of cleaning the gel after the examination (Fig. 5.3). Alternatively, clean gel may be placed directly on the closed eyelid. The patient should be placed in a supine to semi-upright position to maintain the gel's position. Slightly cooling the gel will firm it and further maintain its position. To reduce theoretical iatrogenic injury, the ocular or eye examination setting should be chosen on the ultrasound machine. The examiner can maintain probe stability while scanning by placing the scanning hand on the patient's nasal bridge, forehead, or cheek, and use copious amounts of

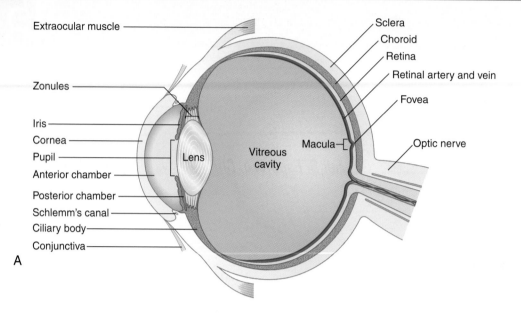

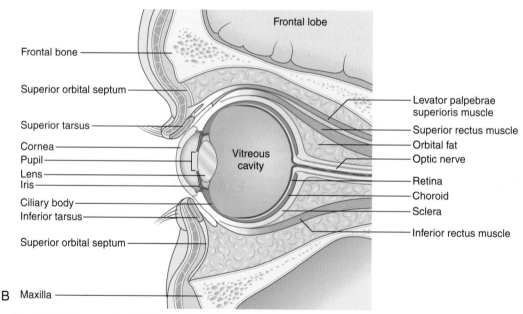

Fig. 5.1 (A) Cross-sectional axial anatomy of the eye. (B) Cross-sectional sagittal anatomy of the eye. (From Kels BD, Grzybowski A, Grant-Kels J. Human ocular anatomy. *Clin Dermatol.* 2015;33(2):140-146, Fig. 1.)

gel to avoid transmitting unnecessary pressure to the eye. Limiting direct pressure on the eye is important for patient comfort, as well as reducing the oculocardiac reflex, which may decrease the patient's heart rate. Use the conventional method of transducer orientation, directing the indicator toward the patient's right in the transverse plane and cephalad in the sagittal plane. Careful methodical scanning of all eye segments in two planes is needed to evaluate pathology. In each orthogonal plane the patient should be asked to move the eyes

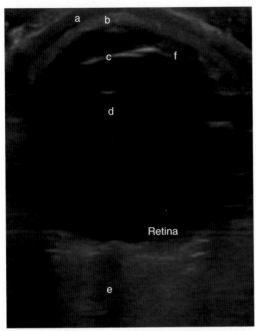

Fig. 5.2 Ultrasound anatomy of the eye. *a,* Eyelid. *b,* Cornea. *c,* Iris. *d,* Lens. *e,* Optic nerve sheath. *f,* Ciliary body.

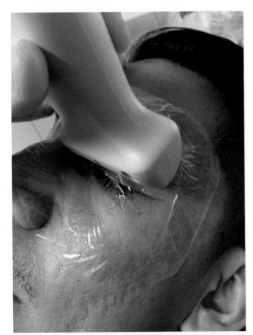

Fig. 5.3 Note the use of the 10-MHz linear array probe. Copious gel is applied over the plastic patch over the eye. Gentle pressure is applied. Follow the conventional probe orientation.

in every direction to allow for full dynamic evaluation of the anterior and posterior chambers, as well as confirm extraocular muscle function. Contraindications include open ocular trauma, periorbital wounds, globe rupture, or retrobulbar hemorrhage.

INDICATIONS AND PATHOLOGY

Acute Loss of Vision

Retinal Detachment. Retinal detachment (RD) has a prevalence of 0.3%, and patients can present with the classic symptoms of sudden, painless loss of vision or a monocular visual field defect, often described as a curtain coming down. Some patients may experience flashers or floaters a few days or weeks before loss of vision. Prompt diagnosis can expedite an ophthalmologic consultation and prevent further vision loss. It is important to assess for a macular-sparing RD, as this will warrant emergent surgery. If the macula is involved, patients may complain of central vision loss, which will require surgery within 1 to 2 weeks. The utility of POCUS in diagnosing RD has been established by several prospective studies, and a 2016 retrospective study of 109 patients by Jacobsen et al. demonstrated a sensitivity and specificity for the use of POCUS to be 91% (95% CI [90–99]) and 96% (95% CI [89–99]), respectively.

The retina is normally anchored to the choroid of the optic nerve and anterolaterally at the ora serrata in the ciliary body. On ultrasound, a RD will appear as a thick, hyperechoic, mobile, membranous flap in the posterior chamber that appears lifted off the posterior surface and moves in conjunction with the patient's eye movements, and is tethered to the optic nerve (Fig. 5.4). The macula is usually seen temporally (lateral) to the optic nerve; thus if there is macular involvement, the retina will appear completely detached up to the optic nerve, resembling a hyperechoic letter "V" in the posterior chamber (Fig. 5.5).

Posterior Vitreous Detachment. A posterior vitreous detachment involves the separation of the vitreous from the underlying retina due to degeneration and/or shrinkage. It can present with similar complaints as an RD with floaters and/or flashes, but may also be insidious. There is typically no mention of a curtain coming down. Floaters are a sensation of gray or dark spots moving in the visual field, and flashes are typically described as monocular repeated flashes of white light in the peripheral visual field. This pathology is more

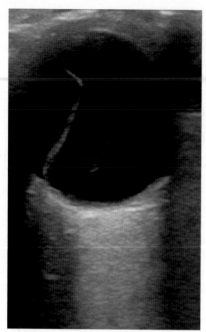

Fig. 5.4 Note the hyperechoic membranous flap. This image is a macula-sparing retinal detachment.

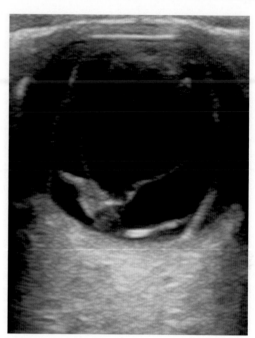

Fig. 5.5 Note the hyperechoic letter "V" that is formed, as this retinal detachment involves the macula.

common with increasing age, with a 24% prevalence in adults 50 to 59 years of age and reaching up to 87% in adults 80 to 89 years of age. Thus suspicion for this pathology should be higher on the differential diagnosis if an elderly patient presents with these symptoms. Other risk factors that may contribute are myopia, trauma, and intraocular infections. On dynamic ultrasound imaging, an undulating, echogenic membrane will be present in the posterior chamber, and it should move freely and swirl in the opposite direction that the eye is turning (Fig. 5.6). Additionally, vitreoretinal adhesions can lead to retinal tears or avulsions of peripheral blood vessels, which may lead to vitreal hemorrhages. Unlike an RD, where the hyperechoic membrane is tethered to the choroid of the optic nerve, a vitreous detachment is free floating. Because a vitreous detachment does not typically lead to permanent vision loss, it is clinically significant to distinguish from an RD.

Vitreous Hemorrhage. Neovascularization from diabetic retinopathy, sickle cell retinopathy, and ocular ischemic syndrome is a vasoproliferative disorder that creates vessels prone to bleeding, leading to vitreous hemorrhage. Normal vessels can be torn in trauma or

due to RD. A final source of hemorrhage can be blood from retinal microaneurysms or age-related macular degeneration. Blood in the posterior chamber causes obstruction of the retina during fundoscopic examination but does not impede the use of ultrasound. The patient may complain of loss of vision, floaters, red cape or hue, or "black rain." The ultrasound characteristics depend on the severity of bleeding and the time course. Of note, the vitreous hemorrhage can also resemble an RD, as there will be echogenic, fibrous membranes floating in the posterior chamber. In the early stages, dynamic imaging can show very subtle low-amplitude echoes. As hemorrhage progresses, fibrinous vitreous echogenic membranes may appear and will be mobile at first, but may stiffen over time (Fig. 5.7). To distinguish it from an RD, observe for any free movement of the echogenic material; this can be referred to as having a "snow globe" or "washing machine" pattern, and is not observed in RD. There will also be absence of any attachment to the optic disc. For hemorrhage associated with RD, urgent surgery is often needed. Hemorrhage without associated RD is treated based on the underlying cause and should be referred urgently to an ocular specialist, as laser therapy or vitrectomy may be needed. Asteroid

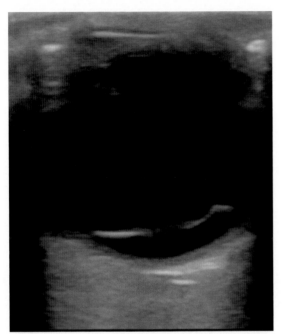

Fig. 5.6 Image of posterior vitreous detachment. Note the undulating hyperechoic membrane in the posterior chamber. This will move freely when the patient is asked to move the eye.

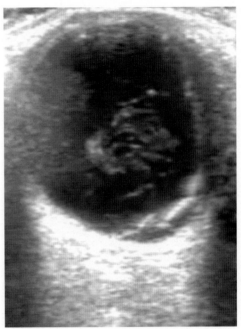

Fig. 5.7 Vitreous hemorrhage. Note the fibrinous echogenic material in the posterior chamber. The material is mobile during dynamic ocular exam.

hyalosis is another condition that may mimic vitreous hemorrhage. It may be present in up to 2% of the population and is caused by vitreal calcium–phosphate crystal deposits that appear as hyperechoic floaters in the posterior chamber. Most patients are asymptomatic, and very few require intervention.

Central Retinal Artery Occlusion. Central retinal artery occlusion (CRAO) is another presentation of painless acute vision loss. Although there are multiple etiologies for CRAO, such as giant cell arteritis, emboli have an associated higher mortality due to cardiovascular risk factors. On POCUS, a long-standing embolus, whether from thrombotic material or cholesterol, will become calcified and demonstrate a "spot sign" if present at the distal aspect of the retinal artery adjacent to the optic nerve. This appears as a small, hyperechoic spot in the central retinal artery adjacent to the optic nerve. Using the color Doppler function allows examination for ocular blood flow in the ophthalmic and central retinal artery and vein. With this function, the examiner may notice a retrobulbar hyperechoic "plaque" suggestive of an embolus. Additionally, with use of the color Doppler,

the examiner can see decreased, or even the absence of, blood flow within the central retinal artery.

Ocular Trauma

Lens Dislocations (Ectopia lentis). Ectopia lentis, a lens dislocation or malposition, is largely due to trauma but can also be seen in patients with collagen disorders (Marfan's and Ehlers-Danlos syndrome). Patients can present with a painful red eye, photosensitivity, diplopia, and partial or complete loss of vision. In a cross-sectional study by Ojaghi Haghighi et al., POCUS use by emergency medicine physicians was shown to have an 84.6% sensitivity (CI 95% [53.7–97.3]) and a 98.3% specificity (CI 95% [93.3–99.7]), respectively. There are two types of dislocations: partial (subluxation) and complete.

- With partial dislocation (subluxation), the lens will be partially attached to the ciliary body, and on dynamic ultrasound imaging can be seen as a convex hyperechoic structure partially attached to the ciliary body. Changing the patient's position during imaging can aid in determining whether the patient presents with a complete or partial dislocation.

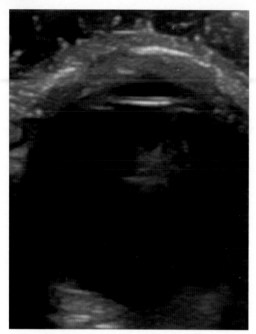

Fig. 5.8 A complete lens dislocation.

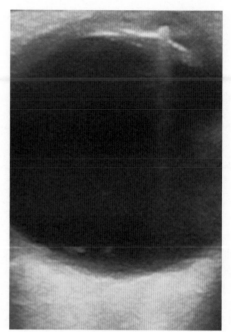

Fig. 5.9 A hyperechoic foreign body is noted in the anterior chamber, with a refractory artifact observed extending to the vitreous.

- With complete dislocation, the lens will appear completely in the vitreous, and on ultrasound imaging may even be overlying the retina (Fig. 5.8).

Foreign Bodies. Intraocular foreign bodies are very common complaints, with an incidence of 18% to 41%. Complaints of sudden eye pain, decreased visual acuity, photophobia, and a history of manual labor or working with power tools should raise the index of suspicion for an intraocular foreign body. The presence of an ocular foreign body may not be evident on physical examination, because those produced from hammering or grinding metal are launched at high speeds with little to no evidence of ocular damage. Although small, they can threaten a patient's vision via scarring of the cornea, cataract formation, endophthalmitis, and RD. In an animal model evaluating the use of ultrasound for detecting intraocular foreign bodies by Shiver et al., the sensitivity and specificity were 87.5% and 95.8%, respectively. Hyperechoic material such as metal or glass may appear in the anterior or posterior chamber. This material can cause bright linear reflections with posterior artifacts due to the high refractory index. Wood can be visualized with ultrasound as well, but is typically less echogenic than metal or glass. At times, an air artifact

can be observed on dynamic oculomotor ultrasound if a significant amount is introduced by the foreign body as it enters the eye (Fig. 5.9). With the use of color Doppler, one can observe for the twinkling artifact—artifactual color appearing behind strongly echogenic structures—which will appear as rapidly changing flashes.

Retrobulbar Hemorrhage/Hematoma. Acute retrobulbar fluid collections, including retrobulbar hematoma (RBH) is a rare complication that can occur after blunt orbital trauma, surgery, or infections. It can lead to an orbital compartment syndrome with increased intraocular pressure and threatened sight due to central retinal artery occlusion, compression of adjacent optic nerve vasculature, or direct optic nerve compression. Patients may present with marked signs of periorbital edema and ecchymosis, proptosis, painful exophthalmos, restriction of extraocular movements, and decreased visual acuity, and an afferent pupillary defect. Most orbital hematomas are commonly seen with nondisplaced orbital wall fractures. Given the presence of facial edema due to trauma or altered mental state, identification of RBH or hemorrhage may be challenging. Although computed tomography (CT) scan is the preferred method for diagnosis of RBH or hemorrhage, POCUS allows for fast evaluation. RBH may appear as a hypoechoic-to-anechoic fluid collection within the hyperechoic retrobulbar area posterior to the retina, with possible distortion of the posterior aspect of the eye (Fig. 5.10). A unilateral hematoma may push the extraocular muscles toward the midline. Blood can coagulate and appear isoechoic, making the diagnosis challenging.

Globe Rupture. Globe rupture is usually due to ocular trauma and is considered an ophthalmologic emergency. It presents with surrounding soft tissue edema, which may prevent direct visualization of the affected eye. Physical examination findings include hyphema, irregular pupils, and a shallow anterior chamber. Use of POCUS is relatively contraindicated for globe rupture. However, if the practitioner's examination is impeded by other trauma, the need for emergent ophthalmologic consultation is suspected, and other imaging options such as CT may be delayed or unavailable, the careful use of POCUS can be indicated. Every effort should be made to not cause further trauma or increase intraocular pressure. The examiner can observe loss of ocular volume, pressure, and vitreous humor, along with distorted size and shape (Fig. 5.11). Chandra et al. used animal models to determine the sensitivity and specificity of this examination to be 64% (95% CI [54%–73%]) and 71% (95% CI [64%–77%]), respectively.

Headache

Giant Cell Arteritis. Giant cell arteritis (GCA) can also cause painless visual disruption due to ischemia from the granulomatous inflammation, resulting in narrowing or occlusion of medium to larger-sized arteries with an internal elastic lamina. All ophthalmic complaints due to GCA are considered medical emergencies; thus practitioners should have a high index of suspicion when patient's present with jaw claudication, headache, diplopia, and/or constitutional symptoms that are suggestive of GCA. Complications of GCA that can lead to vision loss include CRAO, which has been previously described above. Other etiologies of vision loss due to GCA include anterior ischemic optic neuropathy and cilioretinal artery occlusion. Although not a direct ocular ultrasound, the temporal or axillary arteries can be performed when patients present with symptoms suggestive of GCA.

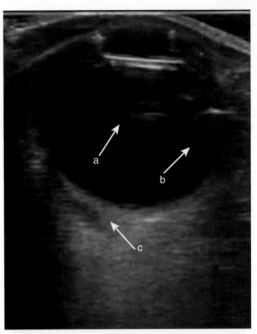

Fig. 5.10 Retrobulbar hematoma. Note the vitreous hemorrhage (*a*), with distortion of part of the orbit (*b*) and some hypoechoic material (*c*) indicative of edema or hematoma in the hyperechoic retrobulbar area posterior to the retina.

Fig. 5.11 Globe rupture. Note the distorted shape of the eye and complete loss of anatomical landmarks.

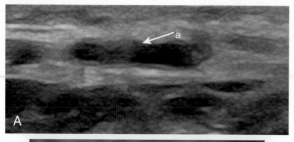

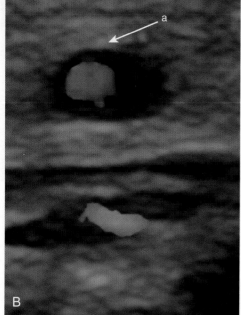

Fig. 5.12 (A) Longitudinal image of a patient's temporal artery concerning for giant cell arteritis (GCA). Note the intimal wall thickening, with decreased compressibility, and appearance of mild edema around the intima. (B) Axial image of the patient's temporal artery concerning for GCA with color Doppler. Note the intimal wall thickening and clear edema around the intima indicative of the "halo sign."

The physician should look for wall thickening (halo sign) or noncompressibility of the temporal or axillary arteries, stenosis, and vessel occlusion (Fig. 5.12A). The halo sign, first mentioned in 1995, was noted as an edematous, hypoechoic material, in contrast the hyperechoic surrounding tissue and anechoic arterial lumen. The halo sign can be best visualized in the transverse view with the color function on (Fig. 5.12B). Cutoff values for the halo diameters for temporal arteries have been shown to be 0.3 to 1.0 mm and for the axillary arteries to be 1.0 to 2.0 mm. According to a meta-analysis performed by Karassa et al., the halo sign has a sensitivity of 69% and a

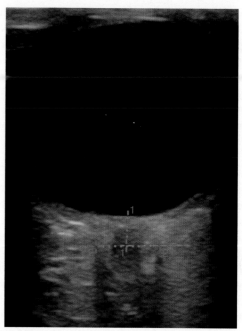

Fig. 5.13 Obtaining the optic nerve sheath diameter. Note the position of the calipers when obtaining these measurements. The optimal distance to obtain the diameter is 3 mm posterior to the retina.

specificity of 82% compared with temporal artery biopsy, which is considered the gold standard for diagnosis.

Increased Intracranial Pressure/Optic Nerve Sheath Diameter

The sheath around the optic nerve is a continuation of the dura, with the subarachnoid space extending along the nerve. Therefore the intraorbital part of the subarachnoid space is distensible and can expand with an increase in intracranial pressure, leading to optic disc edema and papilledema. Due to this, the optic nerve sheath diameter (ONSD) may correlate with intracranial pressure. Measurements of the ONSD are obtained 3 mm behind the retina, in the retrobulbar segment, as this is where cerebrospinal fluid (CSF) can cause the greatest enlargement (Fig. 5.13). Measurements are typically made with the ultrasound in an axial plane, held with the transducer pointed slightly inferior toward the optic nerve (with the patient looking straight ahead). The generally accepted upper limit of ONSD is <5 mm, but some studies suggest a slightly larger value of <5.5 mm (Figs. 5.14 and 5.15). In pediatric patients, the measurements are adjusted to <4.5 mm for children 1 to 15 years of age and <4 mm

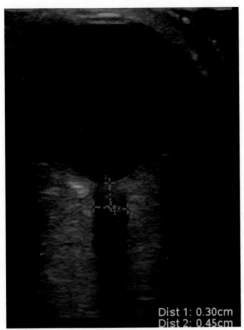

Fig. 5.14 Optic nerve sheath diameter. Note the normal diameter obtained in this image: <5 mm.

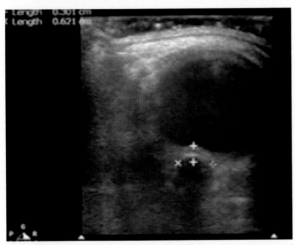

Fig. 5.15 Optic nerve sheath diameter. This sheath is increased and is abnormal, as the value is >5 mm.

for infants. When obtaining dynamic ultrasound imaging, the examiner should be careful to not confuse a hypoechoic artifact that can be seen posterior to the globe with the actual optic nerve sheath. Several investigations have shown good correlation with the use of ocular ultrasound to measure ONSD and its correlation with invasive measurements. Dubourg et al.'s systematic review of six articles summarizing the available evidence and accuracy of ultrasound use for measuring ONSD found a pooled sensitivity and specificity of 90% (95% CI [80%–95%]) and 85% (95% CI [73%–93%]), respectively.

BIBLIOGRAPHY

Bates A, Goett HJ. Ocular Ultrasound. [Updated 2017 Nov 9]. In: *StatPearls [Internet]*. Treasure Island, FL: StatPearls Publishing; 2017. Available from: https://www.ncbi.nlm.nih.gov/books/NBK459120/

Blaivas M, Theodoro D, Sierzenski PR. Elevated intracranial pressure detected by bedside emergency ultrasonography of the optic nerve sheath. *Acad Emerg Med*. 2003;10(4):376–381.

Chandra A, Mastrovitch T, Ladner H, Ting V, Radeos MS, Samudre S. The utility of bedside ultrasound in the detection of a ruptured globe in a porcine model. *West J Emerg Med*. 2009;10(4):263–266.

Crosby Karen S, Kendall John L., In: Gaertner RS, ed. *Practical Guide to Emergency Ultrasound*. Philadelphia, PA: Lipincot Williams & Wilkins; 2014:350–364.

De La Hoz Polo M, Torramilans Lluís A, Pozuelo Segura O, Anguera Bosque A, Esmerado Appiani C, Caminal Mitjana JM. Ocular ultrasonography focused on the posterior eye segment: what radiologists should know. *Insights Imaging*. 2016;7(3):351–364. http://doi.org/10.1007/s13244-016-0471-z.

Dubourg J, et al. Ultrasonography of optic nerve sheath diameter for detection of raised intracranial pressure: a systematic review and meta-analysis. *Intensive Care Med*. 2011;37(7):1059–1068.

Estevez, et al. Ultrasonography evaluation of retrobulbar hematoma in bovine orbits. *Acad Emerg Med*. 2000;7(10):1169–1170.

Foroozan R, Savino PJ, Sergott RC. Embolic central retinal artery occlusion detected by orbital color Doppler imaging. *Ophthalmology*. 2002;109(4):744–747.

Frasure SE, Saul T, Lewiss RE. Bedside ultrasound diagnosis of vitreous hemorrhage and traumatic lens dislocation. *Am J Emerg Med*. 31(6):1002.e1–1002.e2.

Gerbino G, Ramieri GA, Nasi A. Diagnosis and treatment of retrobulbar haematomas following blunt orbital trauma: a description of eight cases. *Int J Oral Maxillofac Surg*. 2005;34(2):127–131.

Hollands H, Johnson D, Brox AC, Almeida D, Simel DL, Sharma S. Acute-Onset Floaters and Flashes: Is This Patient at Risk for Retinal Detachment? *JAMA*. 2009;302(20):2243–2249.

Jacobsen B, Lahham S, Lahham S, Patel A, Spann S, Fox JC. Retrospective review of ocular point-of-care ultrasound for detection of retinal detachment. *West J Emerg Med*. 2016;17(2):196–200. http://doi.org/10.5811/westjem.2015.12.28711.

Kang TL, Seif D, Chilstrom M, Mailhot T. Ocular ultrasound identifies early orbital cellulitis. *West J Emerg Med.* 2014;15(4):394. http://doi.org/10.5811/westjem.2014.4.22007.

Karassa FB, et al. Meta-analysis: test performance of ultrasonography for giant-cell arteritis. *Ann Intern Med.* 2005;142(5):359–369.

Kels BD, Grzybowski A, and JM Grant-Kels JM, Human ocular anatomy. *Clin Dermatol.* 2015;33(2):140–146.

Kniess CK, et al. Early detection of traumatic retrobulbar hemorrhage using bedside ocular ultrasound. *J Emerg Med.* 49(1):58–60.

Mahmoudi S, Almony A. Macula-sparing rhegmatogenous retinal detachment: is emergent surgery necessary? *J Ophthalmic Vis Res.* 2016;11(1):100–107. http://doi.org/10.4103/2008-322X.180696.

Noble VE, Nelson B, Sutingco AN. *Manual of Emergency and Critical Care Ultrasound.* New York NY: Cambridge University Press; 2007:175–181.

Ojaghi Haghighi SH, Morteza Begi HR, Sorkhabi R, et al. Diagnostic accuracy of ultrasound in detection of traumatic lens dislocation. *Emergency.* 2014;2(3):121–124.

Purves D, Augustine GJ, Fitzpatrick D, et al., editors. *Neuroscience.* 2nd edition. Sunderland (MA): Sinauer Associates; 2001. Anatomy of the Eye. Available from: https://www.ncbi.nlm.nih.gov/books/NBK11120/.

Rajajee V, et al. Optic nerve ultrasound for the detection of raised intracranial pressure. *Neurocrit Care.* 2011;15(3):506–515.

Riccardi A, Siniscalchi C, Lerza R. Embolic central retinal artery occlusion detected with point-of-care ultrasonography in the emergency department. *J Emerg Med.* 2016;50(4):e183–e185.

Robba C, Cardim D, Tajsic T, et al. Ultrasound non-invasive measurement of intracranial pressure in neurointensive care: a prospective observational study. *PLoS Medicine.* 2017;14(7):e1002356. http://doi.org/10.1371/journal.pmed.1002356.

Roque PJ, et al. Bedside ocular ultrasound. *Crit Care Clin.* 2014;30(2):227–241.

Schlachetzki F, et al. Titelbildbeitrag – Das retrobulbäre "Spot Sign" – orbitale Sonografie zur Ausschlussdiagnostik der Arteriitis temporalis bei plötzlicher Erblindung. *Ultraschall Med.* 2010;31(06):539–542.

Schmidt WA. Ultrasound in the diagnosis and management of giant cell arteritis. *Rheumatology.* 2018;57(suppl 2):ii22–ii31.

Shek KC, et al. Acute retrobulbar haemorrhage: an ophthalmic emergency. *Emerg Med Australas.* 2006;18(3):299–301.

Shiver SA, Lyon M, Blaivas M. Detection of metallic ocular foreign bodies with handheld sonography in a porcine model. *J Ultrasound Med.* 2005;24:1341–1346. https://doi.org/10.7863/jum.2005.24.10.1341.

Ustymowicz A, Krejza J, Mariak Z. Twinkling artifact in color doppler imaging of the orbit. *J Ultrasound Med.* 2002;21(5):559–563.

Vodopivec I, Rizzo III JF. Ophthalmic manifestations of giant cell arteritis. *Rheumatology.* 2018;57(suppl 2):ii63–ii72.

6

Carotid Artery

William C. Pevec

CLINICAL CORRELATION

The most common disease affecting the carotid arteries is atherosclerosis. Other less common, but clinically important conditions include dissection, trauma, and carotid body tumors.

The carotid bifurcation is a common location for the development of atherosclerotic plaque. Although usually asymptomatic, atherosclerosis of the carotid bifurcation may become unstable and cause monocular blindness, transient cerebral ischemia, or stroke.

Monocular blindness may be temporary (also known as *amaurosis fugax*) or permanent. It is due to embolization of atheromatous debris to the retinal artery. Symptoms are ipsilateral to the arterial source of the emboli. Typically, the patient reports complete blindness in part or all of the visual field of one eye. The blindness is often described as a shade coming across part of the visual field of the eye and may involve a quadrant, half, or all of the visual field. Temporary blindness typically resolves over seconds to a few minutes, with complete resolution. A cholesterol crystal (Hollenhorst's plaque) may be seen on funduscopic examination.

In terms of the carotid arteries, a stroke is defined as a focal, cerebral hemispheric deficit persisting for longer than 24 hours. A transient ischemic attack (TIA) is a focal, cerebral hemispheric deficit persisting less than 24 hours, typically resolving in minutes to a few hours. Symptoms include unilateral motor weakness, unilateral sensory changes (numbness or paresthesia), dysarthria (slurred speech), or language deficit (most typically an expressive dysphasia or aphasia). Motor and sensory deficits occur on the side of the body contralateral to the etiologic carotid artery. Language deficits are due to ischemia of the dominant hemisphere. Dysarthrias may be due to ischemia of either cerebral hemisphere.

Dissection of the carotid artery may occur spontaneously or may be due to trauma, iatrogenic injury, or as a component of aortic dissection. Clinical presentation may include unilateral neck or head pain, Horner's syndrome (decreased diameter of the pupil, drooping of the eyelid, decreased sweating on the side of the face), and/or ipsilateral TIA or stroke.

Penetrating, blunt, or iatrogenic trauma to the neck may cause carotid disruption with hemorrhage and hematoma, carotid occlusion, or carotid dissection. These injuries may present with bleeding, neck fullness, pain, TIA or stroke, or may be asymptomatic.

Carotid body tumors (paragangliomas, glomus tumors, chemodectomas) characteristically present as a painless mass or fullness in the neck. Larger tumors may cause compressive symptoms such as pain, difficulty or pain with swallowing, hoarseness, or stridor.

NORMAL ANATOMY

The right common carotid arises from the brachiocephalic artery. The left common carotid artery arises as the second branch of the aortic arch. The common carotid arteries bifurcate in the midneck into the internal and external carotid arteries. The internal carotid

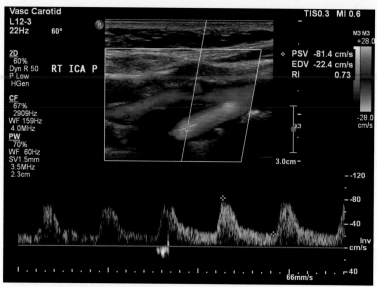

Fig. 6.1 Flow pattern in a normal internal carotid artery.

artery has no branches in the neck. Its terminal branches in the cranial cavity include the ophthalmic, anterior cerebral, middle cerebral, and posterior communicating arteries. The branches of the external carotid artery are the superior thyroid, lingual, facial, occipital, posterior auricular, ascending pharyngeal, superior temporal, and maxillary arteries.

The internal jugular vein lies superficial and postero-lateral to the carotid arteries. The vagus nerve is typi-cally deep to and between the carotid arteries and the jugular vein. The hypoglossal nerve crosses the inter-nal and external carotid arteries from posterolateral to anteromedial. The carotid body lies in the crotch of the internal and external carotid arteries.

IMAGING

Carotid artery evaluation requires high-resolution B-mode imaging and pulsed Doppler with spectral anal-ysis. A linear array scan head with transducer frequen-cies of 5 to 12 MHz is most commonly used. The patient is positioned supine, with the head turned away from the examiner and the neck extended. The examiner is seated at the head of the bed.

The carotid arteries are evaluated in transverse and longitudinal axes with B-mode imaging. Pulse Doppler is performed in the longitudinal axis. Doppler angles should be 60 degrees or less. The sample volume should be moved throughout the long axis of the arteries, par-ticularly at the common carotid bifurcation and in the proximal internal carotid artery, to identify regions of maximal stenosis. Color Doppler may be useful to local-ize areas for more specific assessment with pulse Doppler.

The internal carotid artery typically has low resis-tance to flow, with the spectral waveform showing a brisk upstroke and antegrade flow throughout diastole (Fig. 6.1). The external carotid artery has a smaller diameter than the internal carotid artery at the carotid bulb but a similar diameter more distally (Fig. 6.2). The external carotid artery has flow characteristics similar to most peripheral arteries, with a triphasic spectral waveform: brisk forward upstroke, retrograde flow in early diastole, and antegrade flow in late diastole (Fig. 6.3). The waveform in the external carotid artery may show lower resistance if the external carotid artery has developed collateral flow to the intracranial cir-culation, making it more difficult to tell whether the artery is the internal or external carotid. In this case,

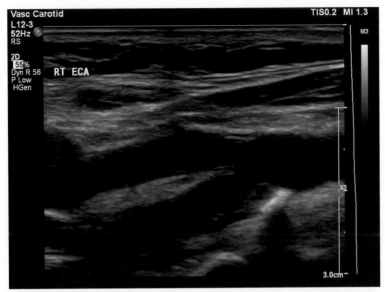

Fig. 6.2 B-mode image of a carotid bifurcation showing the internal (lower in the image) and external (higher in the image) carotid arteries. There is a mild, calcified plaque at the origin of the internal carotid artery.

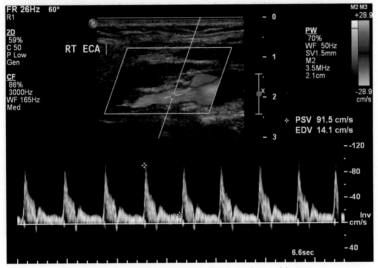

Fig. 6.3 Flow pattern in a normal external carotid artery.

a temporal tap may be used to confirm that the external carotid artery is being evaluated (Fig. 6.4). While monitoring the waveform in the artery, the ipsilateral superficial temporal artery (anterior to the ear) is rapidly compressed with the examiner's finger; oscillations will be visible on the spectral waveform if the artery being evaluated is the external carotid. The common carotid artery supplies flow to both the internal and external carotid arteries; therefore its waveform will be a hybrid between a low-resistance and high-resistance pattern (Fig. 6.5). However, as the internal carotid artery carries much more volume than the external carotid artery, the common carotid artery typically has a relatively low-resistance pattern.

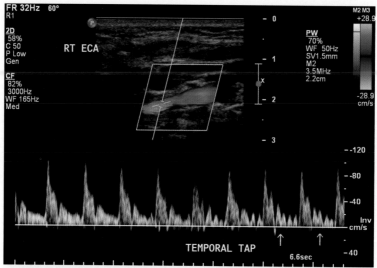

Fig. 6.4 Low-resistance external carotid artery flow with a "temporal tap."

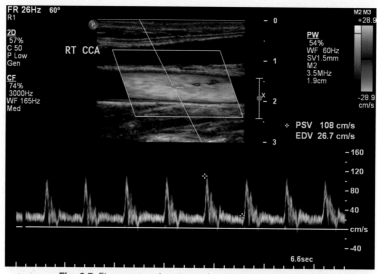

Fig. 6.5 Flow pattern in a normal common carotid artery.

PATHOLOGY

Carotid Stenosis

The diagnosis of carotid stenosis is primary based on spectral analysis for measuring flow velocities. Although B-mode imaging will identify plaque, ultrasound imaging alone is not accurate for measuring carotid stenosis.

A stenosis in the internal carotid artery will lead to turbulent flow patterns. At a moderate degree of stenosis, the peak systolic velocity will be elevated (Fig. 6.6). A more severe stenosis will elevate the end diastolic velocity (Fig. 6.7). The ratio between the peak systolic velocity in the internal carotid artery and the peak systolic velocity in the common carotid artery is also useful. Various criteria have been proposed to define the degree of stenosis in the internal carotid artery; the two most commonly used criteria are presented in Tables 6.1 and 6.2. When the internal carotid artery is occluded, the waveforms in the common carotid artery will assume a pattern similar to that in the external carotid artery (Fig. 6.8). There are no validated criteria to define the degree of stenosis in the common or external carotid arteries.

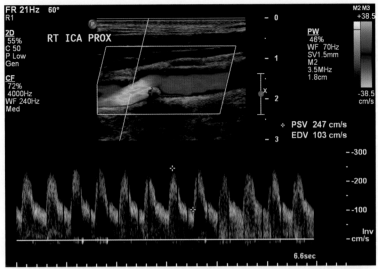

Fig. 6.6 Flow pattern in an internal carotid artery with a 50% to 79% stenosis.

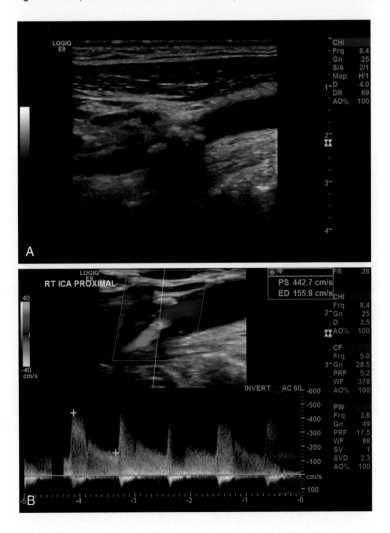

Fig. 6.7 (A) B-mode image of an internal carotid artery with an 80% to 99% stenosis. (B) Flow pattern in an internal carotid artery with an 80% to 99% stenosis.

TABLE 6.1	University of Washington Criteria			
Diameter Reduction	Peak Systolic Velocity	End Diastolic Velocity	Waveform Characteristics
0%	<125 cm/sec	-	Minimal or no spectral broadening
1%–15%	<125 cm/sec	-	Spectral broadening during systolic deceleration
16%–49%	<125 cm/sec	-	Spectral broadening throughout systole
50%–79%	≥125 cm/sec	<140 cm/sec	Marked spectral broadening
80%–99%	≥125 cm/sec	≥140 cm/sec	Marked spectral broadening
100%	-	-	No flow in ICA; decreased diastolic flow in CCA

CCA, Common carotid artery; *ICA*, internal carotid artery.

TABLE 6.2	Consensus Panel Recommendations			
Diameter Reduction	ICA PSV	Plaque Estimate*	ICA:CCA Ratio	ICA EDV
0%	<125 cm/sec	None	<2	<40 cm/sec
<50%	<125 cm/sec	<50%	<2	<40 cm/sec
50%–69%	125–230 cm/sec	≥50%	2–4	40–100 cm/sec
≥70%, not near occlusion	>230 cm/sec	≥50%	>4	>100 cm/sec
Near occlusion	High, low, or undetectable	Visible	Variable	Variable
100%	Undetectable	Visible; no detectable lumen	N/A	N/A

CCA, Common carotid artery; *EDV*, end diastolic velocity; *ICA*, internal carotid artery; *N/A*, not applicable; *PSV*, peak systolic velocity.
*Plaque estimate (diameter reduction) with grayscale and color Duplex ultrasound.

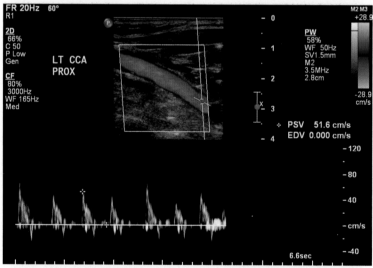

Fig. 6.8 Flow pattern in a common carotid artery with occlusion of the ipsilateral internal carotid artery.

However, a stenosis in these arteries may be inferred by a focal increase in the peak systolic velocity and turbulent flow.

There are conditions that affect the standard diagnostic criteria. In the presence of severe stenosis or occlusion of the contralateral internal carotid artery, the peak systolic velocities in the ipsilateral internal carotid artery may be elevated with no or lesser degrees of stenosis, due to increased volume of the flow in the ipsilateral internal carotid artery if the anterior circle of Willis

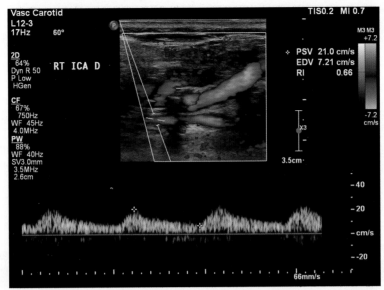

Fig. 6.9 Flow pattern in an internal carotid artery with diffuse, severe narrowing ("string sign").

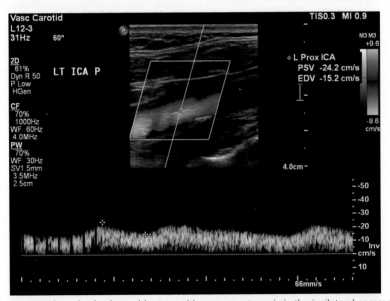

Fig. 6.10 Flow pattern in an internal carotid artery with a severe stenosis in the ipsilateral common carotid or brachiocephalic artery.

is patent and the ipsilateral internal carotid artery is supplying flow to both cerebral hemispheres. If the internal carotid artery is severely narrowed over a long distance, the flow velocities in that internal carotid artery may be low (Fig. 6.9). With more proximal stenoses, in the brachiocephalic or proximal common carotid arteries, a delayed upstroke and low velocity may be seen in the internal carotid artery (Fig. 6.10); a similar pattern may be seen with severe aortic valve stenosis or severe left ventricular heart failure. In the presence of a stent in the carotid artery, the peak systolic velocity criteria to diagnose stenosis need to be adjusted higher; no clear consensus has been reached. Several proposed criteria are displayed in Tables 6.3 to 6.5.

TABLE 6.3   Criteria for Carotid Stenosis After Stenting

Diameter Reduction	PSV	EDV	ICA:CCA Ratio
≥50%	≥225 cm/sec	≥75 cm/sec	≥2.5
≥70%	≥350 cm/sec	≥125 cm/sec	≥4.75

CCA, Common carotid artery; *EDV*, end diastolic velocity; *ICA*, internal carotid artery; *PSV*, peak systolic velocity. From Stanziale SF, Wholey MH, Boules TN, et al. Determining in-stent stenosis of carotid arteries by duplex ultrasound criteria. *J Endovascr Ther.* 2005;12:346–353.

TABLE 6.4   Criteria for Carotid Stenosis After Stenting

Diameter Reduction	PSV	EDV	ICA:CCA
≥30%	>154 cm/sec	>42 cm/sec	>1.5
≥50%	>224 cm/sec	>88 cm/sec	>3.4
≥80%	>325 cm/sec	>119 cm/sec	>4.5

CCA, Common carotid artery; *EDV*, end diastolic velocity; *ICA*, internal carotid artery; *PSV*, peak systolic velocity. From AbuRahma AF, Abu-Halimah S, Bensenhaver J, et al. Optimal carotid duplex velocity criteria for defining the severity of carotid in-stent restenosis. *J Vasc Surg.* 2008;48:589–594.

TABLE 6.5   Criteria for Carotid Stenosis After Stenting

Diameter Reduction	PSV	ICA:CCA
0%–19%	<150 cm/sec	<2.15
20%–49%	150–219 cm/sec	-
50%–79%	220–339 cm/sec	≥2.7
80%–99%	≥340 cm/sec	≥4.15

CCA, Common carotid artery; *ICA*, internal carotid artery; *PSV*, peak systolic velocity. From Lal BK, Hobson RW, Tofighi B, et al. Duplex ultrasound velocity criteria for the stented carotid artery. *J Vasc Surg.* 2008;47:63–73.

Carotid Dissection

Carotid dissection may manifest as an occlusion of the internal carotid artery, typically in the absence of plaque on B-mode imaging (Fig. 6.11). If the artery is patent, the dissection flap may be visible on B-mode imaging, with flow seen in both lumens on color flow imaging, frequently with flow in opposite directions (Fig. 6.12). As fibromuscular dysplasia may predispose to carotid dissection, a "string of beads" pattern may be seen in the mid- and distal contralateral internal carotid artery (Fig. 6.13).

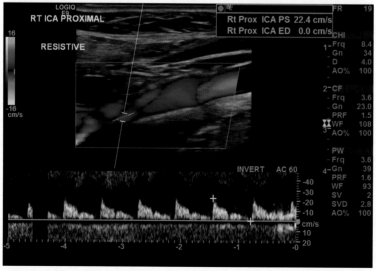

Fig. 6.11 Low-velocity, high-resistance flow pattern in a proximal internal carotid artery, with a more distal occlusion secondary to dissection.

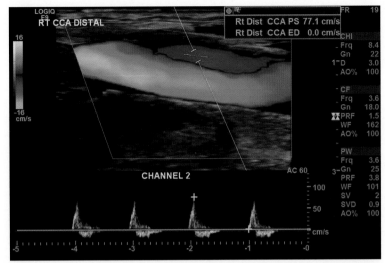

Fig. 6.12 Color flow image of a common carotid artery with dissection and two patent lumens.

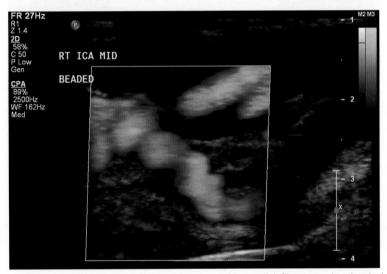

Fig. 6.13 Image of the mid/distal internal carotid artery with medial fibromuscular dysplasia ("string of beads").

Carotid Trauma

Trauma may lead to carotid occlusion or dissection, with findings as noted earlier. Intimal flaps may be seen on B-mode imaging, and the flaps may cause turbulence on color flow imaging and spectral analysis. Carotid disruption may result in a hematoma around the artery (Fig. 6.14), which is seen as a low-density, homogenous or heterogenous fluid collection adjacent to the artery.

Carotid disruption may also cause a pseudoaneurysm, with the presence of flow outside the lumen of the artery on color flow imaging and bidirectional, high-resistance flow signals in the pseudoaneurysm on spectral analysis.

Carotid Body Tumors

Carotid body tumors cause a splaying of the carotid bifurcation on ultrasound imaging.

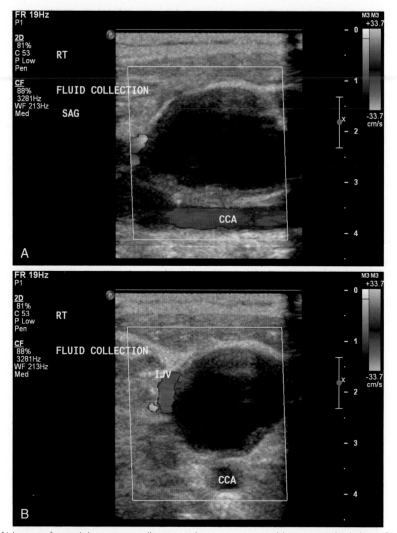

Fig. 6.14 (A) Image of a neck hematoma adjacent to the common carotid artery, sagittal view. (B) Image of a neck hematoma adjacent to the common carotid artery, transverse view.

SUGGESTED READING

Beach KW, Bergelin RO, Primozich JF, et al. *Standardized Ultrasound Evaluation of Carotid Stenosis for Clinical Trials: University of Washington Ultrasound Reading Center.* Cardiovascular Ultrasound; 2010;8:39.

Zierler RE, Dawson DL, eds. *Standness's Duplex Scanning in Vascular Disorders.* 5th ed. Zierler RE, Dawson DL, eds. 5th ed. New York: Wolters Kluver; 2016:91–107.

BIBLIOGRAPHY

AbuRahma AF, Abu-Halimah S, Bensenhaver J, et al. Optimal carotid duplex velocity criteria for defining the severity of carotid in-stent restenosis. *J Vasc Surg.* 2008;48:589–594.

Crafts RC. *A Textbook of Human Anatomy.* 2nd ed. New York: John Wiley and Sons; 1979:585–589.

Cronenwett JL, Johnston KW, eds. *Rutherford's Vascular Surgery.* 8th ed. Philadelphia: Elsevier Saunders; 2014:1578–1579, 1589–1600.

Grant EG, Benson CB, Moneta GL, et al. Carotid artery stenosis: gray-scale and Doppler US diagnosis-society of radiologists in ultrasound consensus conference. *Radiology.* 2003;229:340–346.

Lal BK, Hobson RW, Tofighi B, et al. Duplex ultrasound velocity criteria for the stented carotid artery. *J Vasc Surg.* 2008;47:63–73.

Stanziale SF, Wholey MH, Boules TN, et al. Determining in-stent stenosis of carotid arteries by duplex ultrasound criteria. *J Endovasc Ther.* 2005;12:346–353.

Zierler RE, Dawson DL, eds. *Standness's Duplex Scanning in Vascular Disorders.* 5th ed. New York: Wolters Kluver; 2016:102.

7

Cranial

Rebecca Stein-Wexler

INTRODUCTION

Transcranial ultrasound (US) is commonly used to evaluate complications of prematurity, in which case it may be used as a screening tool, or to evaluate infants with seizures, apnea, bradycardia, or falling hematocrit. When used to screen premature infants, it is often performed around day 5 of life, with further imaging performed as needed. Head US is also useful in older infants presenting with macrocephaly, seizures, or an abnormal neurologic examination. It is especially useful in infants suspected of having meningitis, intracranial hemorrhage, or hydrocephalus.

TECHNIQUE AND NORMAL ANATOMY

Head US is a powerful tool for examining intracranial pathology until about age 12 months, at which time bone maturation limits visualization of intracranial contents. Most imaging is performed in the coronal and sagittal planes with a high-frequency (5–7.5 MHz) linear array transducer at the anterior fontanelle. The complete examination consists of six coronal images (Fig. 7.1), beginning anterior to the frontal horns and ending posterior to the lateral ventricles (Fig. 7.2). The sagittal exam (Fig. 7.3) consists of a single midline image and three additional images on each side (Fig. 7.4).

Grayscale and color Doppler interrogation assess the superficial midline structures, including superior sagittal sinus, gyri, and extraaxial spaces (Fig. 7.5). Linear array 7- to 12-MHz transducers enable high-resolution imaging. In addition, axial images may be obtained through the mastoid and posterior fontanelles, which allow for evaluation of the posterior fossa and provide another plane of imaging. The additional dimension helps elucidate pathology and normal structures.

NORMAL IMAGING APPEARANCE

Surface anatomy changes with age. The brain before 24 weeks is smooth, having no sulci other than the Sylvian fissure. At about 24 weeks, the parieto-occipital fissure forms, and the cingulate gyrus develops at 28 weeks. Additional sulci develop until the term neonate's gyral and sulcal pattern resembles that of an adult.

The lateral ventricles should measure less than 10 mm at the level of the atria, and the third ventricle should measure less than 5 mm transverse. Up to 40% of patients have mildly asymmetric lateral ventricles. The echogenic choroid plexus lies within both lateral ventricles, extending through the foramina of Monroe into the third ventricle. It is not normally seen anterior to the caudothalamic groove in the frontal horn. The choroid plexus may appear lobular or bulbous. However, it should be symmetrical to exclude pathology. Choroid plexus cysts are commonly encountered in normal children. If there are multiple cysts, or if they measure larger than 10 mm, chromosomal abnormalities may be present.

Normal white matter shows uniform, low-level, granular, mild hyperechogenicity predominately brighter than the relatively hypoechoic gray matter, and the transition between white and gray matter is gradual. Artifact or pathology may cause

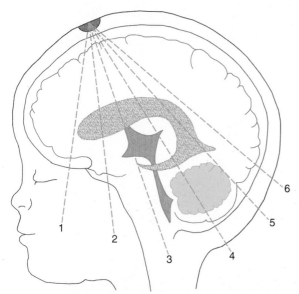

Fig. 7.1 Diagram of standard coronal head ultrasound planes. The transducer is placed over the anterior fontanelle and angled from the front to the back.

periventricular white matter to appear hyperechoic. When pathologic, the white matter is (1) more echogenic than the choroid plexus and (2) abnormal on both sagittal and coronal images, because an artifact is usually only evident in one plane. The normal cortex consists of three layers: echogenic pia (peripheral), hypoechoic gray matter, and hyperechoic white matter (central). Echogenic hemorrhage or ischemia may obscure these layers.

Midline cerebrospinal fluid (CSF) collections are common until about age 6 months, but residual fluid may be seen in adults. The cavum septum pellucidum is a fluid-filled space between the frontal horns bounded by the leaflets of the septum pellucidum. Fluid is found less often within the cavum vergae, between the bodies of the lateral ventricles. The most posterior (and least often encountered) potential fluid collection is at the level of the pineal gland, in the cavum velum interpositum.

In evaluating superficial para-midline extraaxial hemorrhage or other fluid collections, the configuration of bridging vessels is important. Vessels normally course through the subarachnoid space but do not traverse the subdural space, which is deep to the periosteum. Therefore if extraaxial fluid does not contain coursing vessels, subdural fluid, such as subdural hematoma, should be suspected.

Branching echogenic linear foci may be seen in the basal ganglia (Fig. 7.6). This "lenticulostriate vasculopathy" is a common finding in normal patients and in multiple births. The finding may also be identified in infants with infection (especially cytomegalovirus [CMV]), intrauterine drug exposure, hypoxia, and congenital heart disease.

PATHOLOGY

Hemorrhage

Hemorrhage in the brain and in CSF spaces is initially hyperechoic. As blood evolves, it gradually becomes less echogenic as well as more contracted, septated, and nodular. The appearance of evolving hemorrhage depends on location. *Intraventricular* hemorrhage (IVH) initially layers within the affected ventricle and can eventually extend into the rest of the ventricular system. It may later adhere to the ventricular lining, resulting in ependymal irregularities. Alternatively, it may irritate the ependymal lining, resulting in ependymitis, which appears as smooth, echogenic thickening of the ventricular wall. *Parenchymal* hemorrhage may undergo necrosis, leading to porencephaly that often communicates with the adjacent ventricle, appearing as a fluid-filled outpouching from the ventricle. In some cases, parenchyma collapses around the space, resulting in focal volume loss. If identified late, it may be difficult to determine the etiology of the porencephaly. *Extraaxial* hemorrhage demonstrates similar evolution. Minimal hemorrhage may resolve entirely, decreasing in size and becoming anechoic, with subsequent resolution. However, more extensive hemorrhage often demonstrates residual abnormalities.

Hemorrhage in Preterm Infants. The premature infant's inability to autoregulate cerebral blood flow may result in ischemia and/or hemorrhage in metabolically active areas of the brain. This problem is especially severe in infants weighing less than 1500 g (less than 28 weeks estimated gestational age [EGA]). Hemorrhage may also be encountered in term infants who undergo stress, such as hypoxia, hypothermia, and difficult delivery. Complex interplay between various factors determines the location of hemorrhage, which in premature infants is then graded according to a four-tier system.

Grade I IVH is confined to the germinal matrix, which generates neuronal and glial cells. The germinal matrix initially spans the length of the lateral ventricle,

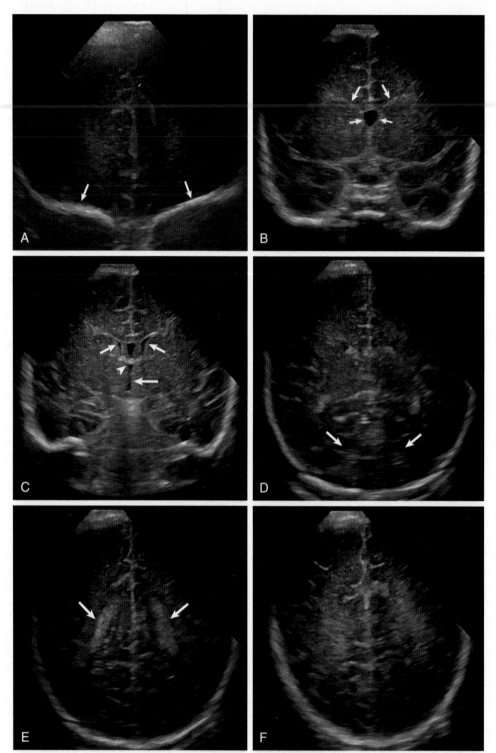

Fig. 7.2 Coronal images obtained from the front to the back in the standard planes. (A) Frontal lobes with orbital roofs (*arrows*). (B) Frontal horns of lateral ventricles (*long arrows*) with cavum septum pellucidum (*short arrows*). (C) Frontal horns (*short arrows*), cavum septum pellucidum, and echogenic choroid plexus (*arrowhead*) in roof of third ventricle (*long arrow*) and in foramina of Monroe. (D) Cerebellum (*arrows*) with portions of lateral ventricles. (E) Choroid plexus (*arrows*) within the atria and posterior horns of the lateral ventricles. (F) Posterior parietal and occipital periventricular white matter.

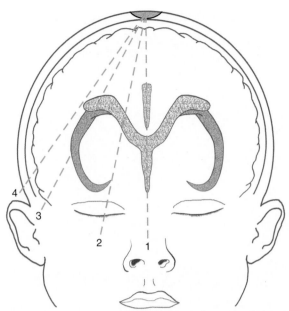

Fig. 7.3 Diagram of standard sagittal head ultrasound planes. The transducer is placed over the anterior fontanelle and angled from the midline to the right and to the left.

involuting by 35 weeks to occupy only the caudothalamic groove. Subependymal in location, it is hypervascular and therefore especially vulnerable to hypoxia. Larger grade I IVH distorts the contour of the floor of the lateral ventricle. It is initially echogenic (Fig. 7.7) but eventually becomes cystic and then resolves. The presence of cystic foci in this area at birth implies evolution of fetal hemorrhage.

Grade II IVH is located within the ventricular system. It results from blood spreading from the germinal matrix across the delicate ependymal lining into the ventricle (or, in term infants, from the choroid plexus). IVH is initially echogenic (Fig. 7.8), and it may be difficult to differentiate from normal choroid plexus. However, because choroid plexus does not extend into either the frontal horns or the occipital horns, echogenic material within these areas can be assumed to represent hemorrhage. Application of color Doppler is also helpful, because IVH is avascular—unlike choroid plexus. Hemorrhage may be confined to the dependent portion of the ventricle and may be identified as a fluid-filled level in the occipital horn. Like hemorrhage elsewhere, grade II IVH evolves, becoming hypoechoic, contracting, and eventually disappearing. Grade II IVH may be accompanied by ventricular

dilatation, but the blood must fill less than 50% of the ventricular volume.

Grade III IVH is also intraventricular in location. However, the affected ventricles are dilated, and echogenic material fills at least 50% of the ventricular volume, almost forming a cast of the ventricle (Fig. 7.9). Diagnosed in the acute phase, grade III IVH should not be confused with posthemorrhagic obstructive hydrocephalus, which may follow a grade II or grade III IVH. Cerebral palsy/developmental delay will be seen in approximately one-half of patients with grade III IVH.

Grade IV IVH extends beyond the germinal matrix into the brain parenchyma. It may result from venous occlusion that can occur if parenchymal draining veins are blocked by either severe grade I IVH or massive ventriculomegaly. It may also result from occlusion of other veins, including the dural venous sinuses. This form of hemorrhage is seen in the periventricular parenchyma (Fig. 7.10). Masslike, it may distort normal structures. Head US may eventually show parenchymal loss at the site of hemorrhage, leading to porencephaly (Fig. 7.11).

Hemorrhage in Term Infants. Although intracranial hemorrhage is especially common in preterm infants, it may be seen in older infants as well. Hemorrhagic infarction may occur in the setting of perinatal ischemia and appears hyperechoic relative to the choroid plexus, often intraparenchymal within the periventricular white matter or the basal ganglia. The hemorrhage tends to have relatively rounded margins, which helps differentiate it from nonhemorrhagic ischemia (Fig. 7.12). Neonates with abnormal clotting mechanisms, such as clotting factor or vitamin K deficiency (Fig. 7.13), may develop extensive parenchymal and extraaxial hemorrhage. When caused by a coagulation disorder, hemorrhage is often large and centered in the deep white matter, basal ganglia, and cerebellum. The echogenicity of extraaxial hemorrhage depends on its phase (Fig. 7.14). Hemorrhage may also be seen in the setting of trauma.

Ventricular Enlargement

Ventricular enlargement occurs in a variety of settings. Obstruction may result from congenital anomalies, hemorrhage, or mass effect. Nonobstructive ventriculomegaly may result from excessive production of CSF or impaired resorption (most often due to sequelae of

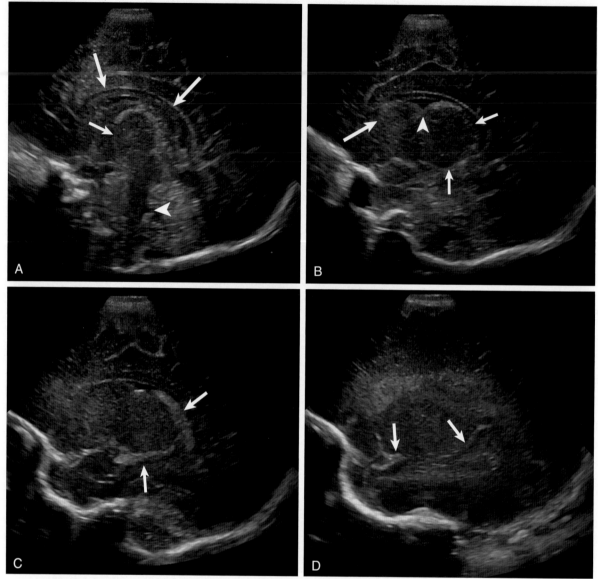

Fig. 7.4 Sagittal images obtained from the midline and to one side. (A) Midline image of corpus callosum (*long arrows*), thalamus (*short arrow*), brainstem, fourth ventricle (*arrowhead*), and cerebellum. (B) Paramedian image showing caudate nucleus (*long arrow*), thalamus (*short arrows*), and caudothalamic groove (*arrowhead*). (C) Choroid plexus (*arrows*) in lateral ventricle. (D) Periventricular white matter lateral to the lateral ventricle, Sylvian sulcus (*arrows*), and temporal lobe.

IVH). Ventricles may also be dilated because of loss of brain tissue, as an *ex vacuo* phenomenon.

Posthemorrhagic Hydrocephalus. In the acute phase, hemorrhage may be so extensive that it fills and dilates the ventricles (in the premature infant, this constitutes grade III IVH, discussed earlier). However, hydrocephalus may also develop as a subacute, posthemorrhagic process, due either to obstruction of ventricular foramina or to impaired resorption of CSF at the arachnoid granulations (Fig. 7.15). The location of the obstruction dictates the pattern of ventricular dilatation.

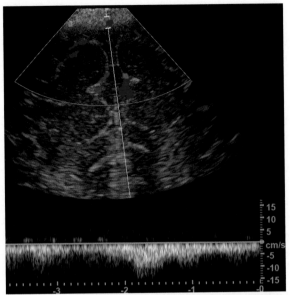

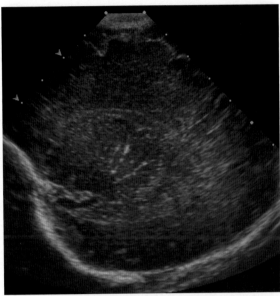

Fig. 7.5 Coronal color Doppler image obtained with a high-frequency probe shows blood flow within the superior sagittal sinus.

Fig. 7.6 Lenticulostriate vasculopathy. Sagittal paramedian image shows linear echogenicity within the basal ganglia.

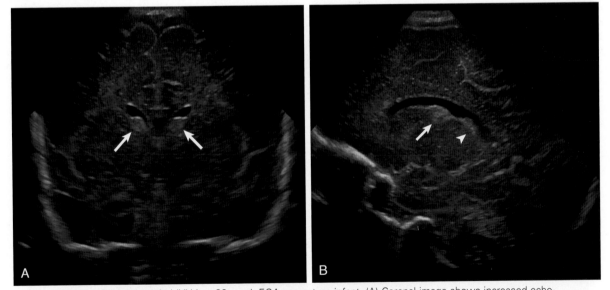

Fig. 7.7 Bilateral grade I IVH in a 32-week EGA premature infant. (A) Coronal image shows increased echogenicity at the inferomedial floor of the lateral ventricles at the foramina of Monroe, with mass effect on the adjacent ventricle (*arrows*). (B) Sagittal view of the right lateral ventricle shows the abnormality is located at the caudothalamic groove (*arrow*); the *arrowhead* delineates the choroid plexus.

Commonly both foramina of Monroe are obstructed, and dilatation is limited to both lateral ventricles, but sometimes only one is affected. If blood deposition obstructs the cerebral aqueduct, the third ventricle dilates as well. In the setting of impaired resorption of CSF, the entire ventricular system dilates, and extraaxial fluid spaces are prominent as well. Serial head US is commonly performed to evaluate increasing hydrocephalus and determine timing for shunt placement (Fig. 7.16).

Ventriculitis/Meningitis. Ventricular dilatation is common in both the acute and chronic phases of ventriculitis/meningitis. The obstruction is often outside the ventricular system, but as with posthemorrhagic hydrocephalus, it may develop at narrow transitions—such as the cerebral aqueduct and the fourth ventricular foramina. Focal ventricular enlargement may result from adhesions that lead to formation of a loculated cyst. In the chronic phase, parenchymal loss may cause ventricular dilatation on an *ex vacuo* basis.

***Ex Vacuo* Ventricular Dilatation.** If brain parenchyma has failed to form or has been destroyed, the adjacent ventricle commonly enlarges to fill the space. This is most often encountered after parenchymal hemorrhage, infarct, or cerebritis. Long after the acute injury, parenchyma may liquefy, forming an area of porencephaly that may or may not merge with the adjacent ventricle (open or closed). *Ex vacuo* ventricular dilatation may be

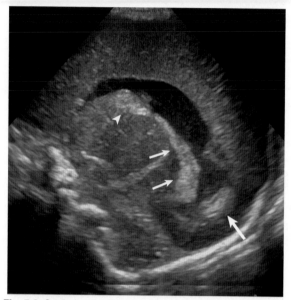

Fig. 7.8 Grade I and II IVH in a premature infant. Sagittal view shows grade I IVH at the caudothalamic groove (*arrowhead*) along with echogenic material within the lateral ventricle (*long arrow*) indicating grade II IVH; the *short arrows* delineate the choroid plexus.

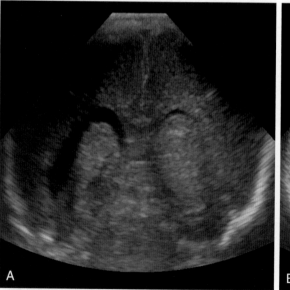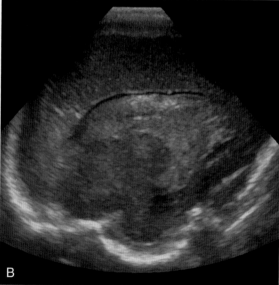

Fig. 7.9 Bilateral grade III IVH in a 25-week EGA infant. (A) Coronal view shows echogenic hemorrhage filling the left lateral ventricle and almost filling the right; both are dilated. (B) Sagittal view shows the echogenic hemorrhage forms a cast of the lateral ventricle.

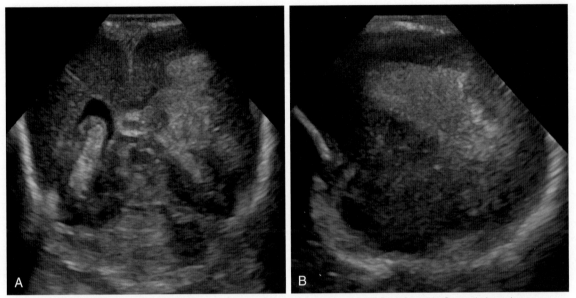

Fig. 7.10 Intraventricular and parenchymal (grade IV) IVH in a 22-week EGA infant. (A) Coronal view shows blood almost filling mildly dilated lateral ventricles and extending into the left parietal parenchyma. (B) Sagittal view shows extensive echogenic parenchymal hemorrhage.

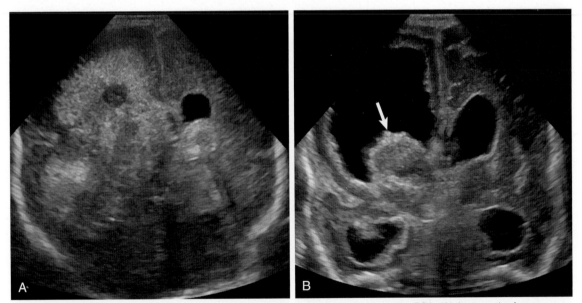

Fig. 7.11 Grade IV IVH evolves to porencephaly in an infant born at 33 weeks EGA. (A) At 1 week of age, coronal view shows grade IV parenchymal IVH on the right as well as blood within dilated lateral ventricles (grade III IVH). (B) At age 7 weeks, hemorrhage has contracted (*arrow*) and parenchyma is replaced with porencephaly that communicates with the dilated ventricular system. Increased ependymal echogenicity indicates ependymitis.

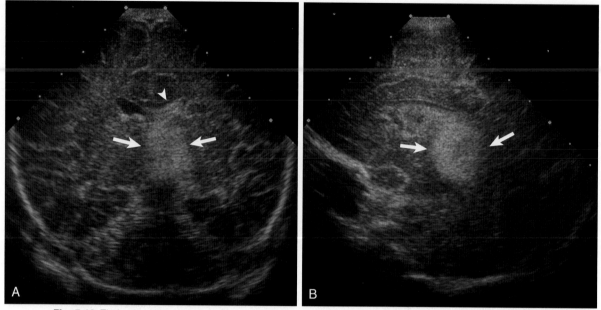

Fig. 7.12 Thalamic and intraventricular hemorrhage in a term infant presenting with seizures. (A) Coronal view shows hemorrhage in the left thalamus (*arrows*) extending into the nondilated left lateral ventricle (*arrowhead*). (B) Sagittal view shows thalamic hemorrhage (*arrows*).

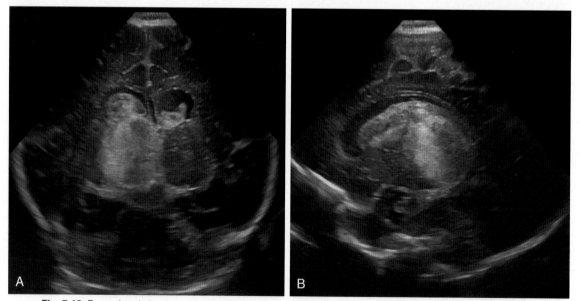

Fig. 7.13 Extensive thalamic and intraventricular hemorrhage in a term infant with vitamin K deficiency who presented at age 3 weeks. (A) Coronal view shows massive right thalamic hemorrhage and a large amount of blood in both lateral ventricles. (B) Sagittal view shows the thalamic and intraventricular hemorrhage.

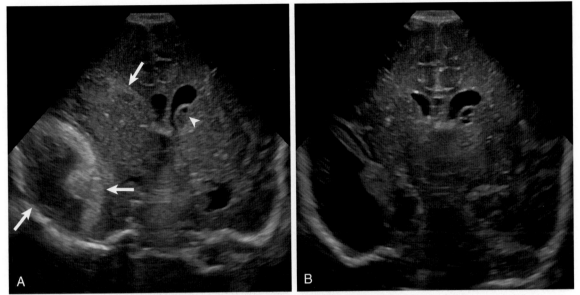

Fig. 7.14 Extraaxial hemorrhage in an infant with trisomy 21 born at 37 weeks EGA. (A) At birth, coronal view shows echogenic parenchymal edema (*long arrow*), mass effect, that effaces the right lateral ventricle, and midline shift secondary to an extraaxial collection of mixed echogenicity on the right (*short arrows*), along with grade I IVH on the left (*arrowhead*); there is also a cavum septum pellucidum. (B) Two months later, the extraaxial fluid has become more hypoechoic, the mass effect has decreased, and the left germinal matrix hemorrhage has evolved.

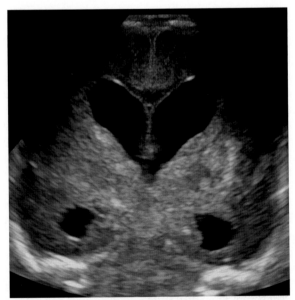

Fig. 7.15 Posthemorrhagic hydrocephalus at age 4 days in a 24-week EGA infant whose postnatal ultrasound showed bilateral grade II IVH. The lateral ventricles are dilated.

differentiated from hydrocephalus by careful evaluation of the ventricular contours. With hydrocephalus, the ventricular wall appears convex and stretched. With *ex vacuo* dilatation, by contrast, the contour of the ventricular lining may be wavier and more irregular. The ventricular wall may also appear floppy after fenestration of a hydrocephalic ventricle by means of a ventriculostomy catheter. After global hypoxic ischemic encephalopathy, profound loss of white and perhaps also gray matter may lead to diffuse parenchymal atrophy and resultant global ventricular dilatation (Fig. 7.17).

Congenital Hydrocephalus. Aqueductal stenosis and Chiari 2 malformation are two relatively common congenital causes of hydrocephalus. Congenital aqueductal stenosis is an X-linked recessive condition that is encountered in boys. It results from severe narrowing of the cerebral aqueduct and presents with enlargement of the lateral and third ventricles. The fourth ventricle is small, but the posterior fossa is otherwise normal. Chiari 2 malformation (Fig. 7.18) occurs in patients

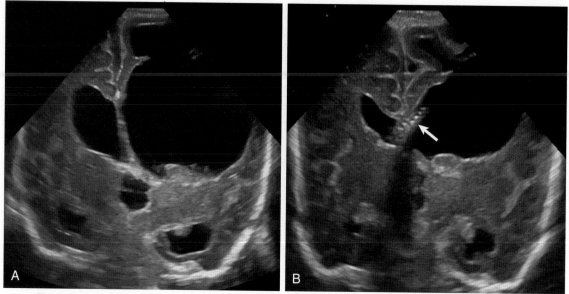

Fig. 7.16 Sequelae of grade III IVH in an ex-27-week EGA infant treated with shunting. (A) Coronal image shows severe hydrocephalus, most pronounced on the left. (B) Seven days later, after placement of a ventricular catheter (*arrow*), the hydrocephalus has improved and the apparent parenchymal thickness has increased.

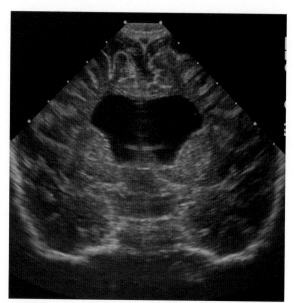

Fig. 7.17 *Ex vacuo* ventricular enlargement in a 4-month-old infant born at term who developed hypoxic-ischemic encephalopathy after cardiac surgery and subsequent white matter loss. Note that the sulci are very close to the lateral ventricles.

with myelomeningocele. The primary abnormality is a small posterior fossa. The fourth ventricle is typically compressed and elongated, whereas the third and lateral ventricles are often enlarged. Additional possible supratentorial abnormalities include a dysmorphic or absent corpus callosum and an irregular, interdigitating appearance of gyri at the midline. In patients with holoprosencephaly, ventricles are enlarged and profoundly deformed (Fig. 7.19). They appear fused to a variable extent into a large monoventricle, and the thalami are fused as well.

Increased Extraaxial Fluid of Infancy (aka Benign Enlargement of the Subarachnoid Space). Infants with macrocephaly who are neurologically normal usually have this common benign condition, which resolves by age 2 years. Fluid in the bifrontal space and interhemispheric fissure appears subjectively more abundant than usual. Some use 5 mm as the cutoff for normal interhemispheric fluid in newborns, allowing up to 8.5 mm in 1-year-olds. The extraaxial fluid must be subarachnoid in location, rather than subdural. This can

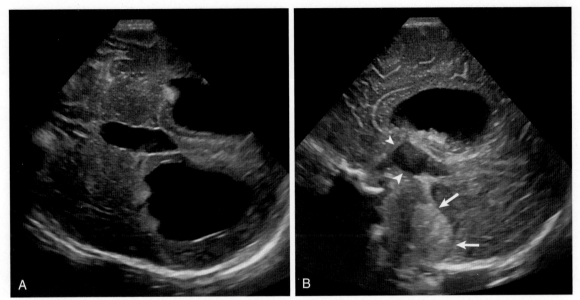

Fig. 7.18 Hydrocephalus in a term baby with Chiari 2 malformation. (A) Transtemporal axial image shows the lateral and third ventricles are dilated. (B) Sagittal midline image shows the small posterior fossa (*arrows*) and fluid within the third ventricle (*arrowheads*).

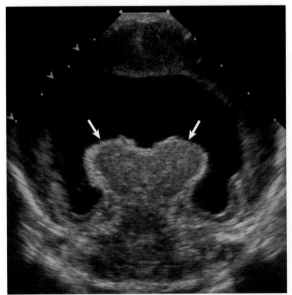

Fig. 7.19 Alobar holoprosencephaly. There is a monoventricle, and the thalami (*arrows*) are fused in the midline.

be confirmed with color Doppler US, because vessels traverse subarachnoid fluid but are compressed by subdural fluid (Fig. 7.20). The ventricles may be prominent, but the brain must appear entirely normal.

Mass. Brain tumors are rare in early infancy, and most are supratentorial. Teratoma is the most common, followed by astrocytoma, lipoma, choroid plexus papilloma, craniopharyngioma, and primitive neuro-ectodermal tumor (Fig. 7.21). Cerebellar tumors often cause hydrocephalus. Thus in the setting of third and lateral ventricular enlargement, the posterior fossa must be carefully evaluated, perhaps by a transmastoid or posterior fontanelle approach. If a normal cerebellum is not identified and common causes of congenital hydrocephalus are not evident, a brain tumor should be considered (Fig. 7.22). Hemorrhage sometimes masks an underlying brain tumor. Factors suggesting the presence of a mass include intense peripheral neovascularity and mass effect. In the posterior fossa, atypical teratoid rhabdoid tumor and teratoma are most frequent.

Infection

Prenatal Infection. Infection of the fetus with TORCH organisms may lead to a variety of abnormalities demonstrable on postnatal head US. Each organism affects the developing brain in specific ways. Toxoplasmosis and CMV cause parenchymal calcifications—typically central (periventricular) for CMV (Fig. 7.23) and scattered for toxoplasmosis. Rubella leads to polymicrogyria

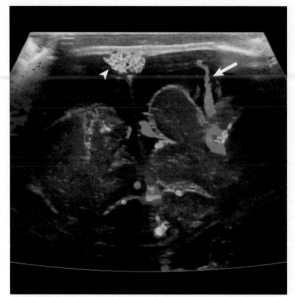

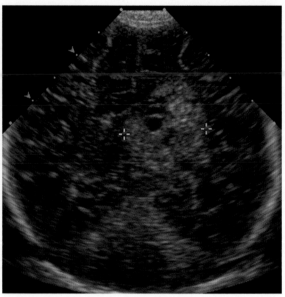

Fig. 7.20 Extraaxial fluid of infancy in a neurologically normal 3-month-old infant with macrocephaly. Coronal image obtained with a high-frequency probe demonstrates a vessel (*arrow*) traversing prominent extraaxial fluid; this indicates that the fluid is subarachnoid. Note flow in the superior sagittal sinus (*arrowhead*).

Fig. 7.21 Primitive neuroectodermal tumor in a term infant. The cursors demarcate an echogenic mass that has several cystic foci.

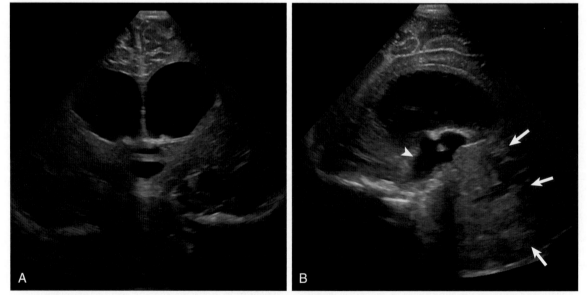

Fig. 7.22 Atypical teratoid rhabdoid tumor causing hydrocephalus in an 8-month-old infant with macrocephaly. (A) Coronal view shows enlarged lateral and third ventricles. (B) Sagittal midline view shows the cerebellum is enlarged and heterogeneous because it is replaced with tumor (*arrows*), and the third ventricle is dilated (*arrowhead*).

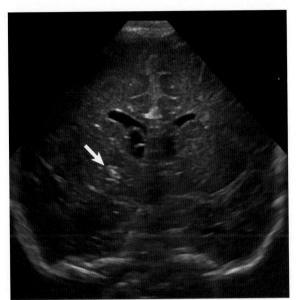

Fig. 7.23 Sequelae of cytomegalovirus infection. Coronal image shows calcification in the right thalamus (*arrow*). There are also postinfectious septations within the right lateral ventricle.

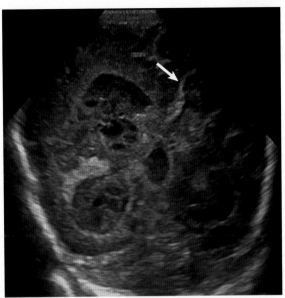

Fig. 7.24 *Escherichia coli* ventriculitis in an ex-27-week EGA infant. The lateral and third ventricles are dilated and filled with heterogeneous debris and lacy septations. Some of the ependyma is strikingly echogenic (*arrow*).

(not usually apparent with head US) and microcephaly (obvious clinically). Herpes may cause ventriculomegaly and multiple scattered echogenic foci with subsequent multicystic cerebral degeneration and eventual porencephaly. Syphilis typically has bony and systemic but not intracranial findings.

Postnatal Meningitis/Ventriculitis. Meningitis is a significant cause of neurologic impairment worldwide, although uncommon in the United States. It usually arises from sepsis and seeding of the choroid plexus. Meningeal inflammation causes vasculitis of the small bridging veins, leading to cortical infarcts. Diffuse cerebral edema develops as well. Group B *streptococcus*, *Escherichia coli*, and *Listeria monocytogenes* are typically responsible for cerebral infection in infants. In the acute phase, head US often shows thick, echogenic meninges; abnormally wide sulci; and prominent cortical vessels. Sterile collections of subarachnoid fluid are common, but subdural empyemas are rare.

The ventricles may eventually fill with exudative material, resulting in intraventricular debris and stranding (Fig. 7.24). This is especially common with *E. coli*. The exudative material is less echogenic than acute hemorrhage and has a more uniformly complex, lacy

appearance than chronic hemorrhage. Adhesions may isolate portions of the ventricular system, leading to intraventricular cysts. In addition, diffuse ventricular dilatation is common in both the acute and chronic phases. Acutely, hydrocephalus results from obstruction, often extraventricular in location. Alternatively this may be due to ependymitis and adhesions at the cerebral aqueduct or fourth ventricular foramina.

There may also be echogenic foci in the parenchyma secondary to focal infection, ischemia, or hemorrhage. Diffuse brain edema results in effacement of fluid spaces, as with diffuse ischemia. Potentially devastating cerebral abscess is most common with *Citrobacter koseri*. This infection evolves from vasculitis to infarction, necrosis, and eventual liquefaction. Early findings of abscess are ill-defined increased echogenicity and hypervascularity, progressing to a well-defined complex mass with echogenic walls and eventual cavitation with markedly hyperemic walls.

Ischemia

The location and appearance of brain ischemia depends on brain maturity, the severity and duration of hypoxia, and the timing of imaging. In general, acute ischemia is echogenic. Normally mildly echogenic white matter becomes more strikingly hyperechoic, and normally hypoechoic gray matter becomes hyperechoic as well. If hemorrhagic conversion has occurred, echogenicity may appear more strikingly increased.

Hypoxic Injury in the Premature Infant. Mild-to-moderate hypoxia may lead to IVH (discussed earlier; see Figs. 7.7–7.11) or periventricular leukomalacia, which is typically seen in infants delivered before 32 weeks of age. The deep periventricular white matter is especially vulnerable in this age group because during development, the brain parenchyma is supplied by vessels that penetrate from the cortex and end in the periventricular white matter. Decreased perfusion leads to ischemia and sometimes hemorrhage. The frontal lobes and peritrigonal area are most often affected, and damage is often symmetric. US initially shows periventricular white matter that is more echogenic than the choroid plexus; cysts may form within several weeks (Fig. 7.25).

In cases of mild-to-moderate hypoxia, deep gray matter is not involved because vascular shunting protects it. However, profound perinatal hypoxia damages gray matter and causes germinal matrix hemorrhage and periventricular leukomalacia. The most myelinated (and hence most metabolically active) areas of gray matter are affected: the thalami, basal ganglia, hippocampi, corticospinal tracts, and cerebellum (Fig. 7.26). Beriberi also preferentially affects the basal ganglia. In this case, thiamine deficiency causes a reversible metabolic abnormality that manifests as symmetric increased echogenicity, usually in the putamina and sometimes caudate nuclei, resembling US findings of profound ischemia (Fig. 7.27). Usually thiamine deficiency is seen in young infants who are breastfed by mothers whose diet consists mostly of polished rice.

Hypoxic Injury in the Term and Postterm Infant. In term and older babies with mild-to-moderate hypotension, ischemia preferentially affects the cortex and parasagittal white matter—the watershed areas between the anterior, middle, and posterior cerebral arteries. As in preterm infants, vascular shunting protects the deep gray matter. However, the white matter is not protected and appears abnormally hyperechoic. The difference between gray and white matter echogenicity becomes more pronounced, and the boundary between the two becomes sharper. If the entire brain is affected, increased

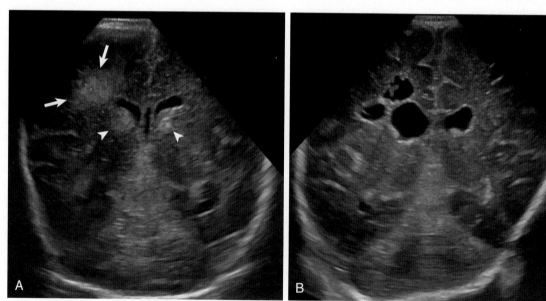

Fig. 7.25 Evolution of periventricular leukomalacia in a preterm infant. (A) At age 1 day, there is increased echogenicity in the right periventricular white matter (*arrows*), along with bilateral grade I IVH (*arrowheads*). Note the narrow cavum septum pellucidum between the frontal horns. (B) Six weeks later, cystic leukomalacia has developed in the right periventricular white matter, and volume loss on the right has caused the right lateral ventricle to enlarge more than the left.

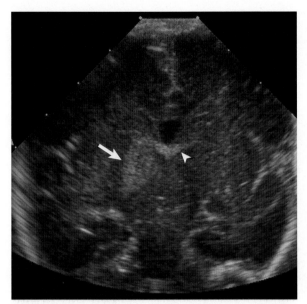

Fig. 7.26 Thalamic infarct in a 28-week EGA infant. There is increased echogenicity in the right thalamus (*arrow*). Note the normal choroid in the roof of the third ventricle (*arrowhead*) below the cavum septum pellucidum.

echogenicity may be blotchy or uniform but is usually relatively well demarcated.

More profound ischemia leads to blurring of gray/white matter differentiation. The cortex may appear echogenic and thickened. Instead of normal, uniform, moderately decreased echogenicity, there are scattered—and sometimes near-confluent—areas of moderately increased echogenicity. If there has been hemorrhagic conversion, there will be more striking, masslike hyperechoic areas (Fig. 7.28). Diffuse brain edema leads to slit-like ventricles and effacement of extraaxial fluid spaces. The interhemispheric fissure may appear blurred and indistinct (Fig. 7.29). Profound prolonged hypoxia also damages the metabolically active gray matter: ventrolateral thalami, posterior putamina, hippocampi, dorsal brainstem, corticospinal tracts, and perirolandic cortex.

Focal Arterial or Venous Infarct. In addition to these global patterns of brain injury, more focal ischemia may occur, usually in infants older than 28 weeks EGA. Perinatal asphyxia, infection, trauma, or coagulation disorders may lead to arterial stroke (usually the left middle cerebral artery) or venous infarction (usually due to superior sagittal sinus thrombosis).

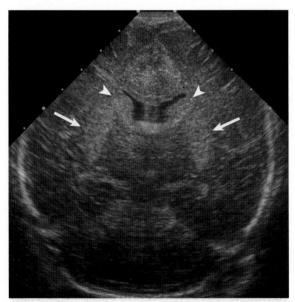

Fig. 7.27 Infarcts from profound hypoxia in a term infant after cardiac surgery. The caudate nuclei (*arrowheads*) and putamina (*arrows*) are preferentially affected. A similar appearance may be seen with beriberi.

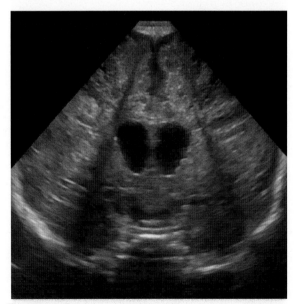

Fig. 7.28 Diffuse hemorrhagic hypoxic-ischemic encephalopathy due to child abuse in a 7-month-old infant, 1 month after trauma. The parenchyma is echogenic and heterogeneous, and the ventricles are mildly dilated due to white matter loss.

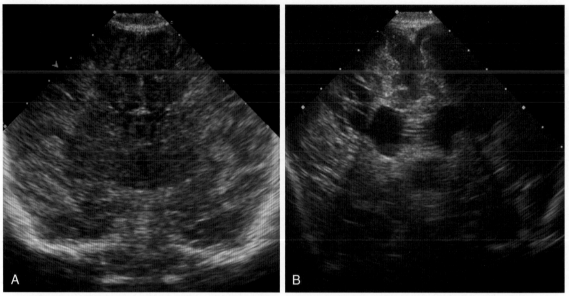

Fig. 7.29 Diffuse hypoxic-ischemic encephalopathy in a term infant who stopped moving 24 hours before delivery. (A) On day 1 of life, gray–white matter differentiation is indistinct, and there are scattered, patchy areas of increased echogenicity. The interhemispheric fissure is indistinct, and the ventricles are slitlike. (B) Seven months later, there is cystic periventricular leukomalacia along with diffuse volume loss.

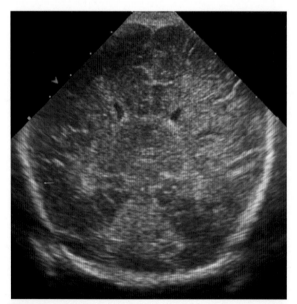

Fig. 7.30 Left middle cerebral artery (MCA) infarct in a term infant who stopped moving the right side. There is loss of gray–white matter differentiation, as well as increased echogenicity in the left MCA territory. The normal hypoechoic subcortical ribbon is accentuated.

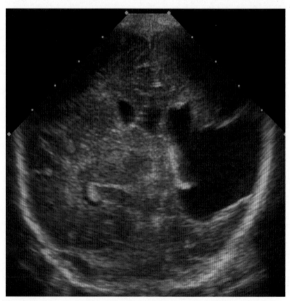

Fig. 7.31 Prenatal left middle cerebral artery (MCA) infarct in a preterm infant has caused left parietal porencephaly.

Focal ischemia may be recognized as a well-defined area of increased echogenicity. If ischemia is extremely severe, heterogeneity becomes more pronounced, and the transition between gray and white matter may be ill-defined. Markedly increased echogenicity suggests superimposed hemorrhage.

Focal lesions may be large or small—restricted to a portion of the basal ganglia or thalamus (see Fig. 7.26) or affecting an entire vascular territory (Figs. 7.30 and 7.31).

BIBLIOGRAPHY

Daneman A, et al. Imaging of the brain in full-term neonates: does sonography still play a role? *Pediatr Radiol.* 2006;36. 346–346.

Daneman A, Epelman M. Neurosonography: in pursuit of an optimized examination. *Pediatr Radiol.* 2015;45:406–412.

Dinan D, Daneman A, Guimaraes CV, et al. Easily overlooked sonographic findings in the evaluation of neonatal encephalopathy: lessons learned from magnetic resonance imaging. *Semin Ultrasound CT MR.* 2014;35:627–651.

Kocaoglu M, Bulakbasi N. Common pitfalls in paediatric imaging: head and spine. *Pediatr Radiol.* 2009;39:347–355.

Lowe LH, Bailey Z. State-of-the-art cranial sonography: part 1, modern techniques and image interpretation. *AJR.* 2011;196:1028–1033.

Lowe LH, Bailey Z. State-of-the-art cranial sonography: part 2, pitfalls and variants. *AJR.* 2011;196:1034–1039.

Maller VV, Cohen HL. Neurosonography: assessing the premature infant. *Pediatr Radiol.* 2017;47:1031–1045.

Vazquez E, Castellote A, Mayolas N, et al. Congenital tumours involving the head, neck and central nervous system. *Pediatr Radiol.* 2009;39:1158.

Wani NA, Qureshi UA, Ahmad K. Cranial ultrasonography in infantile encephalopathic beriberi: a useful first-line imaging tool for screening and diagnosis in suspected cases. *AJNR.* 2016;37:1535–1540.

Yikilmaz A, Taylor GA. Cranial sonography in term and near-term infants. *Pediatr Radiol.* 2008;38:605–616.

Yikilmaz A, Taylor GA. Sonographic findings in bacterial meningitis in neonates and young infants. *Pediatr Radiol.* 2008;38:129–137.

Chest Ultrasound

8

Lung

Kenneth M. Kelley

CLINICAL CORRELATION

Patients who present with undifferentiated shortness of breath can be challenging due to the broad differential diagnosis, which encompasses pulmonary, cardiac, mixed cardiopulmonary, and noncardiopulmonary etiologies. Lung ultrasound has revolutionized the approach to the undifferentiated dyspneic patient. What makes lung ultrasound somewhat unique is that whereas other ultrasound applications use traditional grayscale images of the patient's anatomy to answer focused questions, lung ultrasound looks at changes in expected artifacts, as the pleural interfaces and air-to-water ratio change in the lung during different pathologic processes.

NORMAL ANATOMY

The ultrasound image should include at least two hyperechoic ribs with acoustic shadowing beneath them. The intercostal muscles have a mixed echogenicity, and deep to this is the hyperechoic line that represents the parietal and visceral pleural interface. As the patient breathes, the visceral and parietal pleural move up on one another in opposite directions. The ultrasound representation of this is a "sliding," or movement, artifact at the hyperechoic pleural line. Deep to the pleural interface there are horizontal hyperechoic lines called *A-lines* that are a reverberation artifact between the transducer and the parietal pleural interface and are displayed at equidistant depth intervals in the lung (Fig. 8.1). In addition to A-lines, there is an occasional hyperechoic vertical line that starts at the pleural interface, moves dynamically with lung sliding, and then quickly diminishes or fades. These are referred to as *comet tail artifact* (a type of reverberation artifact). Like lung sliding, comet tail artifacts are an indication that the parietal and visceral pleura are in contact with each other. Lung pulse is a rhythmic shimmering that occurs at the pleural interface due to normal cardiac oscillation when the patient is either breath-holding or poorly ventilating a lung (e.g., mainstem intubation). The M-mode is used to evaluate the lung. M-mode is a focused sector of sound with a display of the reflected images along a time axis. Normal lung where the visceral and parietal pleura are in contact with one another creates a granular artifact at the pleural interface on M-mode that has been described as a *sandy beach*, with the other structures above the pleural interface appearing as a *beach and sky*, making the whole image a *seashore sign* (Fig. 8.2).

IMAGING

Imaging of the lung parenchyma is performed with a low-frequency phased array transducer (microconvex or curvilinear transducers can also be used) with a preset depth range of 12 to 16 cm. In trauma patients who present supine and evaluation for pneumothorax is the primary indication for lung ultrasound, some providers prefer to use a high-frequency linear transducer at 4 to 8 cm depth (depending on the patient's body habitus) for increased resolution of the pleural interface. Each hemithorax is divided into four lung zones (Fig. 8.3). A complete lung exam involves looking at each of the four

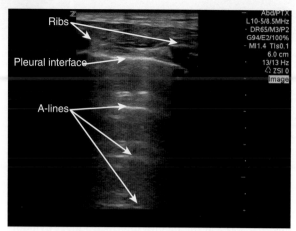

Fig. 8.1 Normal lung with A-lines.

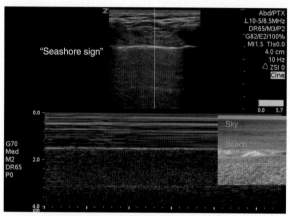

Fig. 8.2 Lung M-mode seashore sign.

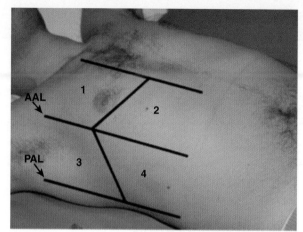

Fig. 8.3 Lung zones hemithorax. (From Volpicelli G, et al. Bedside lung ultrasound in the assessment of alveolar-interstitial syndrome. *Am J Emerg Med.* 2006;24:689-696. Fig. 2.)

zones on both hemithoraces with the patient typically reclined at 30 to 45 degrees.

To start the exam, place the transducer in the second to third intercostal space in the midclavicular line. This is lung zone 1. Direct the probe indicator cephalad. In trauma patients with concern for pneumothorax, place the transducer on the most anterior portion of the chest wall, as this is the most likely spot for air to accumulate.

PATHOLOGY

Pneumothorax

A pneumothorax occurs when the visceral surface of the lung separates from the parietal pleura and air occupies the space in between the two interfaces. This lack of contact between the pleural surfaces leads to the absence of lung "sliding." The absence of expected artifact is a chief indicator of the presence of the pneumothorax. Other criteria that help make the diagnosis of pneumothorax are the absence of comet tail artifact and the absence of lung pulse.

The use of M-mode has also been described in the diagnosis of pneumothorax. When a pneumothorax is present and the transducer is placed over a section of lung where there is no lung sliding, the *sandy beach* of the *seashore sign* will be absent and replaced by horizontal lines similar to the artifact above the pleural interface. This image of a pneumothorax using M-mode is called the *bar code sign* or *stratosphere sign* (Fig. 8.4). In evaluating for a pneumothorax, one can achieve 100% specificity by identifying a "lung point." A lung point is the precise site where the visceral and parietal pleura transition from being in contact with one another to having air between them. The dynamic ultrasound image of this will show an area of lung sliding that abruptly stops. One can liken this image to a curtain that slides across the lung window image but does not make it all the way across (Fig. 8.5). This exact spot where the sliding stops is the edge of the pneumothorax. By following the lung point on the chest wall, one can estimate the size of the pneumothorax. Identifying a lung point rules in the diagnosis

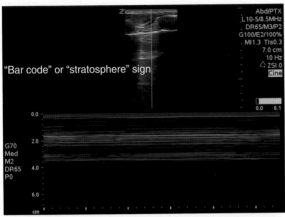

Fig. 8.4 Pneumothorax using M-mode barcode sign.

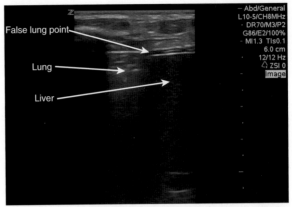

Fig. 8.6 False lung point.

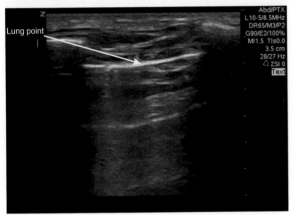

Fig. 8.5 Lung point.

of a pneumothorax. Of note, some anatomic sites can mimic the presence of a lung point. These lung point mimics are termed *false lung points* and occur where the pleural interface ends and either diaphragm or pericardium begins. A false lung point image includes lung sliding that appears to stop; however, when examined closely, the hyperechoic parietal pleura ends and is replaced by the more hypoechoic presence of the pericardium or diaphragm (Fig. 8.6). In a true lung point, the hyperechoic pleural line remains visible. False lung points are normal anatomic interactions that occur in expected places (left side of chest, lower chest wall).

In trauma patients, the sensitivity and specificity of ultrasound for diagnosing pneumothorax ranges from 86% to 98% and 97% to 100%, respectively. In nontrauma

patients, the specificity is decreased, especially in critically ill patients, as conditions such as emphysematous blebs, acute respiratory distress syndrome (ARDS), and pneumonic consolidations can have the appearance of an absent lung slide. In these conditions the visceral and parietal pleura remain in contact with one another; however, there is little movement between them and they can thus appear as though there is no lung sliding. In these situations, despite the absence of easily discernable lung sliding, comet tail artifacts are still present and can be helpful in making a diagnosis that a pneumothorax is not present. Additionally, with processes such as ARDS and pneumonic consolidations, there will be other lung ultrasound findings that help make the diagnosis more apparent.

Interstitial Syndrome

One of the major clinical indications for the use of lung ultrasound is for the assessment of interstitial syndrome. The diagnosis of interstitial syndrome is marked by the presence of B-lines. B-lines are vertical hyperechoic lines that begin at the pleural interface, are dynamic with lung sliding, and are continuous to the bottom of the screen (Fig. 8.7). The presence of multiple B-lines (more than three) in two or more lung fields defines interstitial syndrome. Interstitial syndrome refers to multiple pathologic processes. In a bilateral distribution, pulmonary edema, interstitial pneumonia, and pulmonary fibrosis are the most common etiologies. A unilateral focal appearance of multiple B-lines is more consistent with interstitial pneumonia, pulmonary contusion, atelectasis, infarction, and lung mass.

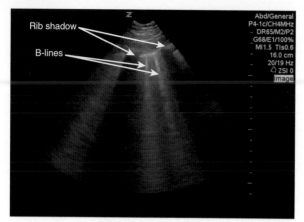

Fig. 8.7 Lung B-lines.

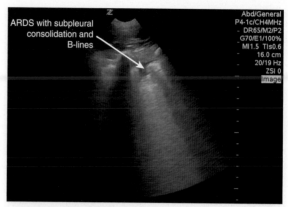

Fig. 8.8 Subpleural consolidation.

Clinically, the most commonly seen interstitial syndrome is pulmonary edema from congestive heart failure. Lung ultrasound has shown in multiple studies to be one of the best tests (positive likelihood ratio) for the diagnosis of congestive heart failure exacerbations—performing better than physical examination findings, laboratory testing, and chest X-ray. There have also been studies looking at the changes in treatment strategies based on lung ultrasound findings and have shown a correlation towards more rapid and accurate diagnosis and treatment when ultrasound is utilized to evaluate acute dyspnea.

Differentiating pulmonary edema from a cardiogenic source versus noncardiogenic process such as ARDS can be challenging. Some lung ultrasound findings are more consistent with ARDS than with cardiogenic pulmonary edema. The inflammatory process that causes ARDS also creates thickening and irregularity of the pleural interface that is visible with ultrasound. In addition, ARDS has a patchy presence in the lungs with spared areas of lung that appear normal. Small subpleural consolidations (Fig. 8.8) may also be present with ARDS, and overall there may appear to be less lung sliding present with ARDS. Lung sliding is unchanged in cardiogenic pulmonary edema. Pulmonary edema of cardiogenic source, on the other hand, tends to have a more uniform distribution of B-lines, especially in dependent areas, and as treatment is rendered, one will dynamically observe a decrease in B-lines.

Pulmonary fibrosis can be differentiated from other interstitial processes with ultrasound. B-lines in pulmonary fibrosis may also have an irregular distribution consistent with the extent of the disease process in the lung. Additionally, there may be thickening and irregularities at the pleural interface with subpleural abnormalities.

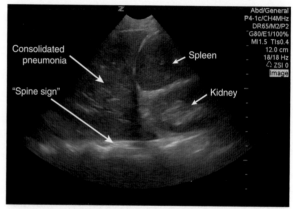

Fig. 8.9 Lung consolidation.

Pneumonia

The disease process of pneumonia usually involves viral or bacterial invasion of the lung. The inflammatory cascade triggered by the infection causes the alveoli to become filled with fluid. As this process reaches the visceral surface of the lung, it initially will appear as B-lines and small subpleural consolidations. As the alveoli consolidate with fluid, the lung develops a similar echotexture as the liver. This phenomenon is called *hepatization* of the lung (Fig. 8.9). In addition to the lung having a liver-like echotexture, there are some other hallmark findings consistent with pneumonia. One pathognomonic finding is the presence of dynamic air bronchograms. Dynamic air bronchograms are the result of air trapped within the bronchioles as the consolidative process occurs. As the patient inhales and exhales, the hyperechoic reflection of air moves much like a meniscus in a branched pattern that follows the pattern of the

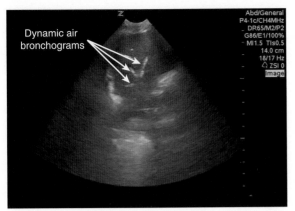

Fig. 8.10 Air bronchograms.

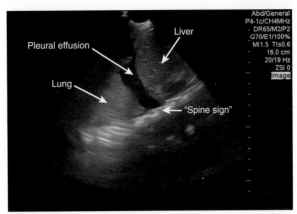

Fig. 8.12 Spine sign.

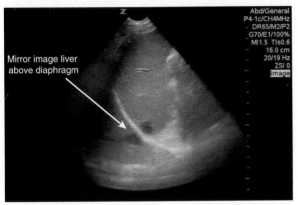

Fig. 8.11 Normal lung with mirror image artifact.

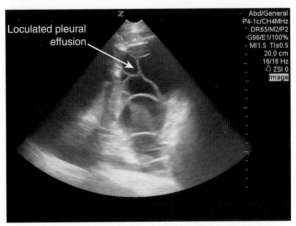

Fig. 8.13 Loculated pleural effusion.

bronchioles (Fig. 8.10). Other lung ultrasound findings are the presence of the *spine sign* when viewing the lower lung field in the midaxillary plane. Normal air-filled lung behind the diaphragm acts as a strong reflector and causes a "mirror image" of the liver or spleen above the diaphragm, which obscures the spine (Fig. 8.11). When a consolidative process or effusion is present above the diaphragm, there is no mirror image artifact present and instead the hyperechoic spine is seen extending past the diaphragm (see Fig. 8.9).

Pleural Effusions

Pleural effusions are readily seen on ultrasound. Pleural effusions generally follow gravity and are located in dependent areas. As a result, they are most readily seen at the lower lung field in the mid-to-posterior axillary line just above the diaphragm. As mentioned previously, the presence of a pleural effusion will produce a positive "spine sign." Effusions are seen as collections above the diaphragm (Fig. 8.12). The echogenicity of the fluid depends on the ratio of fluid to debris in the process. Simple effusions will be hypoechoic. Adjacent to the pleural effusion, consolidative or atelectatic lung is usually visualized. When present, loculations will have hyperechoic, fibrous bands dividing the process into separate collections (Fig. 8.13). In addition to the diagnosis of pleural effusions, ultrasound is considered to improve outcomes in thoracentesis.

BIBLIOGRAPHY

Copetti R, Soldati G, Copetti P. Chest sonograhy: a useful tool to differentiate acute cardiogenic pulmonary edema from acute respiratory distress syndrome. *Cardiovasc Ultrasound.* 2008;6:16.

Cortellaro F, Colombo S, Coen D, et al. Lung ultrasound is an accurate diagnostic tool for the diagnosis of pneumonia in the emergency department. *Emerg Med J.* 2012;29:19–23.

Lichtenstein D, Meziere G. Relevance of lung ultrasound in the diagnosis of acute respiratory failure: the BLUE Protocol. *Chest.* 2008;134:117–125.

Lichtenstein D, Meziere G, Biderman P. The "comet-tail artifact": an ultrasound sign ruling out pneumothorax. *Intensive Care Med.* 1999;25:383–388.

Lichtenstein D, Meziere G, Biderman P. The "lung point": an ultrasound sign specific to pneumothorax. *Intensive Care Med.* 2000;26:1434–1440.

Life in the Fastlane. Comet tail artefact=fatiguing short path reverberation artefact. https://lifeinthefastlane.com/ultrasound/artefacts/comet-tail-artefact/James Rippy, last updated October 23, 2017.

Martindale JL, Wakai A, Collins SP, et al. Diagnosing acute heart failure in the emergency department: a systematic review and meta-analysis. *Acad Emerg Med.* 2016;23: 223–242.

Parlamento S, Copetti R, Di Bartolomeo S. Evaluation of the lung ultrasound for the diagnosis of pneumonia in the ED. *Am J Emerg Med.* 2009;27:379–384.

Pirozzi C, Numis FG, Pagano A, et al. Immediate versus delayed integrated point-of care ultrasonography to manage acute dyspnea in the emergency department. *Crit Ultrasound J.* 2014;6:5.

Prina E, Torres A. Lung ultrasound in the evaluation of pleural effusion. *J Bras Pneumol.* 2014;40(1):1–5.

Stone MB. Ultrasound diagnosis of traumatic pneumothorax. *J Emerg Trauma Shock.* 2008;1(1):19–20.

Volpicelli G, et al. International evidence-based recommendations for point-of-care ultrasound. *Intensive Care Med.* 2012;38:577–591.

Volpicelli G, Mussa A, Garofalo G. Bedside lung ultrasound in the assessment of alveolar-interstitial syndrome. *Am J Emerg Med.* 2006;24:689–696.

Wilkerson RG, Stone MB. Sensitivity of bedside ultrasound and supine anteroposterior chest radiographs for the identification of pneumothorax after blunt trauma. *Acad Emerg Med.* 2010;17:11–17.

9

Transthoracic Echocardiography

Siobhan Smith, Drew Jones, Kathryn Pade, Ryan Horton, Kenton L. Anderson, Laleh Gharahbaghian

BASIC ECHOCARDIOGRAPHY

Clinical Correlation

Point-of-care cardiac ultrasound is indicated for a wide variety of clinical presentations, including cardiac trauma, cardiac arrest, tachycardia, hypotension, shortness of breath, chest pain, and syncope. It requires a minimum of two views of the heart and may also require visualization of the inferior vena cava (IVC) and pulmonary ultrasound to assess for intravascular volume status, associated lung abnormalities, and correlation with the cardiac ultrasound findings. Cardiac sonography is truly a time-sensitive assessment of the undifferentiated symptomatic patient. Some professional societies have published guidelines outlining basic and advanced/expert point-of-care cardiac sonography skills. The basic evaluation usually includes an assessment for pericardial effusion, global cardiac function, relative chamber size, and patient volume status. Other pathologic processes may be demonstrated with more advanced echocardiography skills, but comprehensive echocardiography with cardiology consultation is often recommended, as diagnoses such as wall motion abnormalities, valvular disease, endocarditis, and aortic disease require additional training in comprehensive echocardiography techniques.

Normal Anatomy

Deoxygenated blood flows from the right atrium (RA) across the tricuspid valve to the right ventricle (RV) and then to the lungs via the pulmonary artery. Oxygenated blood returns to the left atrium (LA) via the pulmonary veins, flowing across the mitral valve (MV) into the left ventricle (LV), and finally exiting the heart via the aortic outflow tract through the aortic valve. Parts of the ascending and descending aorta can be seen in basic echocardiography, whereas the aortic arch can be seen with advanced cardiac ultrasound evaluation (Fig. 9.1).

The IVC is a thin-walled, compliant vessel that delivers deoxygenated blood from the lower body back to the heart. The IVC runs inferior to superior in the retroperitoneal space to the right of the spine and crosses the diaphragm to empty into the RA.

Imaging

Bedside Echocardiography. Four cardiac views are used in point-of-care basic cardiac ultrasound: subxiphoid (SX), parasternal long axis (PSL), parasternal short axis (PSS), and apical four-chamber (AP4). All views are obtained using the low-frequency (3–5 MHz) phased array transducer. Patients are typically positioned supine; however, the PSL, PSS, and AP4 views are often more easily obtained with the patient in the left lateral decubitus position (see Fig. 9.1). The transducer's indicator icon may be oriented on the left or right side of the screen, depending on the conventions followed by the specialty/institution. The following basic cardiac ultrasound descriptions are written with the screen's indicator dot on the left side of the screen. (If the screen indicator on the right side is preferred, rotate the transducer 180 degrees from the positions described; Fig. 9.2.)

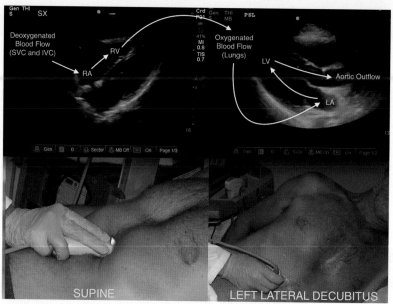

Fig. 9.1 Anatomy: blood flow and patient position for basic echocardiography. The subxiphoid view of the heart is shown to depict how deoxygenated blood flows from the veins of the body to the SVC (upper body) and IVC (lower body) to the RA. It then goes to the RV through the tricuspid valve and to the lungs through the pulmonic valve (not shown). The parasternal long axis view of the heart is shown to depict oxygenated blood flowing to the LA. It then travels to the LV through the mitral valve and then to the aortic outflow tract through the aortic valve. *IVC*, inferior vena cava; *LA*, left atrium; *LV*, left ventricle; *PSL*, parasternal long axis; *RA*, right atrium; *RV*, right ventricle; *SVC*, superior vena cava; *SX*, subxiphoid.

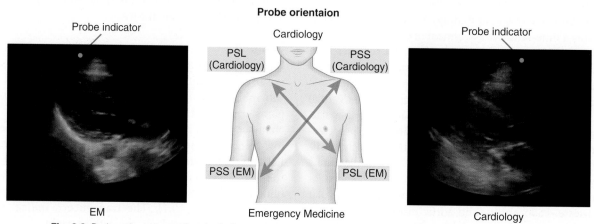

Fig. 9.2 Probe orientation and probe indicator screen icon. The probe indicator icon on the screen can be on either the screen's left or right side. The *red arrows* depict the probe orientation if the screen dot is on the screen's left side for the parasternal long and short axis views of the heart. The *purple arrows* depict the probe orientation if the screen dot is on the screen's right side—the classic orientation used in emergency medicine.

Subxiphoid. Place the transducer on the abdomen just inferior to the xiphoid process in plane with the abdominal wall. The transducer indicator faces the patient's right, and the transducer footprint should be slightly directed toward the patient's left shoulder. Visualize the heart deep to the xiphoid process by applying pressure while flattening the transducer along the patient's abdomen. The liver is used

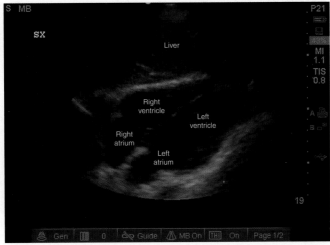

Fig. 9.3 Normal subxiphoid ultrasound anatomy. The subxiphoid is a four-chamber view. The RV is the most inferior and anterior chamber.

as an acoustic window. Adjust the screen depth to include the posterior pericardium. This view can be improved by asking the patient to take and hold a deep breath, as inspiration will lower the diaphragm, causing the heart to move closer to the transducer (Fig. 9.3). This view is traditionally used to evaluate for pericardial effusion; however, other pathologies can also be seen.

Parasternal long axis. Place the transducer perpendicular to the chest wall at the left third or fourth intercostal space adjacent to the sternum, with the transducer indicator pointing toward the patient's left hip. This window is used to visualize the RV, LV, LA, aortic outflow tract, and descending aorta. Adjust the screen depth to include the descending aorta in the inferior aspect of the image (Fig. 9.4). This view is valuable in assessing left ventricular systolic function and to differentiate pericardial effusion from a left-sided pleural effusion.

Parasternal short axis. Rotate the transducer 90 degrees from the PSL view. The indicator should be pointing toward the patient's right hip. The LV can be visualized in cross-section from the level of the MV ("fishmouth" view), to the chordae tendineae and papillary muscles view, and to the LV's apex by sweeping the transducer from its base to its apex (Fig. 9.5). This view allows for assessment of global LV systolic function (LVSF) when visualizing the LV at the level of the papillary muscles and for RV strain.

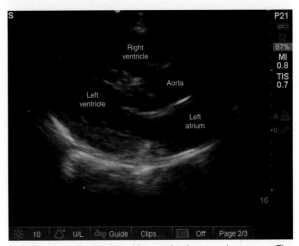

Fig. 9.4 Normal parasternal long axis ultrasound anatomy. The parasternal long axis is a three-chamber view of the heart with visualization of the aortic outflow tract. The RV is the most anterior chamber seen at the top of the screen, whereas the longitudinal view of the LA and LV is seen just deep to the RV.

Apical four-chamber. Place the transducer at the apex of the heart overlying the point of maximal impulse (PMI), typically located in the midclavicular line at approximately the fifth intercostal space. Direct the indicator toward the patient's right, and angle the transducer toward the patient's right shoulder while flattening it in plane with the long axis of the left ventricle (Fig. 9.6). This view is useful to compare ventricular chamber sizes.

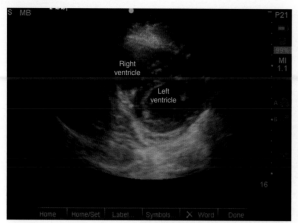

Fig. 9.5 Normal parasternal short axis ultrasound anatomy. The parasternal short axis is a two-chamber view of the heart with partial visualization of the RV and complete visualization of the transverse LV.

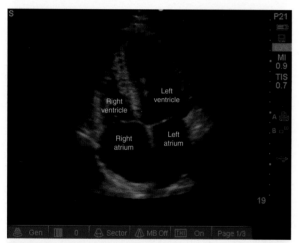

Fig. 9.6 Normal apical four-chamber ultrasound anatomy. The apical four-chamber is a longitudinal view of the heart from its apex. The apex is seen at the top of the screen, closest to the probe location, with the septum shown separating the RV and LV. The RV is two-thirds the size of the LV. The RA and LA are seen at the bottom of the screen.

Inferior Vena Cava Ultrasound. The IVC is thin-walled and compliant and changes diameter according to patient volume status and with variations in intrathoracic pressure during the respiratory cycle. It also reflects changes when there are cardiac flow changes. Sonographic IVC evaluation involves assessment of IVC diameter, as well as collapsibility, during respiration. Position the patient supine and select the low-frequency (3–5 MHz) phased array transducer. Obtain an SX cardiac view, then

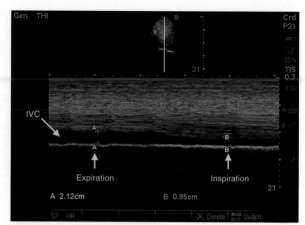

Fig. 9.7 Inferior vena cava ultrasound anatomy with M-mode. The longitudinal IVC is seen entering the right atrium. Using M-mode, which displays motion over time, the respiratory variation of the IVC can been visualized, showing collapse during inspiration. *IVC,* inferior vena cava.

rotate the transducer 90 degrees so that the indicator is directed caudally. With this technique, the IVC can be visualized in the longitudinal plane as it enters the RA. Once the IVC is identified, measure the diameter 2 to 4 cm from where it enters the RA in both expiration and inspiration. Respiratory variation can also be measured in M-mode. With M-mode, the cursor is placed across the IVC. The IVC size variation will be plotted along the time axis. Inspiration causes IVC collapse, as negative intrathoracic pressure draws blood into the thoracic cavity, increasing venous return to the heart (Fig. 9.7). The longitudinal IVC can also be visualized when placing the probe in the right midaxillary line, with the indicator directed cephalad and the transducer angled posteriorly. This view of the IVC, however, has not been proven to correlate with intravascular volume status.

Pathology

Pericardial Effusion. A pericardial effusion appears as an anechoic stripe between the pericardium and the myocardium. Small effusions are seen in dependent areas (posterior and inferior), whereas large effusions may also be seen anteriorly (Fig. 9.8). The epicardial fat pad must be distinguished from a pericardial effusion. Epicardial fat is typically seen anteriorly and appears echogenic. In comparison, a pericardial effusion is visualized posteriorly or inferiorly and appears anechoic. A pleural effusion may also appear as an anechoic area posterior to the heart and is often mistaken for a pericardial effusion.

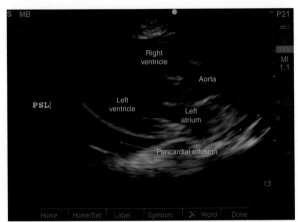

Fig. 9.8 Parasternal long axis view showing a pericardial effusion. Pericardial effusion will be seen in the dependent area of the parasternal view, which lies posterior to the heart, with the anechoic area of fluid being anterior to the descending thoracic aorta.

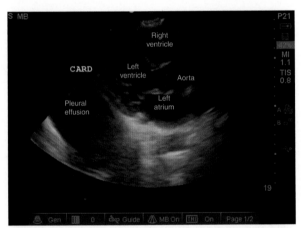

Fig. 9.9 Parasternal long axis view showing pleural effusion. A left-sided pleural effusion will be seen as an anechoic area posterior to the heart and can be distinguished from a pericardial effusion due to the absence of anechoic material anterior to the heart, and the anechoic pleural fluid will traverse posterior to the descending thoracic aorta.

In the PSL view, pleural effusions can be distinguished from pericardial effusions by their location posterior to the descending aorta (Fig. 9.9). Obtain images in at least two cardiac windows for a more accurate evaluation of a pericardial effusion.

Cardiac Tamponade. Cardiac tamponade is a clinical diagnosis involving pericardial fluid, hypotension, tachycardia, pulsus paradoxus, and distended neck veins.

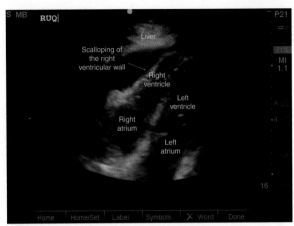

Fig. 9.10 Subxiphoid view showing cardiac tamponade. When the pressure of the pericardial fluid surpasses the ability for the right ventricle (RV) to fill during diastole, RV scalloping and collapse occur with sonographic tamponade physiology.

Sonographic signs of tamponade include pericardial fluid, delayed RV diastolic expansion, and RV diastolic collapse due to increased pericardial pressures on the RV free wall (Fig. 9.10). A dilated IVC with reduced respiratory variation should also be seen in cardiac tamponade.

Left Ventricular Systolic Function. LVSF may be reduced in conditions such as congestive heart failure (CHF), myocardial infarction (MI), and a number of other cardiac pathologies and may correlate with cardiogenic shock in the correct clinical context. LVSF may be increased in conditions with low systemic vascular resistance, cardiac diastolic dysfunction, and hyperautonomic states. Bedside ultrasound assessment of LV function may be achieved by several different methods, outlined next.

Global estimate of left ventricular function. Visual estimation of global LVSF is made by assessing overall endocardial incursion and myocardial thickening. Estimations are categorized as hyperdynamic (corresponds approximately to an ejection fraction [EF] >70%), normal contractility (EF 50%–70%), moderate dysfunction (EF 30%–50%), or severe dysfunction (EF <30%). In an LV with normal function, all walls should thicken and move symmetrically and vigorously toward the center of the chamber during systole. An LV with moderate or severe dysfunction will have decreased myocardial incursion and thickening. A hyperdynamic LV has vigorous myocardial contraction

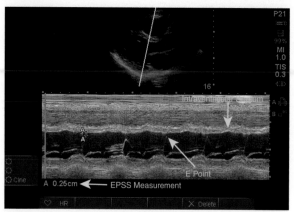

Fig. 9.11 E-point septal separation visualized in M-mode. Placing the M-mode cursor over the anterior mitral valve leaflet and visualizing its motion over time shows ventricular diastole, starting with an E peak. The distance between the anterior mitral valve leaflet and the septum at the E point is an indicator for left ventricular systolic function, with normal measurements being <7 mm in the absence of mitral valve disease and aortic valve regurgitation.

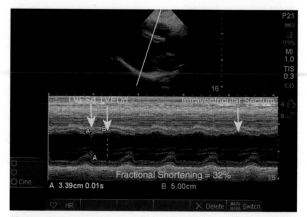

Fig. 9.12 Fractional shortening visualized in M-mode. Noting the percentage difference in ventricular motion during systole and diastole using M-mode, placing the cursor just outside of the mitral valve in the PSL view, can give a quantitative indicator for contractility.

and the LV chamber appears nearly fully contracted during systole. Global LVSF should be estimated in at least two cardiac windows and should be in adjunct to the history, physical examination, and other clinical studies when making a diagnosis.

E-point septal separation. E-point septal separation (EPSS) is a quantitative method for estimating LVSF. EPSS is the minimal distance between the anterior MV leaflet and the interventricular septum (IVS) during diastole. EPSS ≥7mm indicates poor LVSF. EPSS is assessed in the PSL view by placing the M-mode cursor across the anterior MV leaflet and measuring the minimal distance between the anterior MV leaflet and the IVS (Fig. 9.11). In M-mode the first peak will be the E point, which reflects passive left ventricular filling. The peak that follows the E point is the A peak and represents atrial contraction. Valvular disease that restricts mitral leaflet motion or a view that is tangential rather than true PSL may exaggerate EPSS. Aortic regurgitation can also falsely increase the measurement of EPSS. Septal or global LV hypertrophy can lead to underestimation of EPSS.

Fractional shortening. Fractional shortening (FS) is another quantitative method for estimating LVSF. FS is the percentage change in LV chamber size from diastole to systole. FS is measured in the PSL or PSS view by placing the M-mode cursor across the LV just beyond or distal to the MV leaflets (Fig. 9.12). The difference between LV diameter in diastole (LVEDd) and LV diameter in systole (LVESd) is divided by LVEDd to yield FS: (LVEDd – LVESd) / LVEDd. Normal FS is 30% to 45%. FS >45% is hyperdynamic. FS <30% indicates reduced LVSF. Apical wall motion abnormalities will give false FS measurements.

Right Heart Strain. *Right heart strain* is a term used to describe RV dysfunction. Right heart strain may be due to increased pulmonary arterial pressures in conditions such as pulmonary embolism (PE) and pulmonary hypertension, lung disease such as chronic obstructive pulmonary disease (COPD), or due to RV infarction. Signs of right heart strain on echocardiography include dilated RV, paradoxical septal wall motion toward the LV in diastole, and McConnell's sign.

Echocardiography is poorly sensitive for diagnosing PE but useful for risk stratification in patients who are unstable for computed tomography (CT) angiography scanning and for patients who have known PE. Visualization of thrombus in transit (mobile hyperechoic material floating between RA and RV) or new right heart strain may help justify the use of thrombolytics in unstable patients with suspected PE.

Right ventricular dilation. The RV in a normal heart is approximately two-thirds the size of the LV. In moderate right heart strain, the RV is approximately the same size as the LV. In severe right heart strain, the RV is larger than the LV. RV and LV sizes are best compared

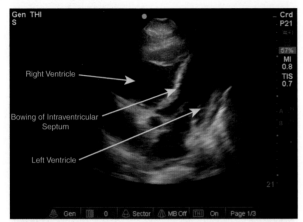

Fig. 9.13 Right ventricular dilation in an apical four-chamber view showing septal bowing into left ventricle. With right heart strain, the right ventricle will be greater than two-thirds of the left ventricle and can result in the septum bowing toward the left ventricle. The figure shows this phenomenon in the apical four-chamber view.

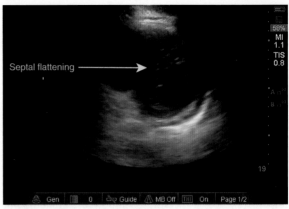

Fig. 9.14 Right ventricular dilation in parasternal short view showing "D" sign. With right heart strain, the right ventricle will result in the septum bowing toward the left ventricle. The figure shows this phenomenon in the parasternal short view, causing a "D" shape of the left ventricle instead of the classic "O" shape.

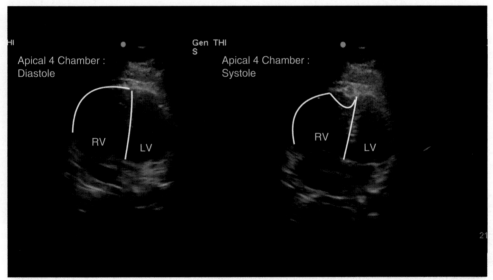

Fig. 9.15 McConnell's sign: right ventricular apical contraction. McConnell's sign depicts a phenomenon seen in acute right heart strain, where the right ventricular apex contracts while the right ventricle free wall remains hypokinetic. *LV*, left ventricle; *RV*, right ventricle.

in the AP4 view at the tip of the mitral and tricuspid valves when valves are fully opened during diastole (Fig. 9.13). RV dilation can also be assessed in the PSS view by appreciating the "D" sign, referring to septal flattening giving the LV a D-shaped appearance instead of a classically relaxed "O" shape (Fig. 9.14).

McConnell's sign. McConnell's sign is mid-RV free-wall hypokinesis with normal contractility of the apex of the RV. This finding is best visualized in the AP4 window and has been shown to be more correlated to pulmonary embolus than a chronic etiology for RV dilation (Fig. 9.15).

Acute versus chronic right heart strain. Right heart strain may be acute or chronic and must be interpreted with clinical context. If a hypertrophic RV myocardium is seen in a heart with right heart strain, this may indicate a more chronic process, such as cor pulmonale or other causes of chronic lung disease.

Abnormal Volume Status. Evaluation of the hypotensive or dyspneic patient should include an assessment of the IVC to correlate it to the echocardiography. Normal IVC diameter in an adult patient is approximately 2 cm with a respiratory cycle variation of approximately 50% from expiration to inspiration during spontaneous respiration. With regard to volume status, patients with normal or high IVC respiratory variation (>50% respiratory collapse) are likely to be tolerant to intravenous fluid resuscitation. Patients with an IVC >2 cm with minimal or no respiratory variation are considered to be in a hypervolemic state. A single IVC evaluation does not determine volume responsiveness, as responsiveness is a measure of improved cardiac output over time. Assessment of fluid tolerance should also involve an evaluation of pulmonary extravascular fluid.

Plethoric noncollapsible inferior vena cava. A plethoric IVC with minimal respiratory variation occurs when the IVC is not cleared of fluid that is returning from the body. This is seen with intravascular volume overload in conditions such as CHF, renal failure, and iatrogenic events. A plethoric, noncollapsible IVC is also seen in cardiogenic shock and obstructive shock states due to conditions such as cardiac tamponade, tension pneumothorax, and PE (Fig. 9.16).

Small collapsible inferior vena cava. A small and collapsible IVC may be seen in distributive shock states due to conditions such as sepsis and in hypovolemic shock states due to conditions such as dehydration or hemorrhage (Fig. 9.17).

ADVANCED ECHOCARDIOGRAPHY

Imaging

The same four cardiac views discussed in the "Basic Echocardiography" section are used (SX, PSL, PSS, AP4). In addition, the apical five-chamber (A5C) and the suprasternal views may provide additional information about thoracic aortic pathology.

Apical Five-Chamber. Once an AP4 view has been obtained, angulation of the transducer more anteriorly produces a "five-chamber" view (Fig. 9.18). The fifth chamber is not an actual chamber, but the left ventricular outflow tract (LVOT), aortic valve (AV), and ascending aorta.

Suprasternal. The suprasternal long view is obtained with the patient in a supine position with the neck extended

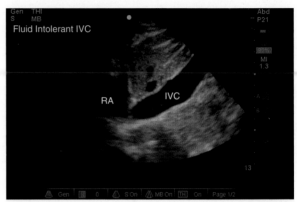

Fig. 9.16 Plethoric IVC. The longitudinal inferior vena cava (*IVC*) is seen traversing into the right atrium (*RA*). Measurements >2 cm with minimal or no respiratory variation are considered a hypervolemic state and can also be seen as a result of various disease processes such as tamponade, pulmonary embolism, and acute pulmonary embolism.

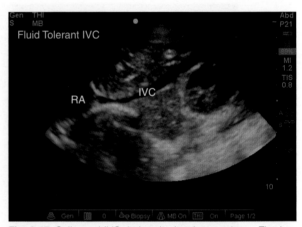

Fig. 9.17 Collapsed IVC during the inspiratory phase. The longitudinal inferior vena cava (*IVC*) is seen traversing into the right atrium (*RA*). Measurements <2 cm with greater than 50% respiratory variation are considered a hypovolemic state and can also be seen as a result of various disease processes causing distributive shock and hypovolemic shock.

(a pillow or towel roll placed behind the shoulders may allow for greater neck extension). Place the phased array transducer in the suprasternal notch, to the left of and parallel to the trachea, with the indicator pointed toward the patient's right side (Fig. 9.19). A suprasternal short axis view can also be obtained by rotating the transducer 90 degrees so that the indicator is aimed toward the patient's head. This results in a cross-section of the aorta located superiorly to the long axis of the right pulmonary

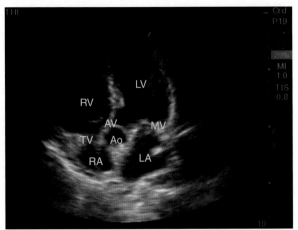

Fig. 9.18 Apical five-chamber (A5C) view. The A5C view is obtained by angling the transducer anteriorly from a four-chamber view to capture the "fifth chamber," which is the left ventricular outflow tract (LVOT) and aorta (*Ao*). *AV*, aortic valve; *LA*, left atrium; *LV*, left ventricle; *RA*, right atrium; *RV*, right ventricle; *TV*, tricuspid valve; *MV*, mitral valve.

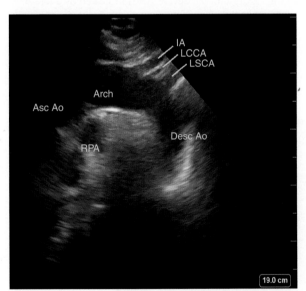

Fig. 9.19 Suprasternal long view. The suprasternal long view demonstrates the aortic arch (*Arch*) and the origin of the three brachiocephalic vessels. *Asc Ao*, ascending aorta; *Desc Ao*, descending aorta; *IA*, innominate artery; *LCCA*, left common carotid artery; *LSCA*, left subclavian artery *RPA*, right pulmonary artery.

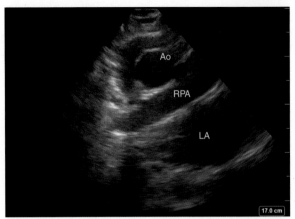

Fig. 9.20 Suprasternal short view. The suprasternal short view demonstrates a transverse view of the aorta (*Ao*) anterior to the right pulmonary artery (*RPA*) and the left atrium (*LA*).

artery and LA (Fig. 9.20). The suprasternal window is often uncomfortable for the patient due to pressure near the trachea and may be impossible in elderly patients who are unable to extend their necks.

Doppler Echo. In addition to the cardiac views described, Doppler allows hemodynamic assessment of the heart and blood vessels by providing the direction and velocity of blood flow through those structures. The three commonly used Doppler echo techniques are described in the following sections.

Continuous wave Doppler. Two crystals are used. One transmits ultrasound continuously, and the other receives continuously. This technique is useful for measuring high velocities but is unable to localize the precise location of those velocities because the signal can originate from any point along the ultrasound beam (Fig. 9.21).

Pulsed wave Doppler. A single crystal is used to transmit and then to receive the ultrasound signal after a preset time delay. This allows velocity to be determined from a small area; the sonologist can move this sample volume, or gate, to the area of interest (Fig. 9.22). Because of the time delay limits, there is a maximum velocity that can be measured before "aliasing" occurs where the displayed velocity "wraps around" the scale.

Color flow mapping. This is an automated two-dimensional (2D) version of pulsed wave Doppler. The velocities and directions of blood flow are represented by color superimposed on a 2D echo image (Fig. 9.23). Typically, velocity toward the transducer is indicated by red color and velocity away from the transducer is blue. Aliasing can also occur in color flow mapping; velocities above the threshold will appear as the opposite color. Areas of high turbulence or acceleration may appear green.

Pathology

Valvular Assessment. In the hemodynamically unstable patient, point-of-care echocardiography can raise suspicion of valvular lesions, especially in patients with new murmurs. Substantial calcifications, vegetations, or reduced valve motion may be noticed by experienced sonologists. However, the evaluation of stable murmurs or mechanical/prosthetic valves requires expert levels of training and is out of the scope of most point-of-care sonologists.

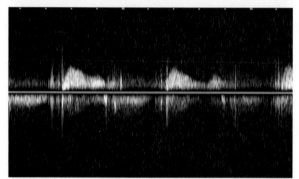

Fig. 9.21 Continuous wave doppler. Continuous wave Doppler tracing over a normal mitral valve.

Stenosis or regurgitation. Visual inspection focused on excursion (ability to open), coaptation (ability to close), and any abnormal masses should occur in all standard cardiac views.

Abnormal coaptation, or flail, can be indicative of regurgitation and can be further evaluated in AP4 (mitral valve) or A5C (aortic valve) using color flow mapping. The assessment of regurgitation severity can be difficult, because it depends on the size of the regurgitant orifice, the length of time the orifice is open, the pressure difference across the valve, and the distensibility of the chambers involved. The severity of mitral regurgitation (MR) can be estimated by obtaining an AP4 view, placing color over the MV and the whole LA, and evaluating the area of the regurgitant jet in the LA. Severe MR is usually holosystolic, is >40% of the total LA area, and may demonstrate eccentric (swirling) jets (see Fig. 9.23). The severity of aortic regurgitation (AR) can be measured by obtaining an A5C view, placing color over the aortic valve and LV, and determining the diameter of the regurgitant jet. Severe AR is indicated by a jet >65% of the LVOT diameter (Fig. 9.24). Appropriate evaluation of AR/MR requires an image with the valve perpendicular to the beam. The severity of MR/AR will be underestimated if the beam is tangential to the valve.

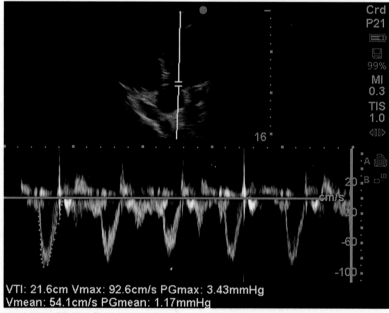

Fig. 9.22 Pulsed wave doppler. Pulsed wave Doppler used to obtain the velocity time integral (*VTI*) across the aortic valve from the apical window.

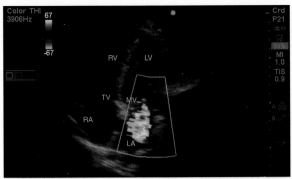

Fig. 9.23 Color flow mapping. Color flow mapping demonstrating mitral regurgitation. *LA,* left atrium; *LV,* left ventricle; *MV,* mitral valve; *RA,* right atrium; *RV,* right ventricle; *TV,* tricuspid valve.

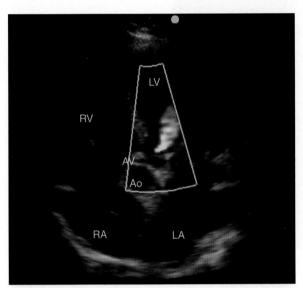

Fig. 9.24 Aortic regurgitation. Color flow mapping demonstrating aortic regurgitation. *Ao,* aorta; *AV,* aortic valve; *LA,* left atrium; *LV,* left ventricle; *RA,* right atrium; *RV,* right ventricle.

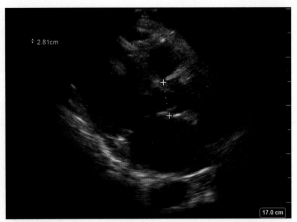

Fig. 9.25 Cardiac output. The cross-sectional area (CSA) of the LVOT is estimated by obtaining the diameter in a parasternal long view, where the aortic cusps meet the septal wall and the mitral valve. Most ultrasound machines calculate the CSA by assuming $CSA = \pi r^2$. Stroke volume = CSA × VTI and Cardiac output = heart rate × stroke volume.

Cardiac output. Cardiac output is the product of stroke volume (SV) and heart rate (HR). Stroke volume may be determined by multiplying the velocity time integral (VTI) of continuous wave Doppler across the LVOT by the cross-sectional area of the LVOT (Fig. 9.25).

Wall Motion Abnormality. In addition to evaluating for global contractility, as discussed in the "Basic Echocardiography" section, marked focal wall motion abnormalities may be detectable by experienced point-of-care sonologists. Ischemia or infarction inhibits the normal contraction of the heart in a predictable fashion, and these changes in contraction may be visualized sonographically. Acute coronary syndrome involves asymmetric occlusion of the coronary vessels, leading to decreased function of the myocardium perfused by the occluded vessel and leading to a regional wall motion abnormality (RWMA). Assessment for RWMA uses the four standard cardiac views.

The LV is the ideal chamber to evaluate RWMA, as it is supplied by all three of the major coronary vessels: the left anterior descending artery (LAD) supplies the anterior wall, distal septum, and apex; the circumflex artery (CRX) supplies the posterior and lateral wall; and the right coronary artery (RCA) supplies the inferior wall and proximal septum. These regions can be differentiated in the PSL, PSS, and AP4 views (Fig. 9.26). The sonologist should evaluate the heart in multiple views to accurately localize an RWMA. In comprehensive echocardiography, shortening of the cardiac walls during contraction is graded as follows: normal (>30%), hypokinetic (10%–30%), akinetic (<10%), and dyskinetic (ballooning during systole). Practically, the point-of-care sonologist will obtain a general gestalt to augment the clinical history and other objective data to make the best management decisions in consultation with cardiology. The difference between acute (ischemia) and chronic (scarring) RWMA cannot be discerned at the bedside, so prior cardiac history must be considered when interpreting RWMA.

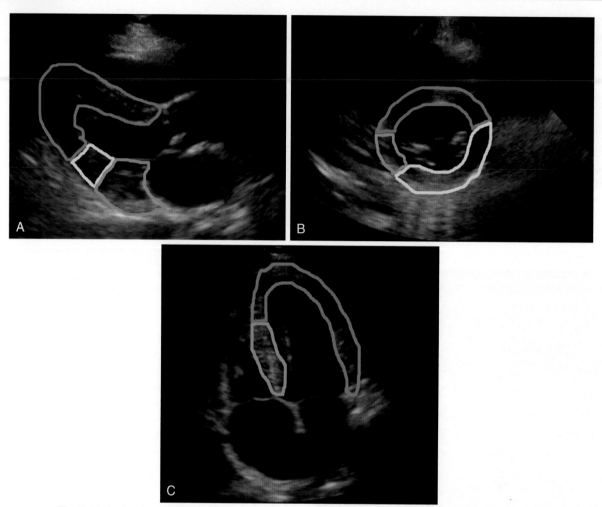

Fig. 9.26 Regional wall motion abnormality. The red region indicates the left anterior descending coronary artery territory (anterior circulation); the green region represents the posterior descending artery territory from the right coronary artery and the left circumflex artery (lateral circulation); and the yellow region represents the left circumflex artery territory (inferior circulation) in (A) parasternal long, (B) parasternal short, and (C) apical four-chamber views.

Tricuspid Annular Plane Systolic Excursion. Tricuspid annular plane systolic excursion (TAPSE) provides an objective measure of RV function. It is one of several objective measurements of RV systolic function that is relatively simple and quick for experienced sonographers to perform and is easily reproducible. Recently, point-of-care TAPSE has been used as an objective measure of RV strain (in addition to the subjective measures described in the "Basic Echocardiography" section) to identify high-risk PE patients.

TAPSE is obtained with an adequate AP4 view, passing an M-mode cursor through the tricuspid lateral annulus and measuring the longitudinal displacement of the annulus during peak systole (Fig. 9.27). As RV function diminishes, the annular displacement decreases. The normal range of TAPSE is unclear and may vary with gender, age, and body surface area. However, a TAPSE less than 16 mm is associated with RV strain and poor outcomes.

TAPSE is only a single measure of RV function and should not be used in isolation. Similar to other measures of RV function, TAPSE will be diminished by conditions that cause increased afterload, such as pulmonary hypertension or severe COPD. TAPSE also

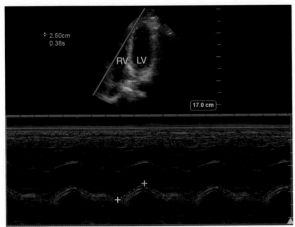

Fig. 9.27 Tricuspid annular plane systolic excursion. TAPSE is measured by passing an M-mode cursor through the tricuspid lateral annulus and measuring the longitudinal displacement of the annulus during peak systole. *LV,* left ventricle; *RV,* right ventricle.

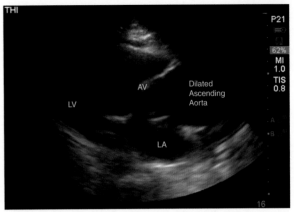

Fig. 9.28 Thoracic aortic dilation. A parasternal long axis view demonstrating ascending aortic dilation. *AV,* aortic valve; *LA,* left atrium; *LV,* left ventricle.

assumes uniform RV contractility and may be inaccurate with RWMA. When performing TAPSE, it is important that an adequate AP4 view be obtained, because a foreshortened view will result in an artificially lower TAPSE measurement. TAPSE can also be falsely augmented by cardiac motion such as a hyperdynamic LV.

Aortic Arch Assessment. The suprasternal notch window allows for visualization of the ascending aorta, aortic arch, and origin of the three brachiocephalic vessels. Although this view is often difficult to obtain, confirmation of aortic dilation, aneurysm, or dissection is possible with an adequate window. The aortic root may be visualized in this view but is usually better visualized in the PSL view, where a cross-section of the descending thoracic aorta is also usually seen posterior to the LV (Fig. 9.28). The aortic root and ascending thoracic aorta are considered dilated at 4 to 5 cm and aneurysmal above 5 cm.

BIBLIOGRAPHY

Burrows B, Kettel LJ, Niden AH, Rabinowitz M, Diener CF. Patterns of cardiovascular dysfunction in chronic obstructive lung disease. *N Engl J Med.* 1972;286(17):912–918.

Dipti A, Soucy Z, Surana A, Chandra S. Role of inferior vena cava diameter in assessment of volume status: a meta-analysis. *Am J Emerg Med.* 2012;30(8):1414–1419.

Dresden S, Mitchell P, Rahimi L, et al. Right ventricular dilatation on bedside echocardiography performed by emergency physicians aids in the diagnosis of pulmonary embolism. *Ann Emerg Med.* 2014;63(1):16–24.

Grifoni S, Olivotto I, Cecchini P, et al. Short-term clinical outcome of patients with acute pulmonary embolism, normal blood pressure, and echocardiographic right ventricular dysfunction. *Circulation.* 2000;101(24):2817–2822.

Henry WL, DeMaria A, Gramiak R, et al. Report of the American Society of Echocardiography committee on nomenclature and standards in two-dimensional echocardiography. *Circulation.* 1980;62(2):212–217.

Horowitz RS, Morganroth J, Parrotto C, Chen CC, Soffer J, Pauletto FJ. Immediate diagnosis of acute myocardial infarction by two-dimensional echocardiography. *Circulation.* 1982;65(2):323–329.

Labovitz AJ, Noble VE, Bierig M, et al. Focused cardiac ultrasound in the emergent setting: a consensus statement of the American Society of Echocardiography and American College of Emergency Physicians. *J Am Soc Echocardiogr.* 2010;23(12):1225–1230.

Lobo JL, Holley A, Tapson V, PROTECT and RIETE investigators, et al. Prognostic significance of tricuspid annular displacement in normotensive patients with acute symptomatic pulmonary embolism. *J Thromb Haemost.* 2014;12(7):1020–1027.

Mark DG, Ku BS, Carr BG, et al. Directed bedside transthoracic echocardiography: preferred cardiac window for left ventricular ejection fraction estimation in critically ill patients. *Am J Emerg Med.* 2007;25(8):894–900.

McConnell MV, Solomon SD, Rayan ME, Come PC, Goldhaber SZ, Lee RT. Regional right ventricular dysfunction detected by echocardiography in acute pulmonary embolism. *Am J Cardiol.* 1996;78(4):469–473.

McKaigney CJ, Krantz MJ, La Rocque CL, Hurst ND, Buchanan MS, Kendall JL. E-point septal separation: a bedside tool for emergency physician assessment of left ventricular ejection fraction. *Am J Emerg Med.* 2014;32(6):493–497.

Moore CL, Rose GA, Tayal VS, Sullivan DM, Arrowood JA, Kline JA. Determination of left ventricular function by emergency physician echocardiography of hypotensive patients. *Acad Emerg Med.* 2002;9(3):186–193. Erratum in: *Acad Emerg Med* 2002;9(6):642.

Pruszczyk P, Goliszek S, Lichodziejewska B, et al. Prognostic value of echocardiography in normotensive patients with acute pulmonary embolism. *JACC Cardiovasc Imaging.* 2014;7(6):553–560.

Randazzo MR, Snoey ER, Levitt MA, Binder K. Accuracy of emergency physician assessment of left ventricular ejection fraction and central venous pressure using echocardiography. *Acad Emerg Med.* 2003;10(9):973–977.

Rudoni RR, Jackson RE, Godfrey GW, Bonfiglio AX, Hussey ME, Hauser AM. Use of two-dimensional echocardiography for the diagnosis of pulmonary embolus. *J Emerg Med.* 1998;16(1):5–8.

Rudski LG, Lai WW, Afilalo J, et al. Guidelines for the echocardiographic assessment of the right heart in adults: a report from the American Society of Echocardiography endorsed by the European Association of Echocardiography, a registered branch of the European Society of Cardiology, and the Canadian Society of Echocardiography. *J Am Soc Echocardiogr.* 2010;23(7):685–713.

Sabia P, Afrookteh A, Touchstone DA, Keller MW, Esquivel L, Kaul S. Value of regional wall motion abnormality in the emergency room diagnosis of acute myocardial infarction. A prospective study using two-dimensional echocardiography. *Circulation.* 1991;84(suppl 3):I85–92.

Schiavone WA, Ghumrawi BK, Catalano DR, et al. The use of echocardiography in the emergency management of nonpenetrating traumatic cardiac rupture. *Ann Emerg Med.* 1991;20(11):1248–1250.

Secko MA, Lazar JM, Salciccioli LA, Stone MB. Can junior emergency physicians use E-point septal separation to accurately estimate left ventricular function in acutely dyspneic patients? *Acad Emerg Med.* 2011;18(11):1223–1226.

Tamborini G, Pepi M, Galli CA, et al. Feasibility and accuracy of a routine echocardiographic assessment of right ventricular function. *Int J Cardiol.* 2007;115(1):86–89.

Taylor RA, Davis J, Liu R, Gupta V, Dziura J, Moore CL. Point-of-care focused cardiac ultrasound for prediction of pulmonary embolism adverse outcomes. *J Emerg Med.* 2013;45(3):392–399.

Vasan RS, Larson MG, Benjamin EJ, Levy D. Echocardiographic reference values for aortic root size: the Framingham Heart Study. *J Am Soc Echocardiogr.* 1995;8(6):793–800.

Zoghbi WA, Enriquez-Sarano M, Foster E, et al. American Society of Echocardiography. Recommendations for evaluation of the severity of native valvular regurgitation with two-dimensional and Doppler echocardiography. *J Am Soc Echocardiogr.* 2003;16(7):777–802.

10

Pediatric Transthoracic Echocardiography

Jay Yeh

CONSIDERATIONS WHEN PERFORMING A PEDIATRIC CARDIAC ULTRASOUND ASSESSMENT

An increasingly used clinical tool for pediatric cardiac assessment is transthoracic echocardiogram (TTE). TTE has the benefits of being noninvasive, portable, and effective in providing detailed anatomic, hemodynamic, and physiologic information about the pediatric heart. A pediatric cardiac ultrasound assessment has some distinctive features and considerations compared with TTE studies performed in adult patients. Pediatric patients are at risk for a wide spectrum of congenital heart defects and cardiac diseases that are unusual in adults. Certain TTE views are of added importance for pediatric assessment. In addition, tremendous patience and special techniques may be required for imaging uncooperative infants and young children. The aim of this section is to provide practical advice and recommendations to persons comfortable with imaging the adult heart but who may lack familiarity with pediatric heart disease.

Unique Differences between Pediatric and Adult Patients

The first noticeable difference in pediatric TTE is that the absolute sizes of cardiac structures are generally smaller. With normal hemodynamics, body size becomes the strongest determinant of the size of cardiovascular structures. All cardiovascular structures increase in size relative to somatic growth, a phenomenon known as *cardiovascular allometry*. Because of the wide range of sizes of pediatric patients, normative values based on body surface area (z-score values) are preferable.

Patience is required when dealing with uncooperative pediatric patients. The examination rooms should be nonthreatening and comfortable. Family members are encouraged to accompany patients during TTE studies. This avoids issues of separation anxiety in both the children and their parents. Providing entertainment and distractions for the pediatric patient is extremely helpful in obtaining a quality study.

Compared with adults, the incidence of heart disease and the types of cardiovascular disease in children are extremely different. In the United States, myocardial infarction is relatively common in adults, with over 700,000 episodes each year. Pediatric patients have a greatly lower incidence of acute myocardial infarction, with an estimated incidence of roughly 157 per year. Congenital heart disease (CHD) is much more commonly encountered in pediatric patients (Table 10.1). The overall incidence of CHD is estimated to be 8 per 1000 live births. The most common forms of CHD are septal defects, such as muscular ventricular septal defects (VSDs), perimembranous VSDs, and secundum atrial septal defects (ASDs) (2.7, 1, and 1 per 1000 births, respectively). The incidence for clinically severe conditions is

TABLE 10.1   Common Pediatric Cardiac Diseases to Consider Echocardiographic Evaluation in the Emergency Department

Congenital	Left heart obstruction—one of the most common reasons for heart failure presenting in the first month of life	Aortic stenosis (Fig. 10.4) Coarctation of the aorta (see Fig. 10.2) Mitral stenosis Shone's complex HLHS
	Cyanotic heart conditions	Tetralogy of Fallot (pulmonary atresia with VSD) Transposition of the great arteries Single ventricles (HLHS, DILV, PAIVS) Total anomalous pulmonary venous return
	Left-to-right shunts or septal defects	VSD (CHF usually develops at about 6 weeks) (see Fig. 10.3) Atrioventricular septal defects PDA (variable depending on size) ASD (CHF symptoms in years, maybe decades of life)
Noncongen-ital		Kawasaki's disease Various forms of cardiomyopathy Myocarditis and pericarditis

Etiology of Heart Failure in Pediatrics

Prenatal	Causes of hydrops fetalis (immune 10%–20% and nonimmune 80%–90%) Cardiovascular disorders represent about 20% of nonimmune hydrops fetalis • AV valve regurgitation (severe Ebstein's anomaly) • AVMs (vein of Galen) • Arrhythmia (SVT, atrial flutter, or severe bradycardia) • Various cardiomyopathies Chromosomal/genetic syndromes • T13, T18, T21, Turner's syndrome, Noonan's syndrome Fetal anemia • α-Thalassemia, parvovirus, fetal hemorrhage, G6PD deficiency Infection • Parvovirus, CMV, syphilis, coxsackie virus, rubella, toxoplasmosis, HSV, VZV, adenovirus, enterovirus, influenza, *Listeria* Thoracic abnormalities • CCAM, chylothorax, diaphragmatic hernia, mediastinal tumor, skeletal dysplasias Twinning • Twin-to-twin transfusion syndrome Tumors • Sacrococcygeal teratoma, hemangiomas, adrenal neuroblastoma, chorioangioma Miscellaneous • Cystic hygromas, inheritable disorders of metabolism (lysosomal storage diseases), maternal thyroid disease, congenital nephrotic syndrome
Newborns	Left-sided obstructive lesions • HLHS • Interrupted aortic arch • Coarctation of the aorta • Shone's complex • Critical aortic stenosis Critical pulmonary stenosis d-TGA PDA (left-to-right shunt)—preterm infants Obstructed TAPVR

TABLE 10.1 Common Pediatric Cardiac Diseases to Consider Echocardiographic Evaluation in the Emergency Department—cont'd

	Sepsis
	Birth asphyxia with myocardial ischemia
	Hypoglycemia
	Hypocalcemia
	Hypothyroidism
	Severe anemia
	Arrhythmias
	Myocarditis
	Cardiomyopathy
2–6 weeks	Left-to-right shunts predominate (due to decrease in pulmonary vascular resistance)
	VSDs
	AVSDs
	Others: PDA, AP window, unobstructed TAPVR, truncus arteriosus
Infants and toddlers	Typically present with failure to thrive
	Left-to-right shunts
	Less severe left-sided obstruction
	ALCAPA
	Cardiomyopathies/myocarditis
Adolescents	Typically present with exercise intolerance, dyspnea, and excessive fatigue
	Cardiomyopathy
	Aortic regurgitation
	Mitral regurgitation or stenosis
	Systemic or pulmonary hypertension
	Acquired heart disease
	Myocarditis, rheumatic, cardiotoxic drugs

ALCAPA, Anomalous left coronary artery from the pulmonary artery; *AP*, aortopulmonary; *AV*, atrioventricular; *AVM*, arteriovenous malformation; *AVSD*, atrioventricular septal defect; *CCAM*, congenital cystic adenomatoid malformation; *CHF*, congestive heart failure; *CMV*, cytomegalovirus; *DILV*, double inlet left ventricle; *d-TGA*, dextro-transposition of the great arteries; *HLHS*, Hypoplastic left heart syndrome; *HSV*, herpes simplex virus; *PAIVS*, pulmonary atresia with intact ventricular septum; *PDA*, patent ductus arteriosus; *SVT*, supraventricular tachycardia; *TAPVR*, total anomalous pulmonary venous return; *VSD*, ventricular septal defect; *VZV*, varicella zoster virus.

approximately 3 per 1000 births, and when including moderately serious conditions is 6 per 1000 births. The incidence of tetralogy of Fallot (the most common cyanotic form of CHD) is twice that of dextro-transposition of the great arteries (0.47 versus 0.23 per 1000 births).

Subcostal imaging is superior and often optimal for viewing cardiac structures in children (Table 10.2). This window normally provides detailed visualization of nearly the entire cardiac anatomy. The relatively large liver also acts as a helpful medium for imaging the heart from the subcostal position, similar to the concept of stand-off pads or gel pads. A well-performed subcostal sweep from the transverse to coronal planes can diagnose a majority of congenital heart defects. Visceral and cardiac situs can be quickly obtained. In most cases,

images from the subcostal position will focus on the inferior and superior venae cavae, the atrial septum, and the ventricles. The great arteries can also be assessed with the imaging plane angled anteriorly. Interrogation of the atrial septum for ASDs is best performed from the subcostal views. The pulmonary veins may also be visualized from subcostal imaging. Rapid evaluation for pericardial (Fig. 10.1) and pleural effusions (or ascites) can also be easily performed. For echocardiographic guidance of venous cannula placement (e.g., cannulation for extracorporeal life support), the subcostal imaging position is preferred, as it is away from sterile procedure sites and may even be performed underneath a sterile drape.

The suprasternal notch imaging position is of increased importance in pediatric patients. It is necessary for

TABLE 10.2	**Tips and Comments on Standard Pediatric Echocardiographic Views**
Subcostal	• Use the liver as a medium for imaging, moving lower into the abdomen and slightly away from the heart
	• Optimal imaging for visceral situs and segmental anatomy
	• Often the ideal angle for measuring VSD shunt flow
	• Optimal position for imaging the interatrial septum
	• Ideal position for Doppler interrogation of descending aorta flow
	• Routine position for evaluating effusions or ascites (see Fig. 10.1)
	• Often preferred for echocardiographic assistance during sterile procedures
Parasternal	• Complete sweep in short axis (with color) of interventricular septum is mandatory for ruling out VSDs (see Fig. 10.3)
	• Optimal imaging planes for assessing ventricular systolic function and hypertrophy (see Fig. 10.4)
	• Mandatory imaging plane for aortic valve morphology and visualizing the coronary arteries
	• Routine position for evaluating pericardial effusions (Fig. 10.5)
Apical	• Optimal imaging planes for AV valve interrogation
	• Optimal position for measuring TR maximum velocity
	• Additional imaging plane for assessing ventricular systolic function and hypertrophy
Suprasternal	• Left aortic arch is often easiest to image with transducer slightly on patient right and imaging plane angled left
	• Optimal imaging position for aortic arch obstruction (see Fig. 10.2)
High left parasternal	• Also known as the *ductal view*
	• Optimal imaging position to assess PDA anatomy
	• Also a helpful view for assessing juxtaductal coarctation of the aorta
Suprasternal or high parasternal coronal	• Also known as the *crab view*
	• Ideal view for assessment of pulmonary venous connections

AV, atrioventricular; *PDA,* patent ductus arteriosus; *TR,* tricuspid regurgitation; *VSD,* ventricular septal defect.

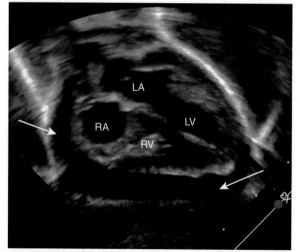

Fig. 10.1 Pericardial effusion. Subcostal coronal view. *Arrows* point to inferior and lateral pericardial effusion. *LA,* Left atrium; *LV,* left ventricle; *RA,* right atrium; *RV,* right ventricle.

assessing the aortic arch anatomy. In young children, this is also the most anxiety-provoking and fearful part of the TTE. Extension of the neck and having a few towels raising the upper back yields improved images. Evaluation for possible coarctation of the aorta is best performed in this position (Fig. 10.2). Aortic arch sidedness and vessel branching are also best obtained from suprasternal images. A patent ductus arteriosus can also be evaluated from suprasternal windows, though it is usually best visualized in a high left parasternal position (often referred to as a *ductal view*).

Similar to adults, the right parasternal view is optimal for assessing the proximal ascending aorta and spectral Doppler interrogation of left ventricular outflow tract stenosis. It is also a unique position for assessing the inferior and superior venae cavae connections to the right atrium, the upper interatrial septum, and the right upper pulmonary vein as it connects to the left atrium.

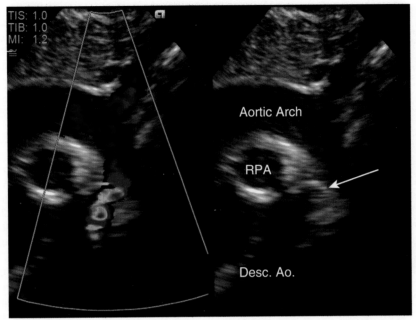

Fig. 10.2 Coarctation of the aorta. Long-axis view of the aortic arch from the suprasternal notch with color compare. Note the turbulent color flow at the site of coarctation. *Arrow* points to location of aortic coarctation. *Desc. Ao.,* Descending aorta; *RPA,* right pulmonary artery.

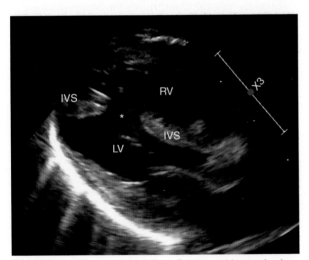

Fig. 10.3 Ventricular septal defect. Parasternal long-axis view. *Asterisk* at location of large ventricular septal defect. *IVS,* Interventricular septum; *LV,* left ventricle; *RV,* right ventricle.

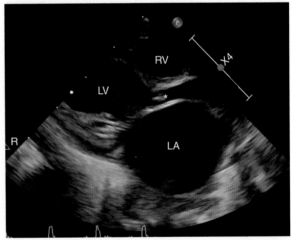

Fig. 10.4 Critical aortic valve stenosis. Parasternal long-axis view. Note the severely dilated left atrium and left ventricle. *Asterisk,* Small aortic valve; *LA,* left atrium; *LV,* left ventricle; *RV,* right ventricle.

In pediatric and adult patients, tricuspid valve regurgitation velocity is the most reliable echocardiographic surrogate for estimating right ventricular systolic pressure. The persons performing and interpreting pediatric TTE should understand the significant physiologic changes in transitions from fetal to newborn circulations. There may be a relatively high tricuspid regurgitation velocity in a newborn infant that should be considered normal. The presence of left-to-right cardiac shunts such as a large VSD (Fig. 10.3) or patent

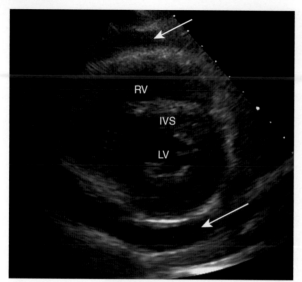

Fig. 10.5 Pericardial effusion. Parasternal short-axis view. *Arrows* point to anterior and posterior pericardial effusion. *IVS,* Interventricular septum; *LV,* left ventricle; *RV,* right ventricle.

ductus arteriosus may also lead to high tricuspid regurgitation velocities. In this setting, the high right ventricular systolic pressure is secondary to excess pulmonary blood flow and not necessarily due to abnormally high pulmonary vascular resistance.

BIBLIOGRAPHY

Hoffman JI, Kaplan S. The incidence of congenital heart disease. *J Am Coll Cardiol.* 2002;39:1890–1900.

Lai WW, Geva T, Shirali GS, et al. Guidelines and standards for performance of a pediatric echocardiogram: a report from the Task Force of the Pediatric Council of the American Society of Echocardiography. *J Am Soc Echocardiogr.* 2006;19:1413–1430.

Lopez L, Colan SD, Frommelt PC, et al. Recommendations for quantification methods during the performance of a pediatric echocardiogram: a report from the Pediatric Measurements Writing Group of the American Society of Echocardiography Pediatric and Congenital Heart Disease Council. *J Am Soc Echocardiogr.* 2010;23:465–495.

Mahle WT, Campbell RM, Favaloro-Sabatier J. Myocardial infarction in adolescents. *J Pediatr.* 2007;151(2):150–154.

Mozaffarian D, Benjamin EJ, Go AS, et al. Heart disease and stroke statistics—2015 update: a report from the American Heart Association. *Circulation.* 2015;131:e29–322.

Reller MD, Strickland MJ, Riehle-Colarusso T, Mahle WT, Correa A. Prevalence of congenital heart defects in metropolitan Atlanta, 1998-2005. *J Pediatr.* 2008;153(6):807–813.

Sluysmans T, Colan SD. Theoretical and empirical derivation of cardio- vascular allometric relationships in children. *J Appl Physiol.* 2005;99:445–457.

Yock PG, Popp RL. Noninvasive estimation of right ventricular systolic pressure by Doppler ultrasound in patients with tricuspid regurgitation. *Circulation.* 1984;70:657–662.

11

Focused Transesophageal Echocardiography

Orode Badakhsh, David Li

INTRODUCTION

Long considered to be a vital diagnostic tool utilized exclusively within the realm of cardiology, transesophageal echocardiography (TEE) is being used safely and effectively within the perioperative, critical care, and emergency room settings. Of particular importance is the ability to diagnose a vast array of diverse pathologies causing hemodynamic instability. In this capacity, a focused TEE examination has been proven to serve as an important adjunct to the history and physical examination to aid in the clinical decision-making process and to help guide treatment strategies.

COMPARING TEE TO TTE

The transducers utilized in transthoracic echocardiography (TTE) are typically single-plane phased array probes, requiring the sonographer to physically manipulate the probe to move from one view to the next. On the other hand, most TEE probes, and for the purposes of the discussion in this chapter, are multiplane phased array probes. Several thousand piezoelectric crystal elements are assembled in a matrix configuration (Fig. 11.1) and mounted to the distal tip of an endoscope. This arrangement allows a linear scan line to be created that can be electronically rotated from 0 toward 180 degrees using two buttons on the handle of the ultrasound probe (Fig. 11.2). As such, multiple views are able to be created without any physical probe manipulation. Rotating the scan line (also called the *omniplane angle*) in the direction of 180 degrees is termed *rotating forward*, whereas rotating back to 0 degrees is termed *rotating backward*. Physical probe manipulation can be performed by turning the large control wheel on the handle to anteflex (anteriorly) or retroflex (posteriorly) the probe. Furthermore, the tip of the probe can be flexed left or right by rotating the smaller control wheel. The shaft of the probe can be advanced, withdrawn, turned clockwise to image right-sided structures, or turned counterclockwise to image left-sided structures (Fig. 11.3).

The transducers used in TEE can generally operate at a higher frequency, as high as 8 MHz in some cases, compared with the typical 1 to 5 MHz of TTE probes. Although this leads to less depth of penetration, the overall resolution and image quality are better than TTE. Additionally, the TEE probe sits in the esophagus in close proximity to the heart, unlike in TTE, where the ultrasound waves must travel through multiple layers of tissue, ribs, and potentially aerated lung before reaching the heart.

Given the relative position of the esophagus to the heart, specific structures are better visualized with TEE compared with TTE. Anterior structures tend to be imaged better using TTE, and posterior structures tend to be better imaged using TEE. One caveat, however, is that the left atrium sits next to the TEE transducer. Because the ultrasound beam of a phased array probe starts at a narrower origin and fans out (just as it appears on the screen of the machine), the entire left atrium can generally not be visualized using TEE. However, the mitral valve (MV), aortic valve (AV), and left atrial appendage (LAA) are visualized well. TTE, on the other hand, provides better imaging of the left ventricular (LV) apex and more optimal Doppler alignment through both the aortic and tricuspid valves, allowing for more accurate calculations of cardiac output and right ventricular (RV) systolic pressures, respectively.

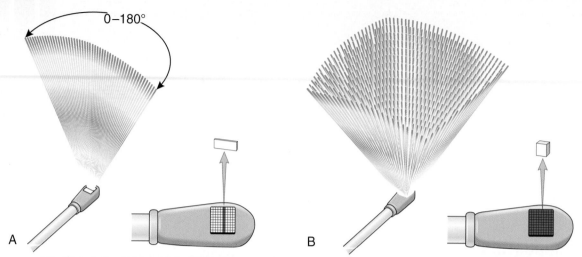

Fig. 11.1 At the distal tip of the TEE probe, several thousand piezoelectric crystal elements are arranged in a matrix configuration. The crystals can be sequentially activated to create a linear scan line depicted in red (A) that can be rotated 0 to 180 degrees via the omniplane functionality of the probe. Alternatively, some probes can activate all of their crystal elements (B) to create a three-dimensional image.

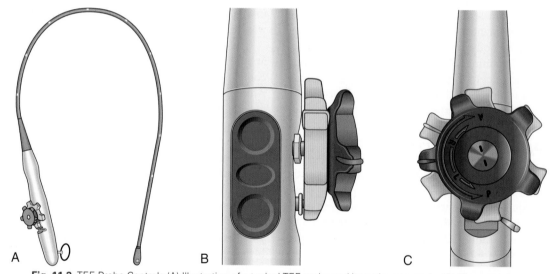

Fig. 11.2 TEE Probe Controls (A) Illustration of a typical TEE probe and its various controls. (B) The omniplane controls are depicted by the two circular buttons that rotate the angle either forward or back. (C) Furthermore, the probe can be anteflexed or retroflexed by the large internal control wheel (*cream wheel*) or turned left or right with the small external control wheel (*dark gray wheel*).

A standard nomenclature is used to name all of the TEE views that varies slightly from the TTE nomenclature. The first portion of the naming format refers to the transducer location (upper esophageal, midesophageal, transgastric). This is followed by the primary anatomic structure of interest and then the imaging plane (short axis versus long axis). For instance, the midesophageal

aortic valve short axis (TEE) corresponds to the parasternal aortic valve short axis (TTE).

Although TTE remains a powerful diagnostic tool in the assessment of critically ill patients, it has several limitations. Unlike TEE, TTE is dependent on patient positioning and body habitus and is difficult in patients with emphysematous lung disease. Imaging can also be

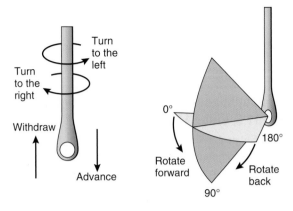

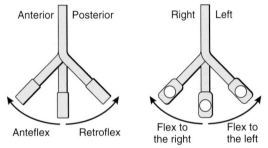

Fig. 11.3 Probe Manipulation This image depicts the various probe manipulation maneuvers. (Redrawn with permission from Shanewise JS, Cheung AT, Aronson S, et al. ASE/SCA guidelines for performing a comprehensive intraoperative multiplane transesophageal echocardiography examination: recommendations of the American Society of Echocardiography Council for Intraoperative Echocardiography and the Society of Cardiovascular Anesthesiologists. *Anesth Analg.* 1999;89(4):870–884, Fig. 1.)

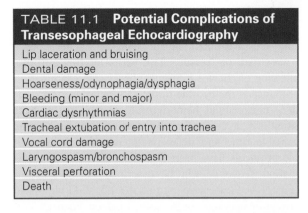

TABLE 11.1 Potential Complications of Transesophageal Echocardiography
Lip laceration and bruising
Dental damage
Hoarseness/odynophagia/dysphagia
Bleeding (minor and major)
Cardiac dysrhythmias
Tracheal extubation or entry into trachea
Vocal cord damage
Laryngospasm/bronchospasm
Visceral perforation
Death

TABLE 11.2 Contraindications to Transesophageal Echocardiography	
Absolute	**Relative**
Patient refusal	Hiatal hernia
History of esophagectomy	Cervical spine instability
Significant esophageal pathology/injury	Esophageal varices
Perforation	Barret's esophagus/peptic ulcer disease/esophagitis
Tumor	Unilateral vocal cord paralysis
Diverticulum	History of bariatric surgery more than 6 months
Scleroderma	Dysphagia
Tracheoesophageal fistula	Coagulopathy/thrombocytopenia
Stricture	Thoracoabdominal aortic aneurysm
Esophageal webs	
Active bleeding	
Recent upper gastrointestinal surgery within the last 6 months	

difficult in patients with dressings or chest tubes in place and also suboptimal in mechanically ventilated patients in the intensive care unit (ICU) compared with TEE. Conducting a TTE examination in patients undergoing cardiopulmonary resuscitation (CPR) is technically challenging. However, due to TEE's semiinvasive nature, it is generally not tolerated as well in awake patients. TEE remains an overall safe imaging modality, with an overall complication rate of 0.2% to 1.2% and a risk of injury leading to death of less than 0.01%.

Careful consideration must be given to the associated risks of TEE (Table 11.1), as well as the appropriate indications and contraindications to the placement of a TEE probe (Table 11.2). A TEE examination should only be performed in patients in whom a transthoracic examination is thought to be suboptimal and in whom the benefits are deemed to outweigh the overall risks of probe placement.

THE TEE EXAMINATION

Multiple medical societies encourage the use of ultrasound and have created various position papers regarding both the training requirements and educational curricula needed to achieve proficiency. Moreover, many of these societies advocate for focused or goal-directed examination protocols to help physicians make time-sensitive, potentially lifesaving clinical decisions.

Focused, or "rescue," TEE exists for this purpose, allowing physicians to use an abbreviated examination sequence at the bedside in patients suffering from sudden, unexplained hemodynamic instability. In these situations, a comprehensive examination may waste valuable time and delay treatment. Although multiple protocols have been described, an 11-view examination sequence will be described in this chapter (Fig. 11.4). Please keep in mind that not all 11 views will always be necessary or be easily obtained. Focused TEE emphasizes speed and efficiency by using a qualitative and dichotomous approach. Usually, a diagnosis can be elucidated with a select number of views. One must keep in mind that due to anatomic variations from patient to patient and the potential for pathology to distort cardiac anatomy, the described approaches for obtaining the views as they relate to both imaging depth and omniplane angle can vary considerably.

Great care must be given during both probe placement and manipulation. Before placement, the oral cavity should be inspected for signs of obvious dental damage or previous injury. A dental guard should always be used to minimize the risk of dental trauma and probe damage. The probe control lock should always be in a neutral position and never engaged during probe placement or manipulation, although slight anteflexion of the tip with the control wheel may be helpful during insertion. A generous amount of lubrication should be applied to the probe before placement in the oropharynx. The probe should never be forced if met with resistance. Gently lifting the mandible anteriorly may be helpful in placement, as is occasionally either neck flexion or extension. Direct laryngoscopy may also be used. The exam should be performed in a manner that minimizes overall probe manipulation, including minimizing the number of times the probe is advanced and withdrawn.

When performing an examination, a few basic rules optimize image quality. First, the focal zone should be set at or slightly above the anatomic structure of interest. The resolution will be the highest in this zone. Furthermore, the depth should also consider the structure of interest so as to further enhance resolution and detail. The greater the depth, the lower the overall resolution. To image deeper structures, the frequency may need to be decreased. Finally, the gain is the amplification of the ultrasound signal and should be set in a manner to improve contrast between fluid and tissues.

TEE VIEWS

Midesophageal Four-Chamber View (ME 4C) (Fig. 11.5, Video 11.1)

The TEE probe should be advanced into the esophagus approximately 30 to 40 cm. The omniplane angle should be set to between 0 and 20 degrees. Often, some slight retroflexion of the probe may help to develop the view to open all four chambers. This is due to the LV apex being positioned slightly inferiorly and laterally relative to the base of the heart. In the adult chest, the imaging depth should initially be set to about 16 cm to ensure the entirety of the heart is visualized. If the AV and left ventricular outflow tract (LVOT) are still visible (informally called a *five-chamber view*), the probe should be advanced slightly into the esophagus until the LVOT disappears, only the four chambers are visible, and the annulus of the tricuspid valve is maximized.

The right heart will appear on the left side of the screen, and the left heart will appear on the right. Both the atria will be at the top of the screen closest to the TEE probe separated by the interatrial septum. The ventricles reside on the bottom of the screen separated by the interventricular septum. The tricuspid and MVs are visible on the left and right, respectively. Furthermore, the anterolateral and inferoseptal walls of the left ventricle appear in this view.

Midesophageal Two-Chamber View (ME 2C) (Fig. 11.6, Video 11.2)

With only minor physical manipulation of the probe, the omniplane angle should be rotated forward to between 80 and 100 degrees. The left atrium (top) and left ventricle (bottom) will both be visible. The anterior and inferior walls of the left ventricle will appear on the right and left of the screen, respectively. The left atrial appendage will be visible and can be assessed for clots.

Midesophageal Long-Axis View (ME LAX) (Fig. 11.7, Video 11.3)

The omniplane angle is further rotated from the ME 2C view to between 120 and 160 degrees. Again, both the left atrium and left ventricle are visible. The MV resides

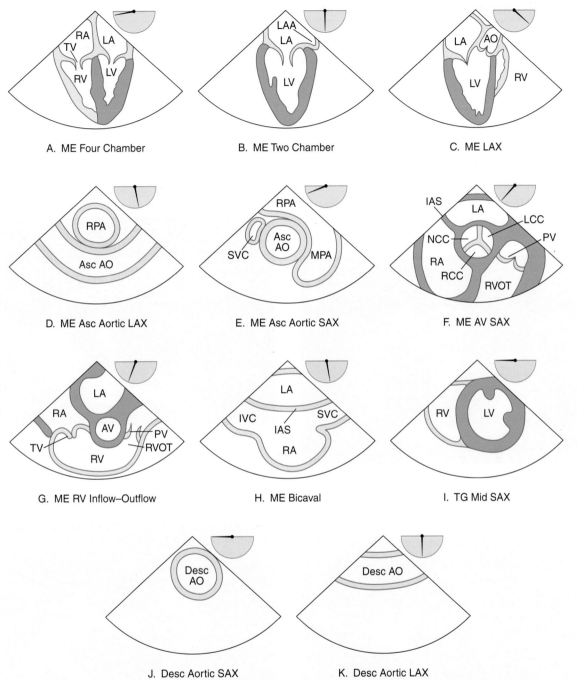

Fig. 11.4 TEE Views (A–K) This is a depiction of the 11 cross-sectional views endorsed by the American Society of Echocardiography (ASE) and Society of Cardiovascular Anesthesiologists (SCA) as part of a basic perioperative transesophageal echocardiography examination. *Asc*, ascending; *AV*, aortic valve; *Desc*, descending; *LAX*, long axis; *ME*, midesophageal; *SAX*, short axis; *TG*, transgastric; *RA*, right atrium; *LA*, left atrium, *RV*, right ventricle; *LV*, left ventricle; *TV*, tricuspid valve; *MV*, *LAA*, left atrial appendage; *AO*, aorta; *RPA*, right pulmonary artery; *Asc AO*, ascending aorta; *SVC*, superior vena cava; *MPA*, main pulmonary arty; *IAS*, interatrial septum; *RVOT*, right ventricular outflow tract; *PV*, pulmonic valve; *LCC*, left coronary cusp; *RCC*, right coronary cusp; *NCC*, non-coronary cusp; *AV*, aortic valve; *IVC*, inferior vena cava; *Desc AO*, descending aorta. (Redrawn with permission from Reeves ST, Finley AC, Skubas NJ, et al., Basic perioperative transesophageal echocardiography examination: a consensus statement of the American Society of Echocardiography and the Society of Cardiovascular Anesthesiologists. *J Am Soc Echocardiogr.* 2013;26(5):443–446.)

on the left side of the screen, and the long axis of the AV can be visualized on the right side of the screen at the distal end of the LVOT as it opens to the proximal ascending aorta. The anteroseptal wall separates the left ventricle from the RV outflow tract. The inferolateral wall of the left ventricle is visible on the left side of the screen.

Midesophageal Bicaval View (ME Bicaval) (Fig. 11.8, Video 11.4)

From the ME LAX view, the shaft of the probe should be turned clockwise and the omniplane angle rotated backward to between 80 and 110 degrees. The depth should be decreased to maximize visualization of all the relevant structures.

The superior vena cava (SVC) will appear on the right side of the screen, and the inferior vena cava (IVC) will appear on the left. The interatrial septum can be visualized separating the left atrium (top of screen) from the right atrium (bottom of screen) and consists of a thinner region termed the *fossa ovalis* flanked by thicker limbus regions both anteriorly and inferiorly. Assessments for the presence

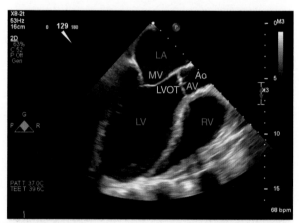

Fig. 11.7 Midesophageal Long-Axis View ME LAX view displaying the left atrium (*LA*), mitral valve (*MV*), left ventricle (*LV*), and right ventricle (*RV*). Additional significant structures include the left ventricular outflow tract (*LVOT*), aortic valve (*AV*), and proximal ascending aorta (*Ao*).

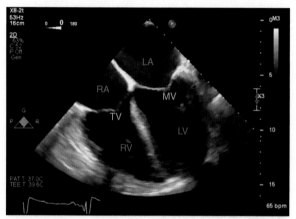

Fig. 11.5 Midesophageal Four-Chamber View ME 4C view depicting the left atrium (*LA*), right atrium (*RA*), left ventricle (*LV*), and right ventricle (*RV*). Additionally, the tricuspid valve (*TV*) and mitral valve (*MV*) are visualized.

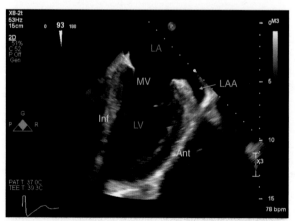

Fig. 11.6 Midesophageal Two-Chamber View ME 2C view displaying the left atrium (*LA*), mitral valve (*MV*), left ventricle (*LV*), and left atrial appendage (*LAA*). Also visible are the anterior (*Ant*) and inferior (*Inf*) walls of the LV.

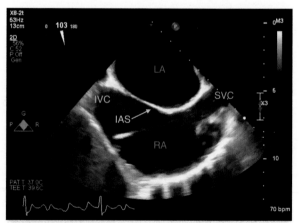

Fig. 11.8 Midesophageal Bicaval View ME bicaval view displaying the left atrium (*LA*), interatrial septum (*IAS*), and right atrium (*RA*). Additionally, the superior vena cava (*SVC*) can be seen entering from the right side of the screen and the inferior vena cava (*IVC*) from the left.

of a patent foramen ovale or interatrial shunt should be made utilizing color flow Doppler (CFD) with the Nyquist limit decreased to detect lower-velocity blood. Occasionally, a eustachian valve and crista terminalis are visible at the inlets of the IVC and SVC, respectively. These normal anatomic variants are embryologic remnants and appear as a fluttering flap, not to be confused with a vegetation.

Midesophageal Right Ventricular Inflow–Outflow View (ME RV Inflow–Outflow) (Fig. 11.9, Video 11.5)

Without moving the probe, the omniplane angle should be decreased even farther to approximately 50 and 90 degrees. The valve on the left is the tricuspid valve as blood inflows into the right ventricle. Toward the right of the screen, the long axis of the pulmonic valve appears and serves as the outflow of blood from the right ventricle, hence the name of this view. Although, the aortic valve short axis often can be visualized in this view, emphasis should be placed on identifying both the pulmonic and tricuspid valves. The left atrium appears as the chamber closest to the probe near the top of the screen.

Midesophageal Aortic Valve Short-Axis View (ME AV SAX) (Fig. 11.10, Video 11.6)

Decreasing the omniplane angle from the RV inflow–outflow view to between 30 and 60 degrees will help to visualize all three leaflets of the AV in short axis.

Typically, this involves only a slight decrease in the omniplane angle, if at all. Not uncommonly, all three valves can be seen in the same view. Furthermore, the same chambers as in the ME RV inflow–outflow view are also visible.

Midesophageal Ascending Aortic Short-Axis View (ME Asc Ao SAX) (Fig. 11.11, Video 11.7)

From the ME 4C view, the probe should be withdrawn until a "five-chamber view" develops. The LVOT and the AV should be centered. The probe should be withdrawn slightly farther (approximately 30–35 cm), and with some slight anteflexion, the view will develop.

The vascular structure in the middle of the view is the short axis of the aorta and may appear pulsatile. To the left of the aorta is the short axis of the SVC. To the right of the aorta in this view, the main pulmonary artery (PA) can be visualized as it divides into the left and right branches. The right PA branches off the main and progresses to the left side of the screen, whereas the left PA is often difficult to visualize due to the interposition of the left mainstem bronchus between the left PA and the esophagus.

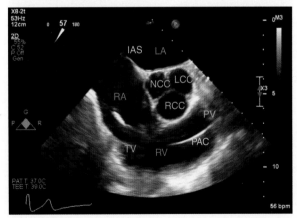

Fig. 11.10 Midesophageal Aortic Valve Short-Axis View ME AV SAX view displaying the aortic valve. Although this view differs only slightly from the ME RV inflow–outflow view, the primary anatomic area of interest is the aortic valve and the individual leaflet cusps that comprise it. The left coronary cusp (*LCC*), right coronary cusp (*RCC*), and noncoronary cusp (*NCC*) should all be visible. Also visible are the left atrium (*LA*), right atrium (*RA*), right ventricle (*RV*), tricuspid valve (*TV*), occasionally the pulmonic valve (*PV*), and the interatrial septum (*IAS*). Please note that a pulmonary artery catheter (PAC) depicted by a hyperechoic line is also visible in this view entering and exiting the RV.

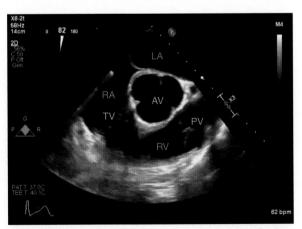

Fig. 11.9 Midesophageal Right Ventricular Inflow-Outflow View ME RV inflow–outflow view displaying RV inflow from the right atrium (*RA*) through the tricuspid valve (*TV*) to the right ventricle (*RV*) and RV outflow from the RV through the pulmonic valve (*PV*) to the main pulmonary artery. The left atrium (*LA*) and aortic valve (*AV*) are also visible in this view.

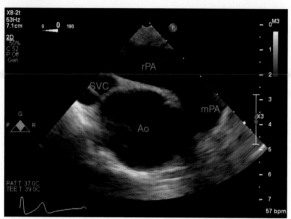

Fig. 11.11 Midesophageal Aortic Valve Short-Axis View ME Asc Ao SAX view displaying the superior vena cava (*SVC*) in short axis, ascending aorta (*Ao*) in short axis, main pulmonary artery (*mPA*), and right pulmonary artery (*rPA*). Note: Artifact from PA catheter can be seen in the ascending aorta.

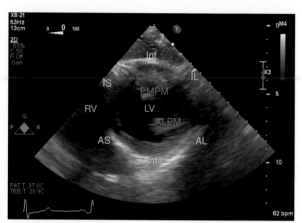

Fig. 11.13 Transgastric Midpapillary Short-Axis View TG Mid SAX view displaying the right ventricle (*RV*), left ventricle (*LV*), and its six segments: the anterior (*Ant*), anteroseptal (*AS*), inferoseptal (*IS*), inferior (*Inf*), inferolateral (*IL*), and anterolateral (*AL*) walls. The anterolateral and posteromedial papillary muscles (*ALPM* and *PMPM*, respectively) are also visible.

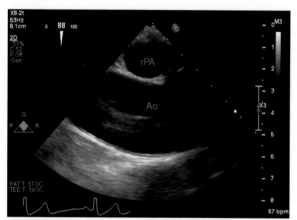

Fig. 11.12 Midesophageal Aortic Valve Long-Axis View ME Asc Ao LAX view displaying the right pulmonary artery (*rPA*) in short axis and ascending aorta (*Ao*) in long axis. Note: Artifact from PA catheter can be seen in the ascending aorta.

Midesophageal Ascending Aortic Long-Axis View (ME Asc Ao LAX) (Fig. 11.12, Video 11.8)

This view is obtained by simply rotating the omniplane angle forward to approximately 100 to 150 degrees from the ascending aortic short-axis view. In the near field at the top of the screen, the short axis of the right PA becomes visible, and distal to that resides the long axis of the aorta.

Transgastric Midpapillary Short-Axis View (TG Midpap SAX) (Fig. 11.13, Video 11.9)

From the ME 4C view, the probe should be advanced to an approximate depth of 40 to 45 centimeters and then slightly anteflexed at an omniplane angle of 0 to 20 degrees until both papillary muscles are visible and the circular symmetry of the left ventricle is optimized. The imaging depth should be decreased to maximize the size of the left ventricle.

Both the left and right ventricles are depicted in this view. Furthermore, the transgastric short axis is the only view that allows for assessment of LV segmental wall motion as it correlates to the distribution of all three coronary arteries in a single plane. Both the posteromedial and anterolateral papillary muscles are visible.

Descending Aortic Short-Axis View (Desc Ao SAX) (Fig. 11.14, Video 11.10)

Withdraw the probe back to the ME 4C view and rotate the shaft of the probe 180 degrees until the descending aorta comes into view. The depth should be decreased to approximately 6 to 8 cm to maximize the size of the aorta. The probe should be advanced and withdrawn to scan as much of the descending aorta as possible starting from the proximal descending arch. The short axis of the aorta is visualized and should appear circular.

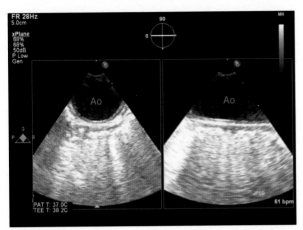

Fig. 11.14 Descending Aortic Short-Axis View On the left half of the screen, the aorta (*Ao*) is depicted in its short axis and the long axis on the right.

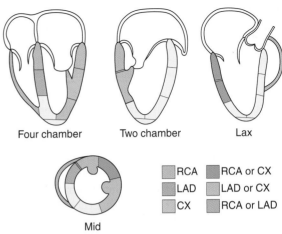

Fig. 11.15 Coronary Artery Distribution This figure depicts the typical distribution of the coronary arteries as they relate to the various segments of the heart. *CX,* Circumflex; *LAD,* left anterior descending; *RCA,* right coronary artery. (Redrawn with permission from Lang RM, Badano LP, Mor-Avi V, et al. Chamber Quantification Writing Group; American Society of Echocardiography's Guidelines and Standards Committee; European Association of Echocardiography. Recommendations for chamber quantification: a report from the American Society of Echocardiography's Guidelines and Standards Committee and the Chamber Quantification Writing Group, developed in conjunction with the European Association of Echocardiography, a branch of the European Society of Cardiology. *J Am Soc Echocardiogr.* 2005;18:1440–1463, Fig. 9.)

Descending Aortic Long-Axis View (Desc Ao LAX) (see Fig. 11.14, Video 11.10)

From the short axis of the aorta, the omniplane angle should be increased to approximately 90 to 110 degrees. The aorta is now visualized in its long axis, with blood flowing proximally from the right side of the screen distally to the left.

PATHOLOGIES

Left Ventricular Dysfunction and Myocardial Ischemia (Video 11.11)

Left Ventricular wall motion can be assessed in multiple views, including those in the midesophagus. However, the transgastric midpapillary short-axis view is arguably the single best view to do so. The advantage of this view over others rests in the ability to simultaneously visualize all the myocardial walls with respect to the distribution of all three coronary arteries in a single plane: the left anterior descending (LAD), the left circumflex (LCX), and the right coronary artery (RCA) (Fig. 11.15). Although only 6 LV segments are visualized in this view, the prognostic value is similar to that of assessing all 17 segments.

Special attention must be paid to the wall motion of each individual segment. Reduced, absent, and/or paradoxical motion may be indicative of LV ischemia or failure. It must be noted, however, that echocardiography can overestimate wall motion in some patients with segmental wall motion abnormalities. This is due to the

wall motion of normal segments affecting the motion of adjacent failing or ischemic segments. Therefore it is important to assess both systolic wall thickening (endocardial thickening) and wall motion.

Right Ventricular Dysfunction

Multiple methodologies exist for the quantification of RV function; however in the context of the unstable patient, the most feasible approach is still a visual or qualitative one. One must consider the potential for both ischemic changes and scenarios in which there are either acute or chronic increases in RV afterload. The right ventricle is less capable of compensating for such changes than the more muscular left ventricle.

Assessment of RV function most frequently occurs in the ME 4C view. Due to a greater number of longitudinal muscle fibers, the right ventricle tends to move up and down in this view, as opposed to inwards like the left ventricle. As such, one must pay attention to the distance the lateral annulus of the tricuspid valve travels from the annular base at end diastole toward the RV apex in systole, formally termed the *tricuspid annular plane systolic excursion* (TAPSE). Excursion of less than 16 mm may be indicative of RV dysfunction. Another echocardiographic sign of RV dysfunction is assessment of tricuspid regurgitation, as both increases in pressure and annular dilatation can increase regurgitation occurrence and severity.

Although pericardial effusions can affect both the left and right heart, the right heart is much more susceptible to tamponade. Its chambers generally have lower baseline pressures than those on the left, rendering them more sensitive to external pressure. Echocardiographic evidence of cardiac tamponade includes a collapsed right atrium, RV end-diastolic collapse, dilatation of the IVC, and a potentially underfilled left ventricle, leading to compromised stroke volume and hypotension. The ME 4C view can assist in determining if there is evidence of right atrial or ventricular compression (Video 11.12). The transgastric midpapillary short axis can aid in determining the location of the effusion (Video 11.13). Pericardial fluid will appear between the heart and pericardium as black or echolucent. Pericardial effusions are graded as small (<0.5 cm), moderate (0.5–2.0 cm), and large (>2.0 cm).

Although not the gold standard for the diagnosis of pulmonary embolism (PE), TEE has a relatively high diagnostic sensitivity and specificity so long as a PE is acute and central. Although there may sometimes be echocardiographic evidence of echogenic embolic phenomenon either in the right atrium or ventricle on the ME 4C view or midesophageal RV inflow–outflow view, the most useful views for the visualization of a PE in the pulmonary vascular tree are the midesophageal ascending short- and long-axis views (Videos 11.14–11.16). Unfortunately, visualization remains limited to areas of the main pulmonary and proximal right pulmonary arteries. Visualization of a clot can prove difficult in the left PA, due to the interposition of the left mainstem bronchus between the probe and the artery itself. Aside from visualization of a discrete clot, secondary echocardiographic findings of PE include RV dilatation, tricuspid regurgitation, and RV systolic dysfunction with resultant motion abnormalities of the RV free wall. Furthermore, there may also be evidence of leftward deviation of the interatrial or interventricular septa. In the absence of echocardiographic embolic evidence, it is important to keep in mind that PE cannot be

completely ruled out if clinical suspicion remains high. As such, more distal clots may not be easily detected, and the patient should be referred to computed tomography (CT) in such cases.

Valvular Abnormalities

Aortic Stenosis. Visual inspection of AV leaflet morphology should be made within the midesophageal long-axis view. The valve may appear heavily calcified, and its leaflets may display severely restricted mobility (Videos 11.17 and 11.18). Assessing AV mobility, however, may be difficult in patients with severely compromised LV systolic function, as the LV may not be able to generate a sufficient gradient to adequately open the AV leaflets. In addition to assessing leaflet motion, CFD may display evidence of flow acceleration distal to the AV (Video 11.19).

The severity of aortic stenosis can be quantified utilizing continuous wave Doppler to generate a transvalvular pressure gradient (Fig. 11.16). This is ideally performed in the deep transgastric long-axis view, which allows for optimal alignment of the Doppler beam in parallel with blood flow through the AV. It is obtained by advancing the probe even farther than with the transgastric midpapillary short-axis view, usually to between 45 and 50 cm, until the LV disappears. The probe tip is then anteflexed until the LV apex comes into view near the top of the screen and one is looking back toward the base of

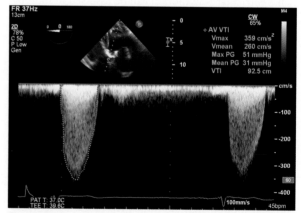

Fig. 11.16 Deep Transgastric Long-Axis View with Continuous Wave Doppler (CWD) In this view, the spectral Doppler beam (CWD) can be placed through the aortic valve to assess transvalvular pressure gradients to quantify the degree of severity of aortic stenosis.

the heart. The AV and aorta will appear near the middle of the screen, and the MV will appear to the right (Video 11.20). A pressure gradient of >40 mm Hg and peak aortic velocity >4.0 m/sec are suggestive of severe aortic stenosis.

Left Ventricular Outflow Tract Obstruction. LVOT obstruction is commonly seen in patients with hypertrophic cardiomyopathy (HCM). In these patients, the upper basal portion of the interventricular septum becomes hypertrophied, narrowing the overall diameter of the LVOT. As such, there is obstruction to flow, creating turbulence within the LVOT that can be detected using color Doppler in the midesophageal long-axis or "five-chamber" views. These patients are also at increased risk for systolic anterior motion (SAM) of the anterior MV leaflet. This occurs when, during systole, the anterior MV leaflet becomes entrained via a Venturi effect into the LVOT with resultant obstruction to blood flow and severe mitral regurgitation, both detectable with CFD (Video 11.21). This is a dynamic process and is exacerbated by hypovolemia, tachycardia, increased cardiac inotropy, and vasodilatation.

Aortic Insufficiency (Video 11.22). Acute aortic insufficiency can lead to profound hemodynamic instability. Common causes of aortic insufficiency include dehiscence or malfunction of surgically implanted valves, aortic dissection, endocarditis, and chest trauma leading to valve rupture.

The degree of severity is best assessed in the midesophageal long-axis view using color flow Doppler. The length of the jet into the left ventricle should be assessed. A jet that extends beyond the papillary muscles is likely indicative of severe AI. Additionally, if the jet is central, the width of the jet relative to the diameter of the LVOT within 1 cm of the AV should be assessed. If the jet occupies >65% of the LVOT diameter, it is considered severe, whereas if it occupies <25%, it is considered mild. Finally, holodiastolic flow reversal in the descending aorta is both highly sensitive and specific for severe aortic insufficiency, at 100% and 97%, respectively. This should be assessed in the descending aortic long-axis view utilizing pulse wave Doppler (Fig. 11.17).

Mitral Stenosis (Videos 11.23 and 11.24). Rheumatic heart disease remains the most common etiology for mitral stenosis in developing countries. Mitral stenosis

may also occur as a complication after surgical valve repair, severe mitral annular calcification, pulmonary vein obstruction, and congenital heart disease.

Severe mitral stenosis is best identified with TEE using the ME 4C view by noting a thickened, highly echogenic MV with reduced leaflet mobility. Utilizing CFD, a high-velocity LV inflow jet distal to the MV can usually be seen. Additionally, continuous wave Doppler interrogation of the mitral inflow can be used to measure the transvalvular gradient (Fig. 11.18). The Doppler diastolic mitral flow profile is traced, and the maximal and mean gradients are subsequently calculated automatically by integrated software on the machine. A mean gradient of <5 mm Hg is considered mild, 5 to 10 mm Hg moderate, and >10 mm Hg severe.

Mitral Regurgitation (Video 11.25). Acute mitral regurgitation can lead to profound hemodynamic instability and should be considered in patients in whom myocardial ischemia is highly suspected. Acute myocardial ischemia leading to LV dysfunction can cause wall motion abnormalities and papillary muscle dysfunction, causing leaflet tenting and restricting the ability of the MV leaflets to coapt. This is termed *functional mitral regurgitation*. Furthermore, acute ischemia may also lead to infarction of papillary muscles that could also result in acute mitral regurgitation. Chronic ischemia may lead to dilation of

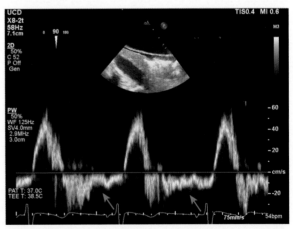

Fig. 11.17 Holodiastolic Flow Reversal Descending aortic long-axis view with pulse wave Doppler in the proximal descending aorta. Holodiastolic flow reversal represented by flow below the baseline in the descending aorta is seen here (*red arrows*), which is both highly sensitive and specific for severe aortic insufficiency.

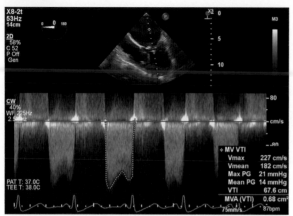

Fig. 11.18 Mitral Valve Pressure Gradient Continuous wave Doppler is used to measure the transvalvular pressure gradient through the mitral valve. This patient's mean pressure gradient through the mitral valve is 14 mm Hg, consistent with severe mitral stenosis. Furthermore, the integrated software of the TEE machine has calculated the mitral valve area to be 0.68 cm².

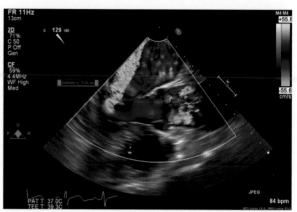

Fig. 11.19 Vena Contracta The vena contracta, the narrowest central point in the regurgitant jet during end systole, is depicted in this image. Here, the vena contracta is 9.1 mm, consistent with severe mitral regurgitation.

the left ventricle and mitral annuls. The leaflets would no longer be able to coapt effectively. Other causes include myxomatous MV disease with or without chordal rupture, rheumatic disease, endocarditis, and SAM associated with HCM.

The severity of mitral regurgitation is primarily assessed using CFD visualization of the regurgitant jet, focusing mainly on evaluating the length, height, area, and direction of the regurgitant jet. Another major component in the evaluation of mitral regurgitation is assessing the width of the vena contracta, the narrowest central point in the regurgitant jet during end systole (Fig. 11.19). The vena contracta is reported to be mostly independent of loading conditions and represents a good method of assessing the severity of mitral regurgitation. A vena contracta of <3 mm is indicative of mild mitral regurgitation, whereas a vena contracta >7 mm indicates the mitral regurgitation is severe.

Hypovolemia (Hemorrhagic Shock) (Video 11.26). The assessment of volume status is essential in managing hemodynamically unstable patients. Hypovolemia due to hemorrhage is characterized by intravascular volume depletion resulting in decreased preload and cardiac output. In patients with normal systolic function, hypovolemia manifests as a hyperdynamic

left ventricle with a reduced left ventricular end-diastolic area (LVEDA) and left ventricular end-systolic area (LVESA). The percentage difference in area between end diastole and end systole is termed the *fractional area change* (FAC) and correlates well with assessments of decreased intravascular volume. The FAC is typically low in hypovolemic patients. This can be readily assessed in the TG midpapillary SAX view. Additionally, it may be such that the LV cavity becomes obliterated with near contact of the papillary muscles. The papillary muscles are described as "kissing" each other. Care must be taken in patients with dilated cardiomyopathies, as their baseline LVEDA may be large in spite of depletions in intravascular volume. On the other hand, patients with hypertrophic left ventricles and significant diastolic dysfunction may appear empty at baseline in spite of being euvolemic.

Distributive Shock. Distributive shock is characterized by low systemic vascular resistance (SVR) leading to hypotension and compromised tissue perfusion. Common causes include sepsis from infection as well as noninfectious etiologies leading to systemic inflammatory response syndrome such as pancreatitis, trauma, and burn injuries. Anaphylaxis, medication reactions, adrenal or hepatic insufficiency, and damage to the central nervous system can also lead to profound decreases in SVR.

Similar to hypovolemia, distributive shock also presents with a hyperdynamic left ventricle and a decreased LVESA on the TG LV SAX view. Unlike in hypovolemia, however, where the LVEDA is also decreased, the LVEDA in distributive shock is usually normal. Therefore the FAC is usually normal to high. It is therefore crucial to assess the internal LV area at both end systole and end diastole.

▶ **Aortic Dissection (Video 11.27).** Aortic dissection is characterized by a tear in the intimal lining. With the subsequent separation of the intima and media, a false lumen is created, allowing blood to enter. The dissection can propagate anywhere along the length of the aorta or branching arteries. Hypotension may occur secondary to myocardial ischemia and LV dysfunction from dissection into the coronary arteries, tamponade, aortic insufficiency, or even aortic rupture.

TEE is an extremely useful imaging modality in the setting of aortic dissection. Its diagnostic accuracy is similar to that of helical CT and magnetic resonance imaging (MRI), with a sensitivity and specificity greater than 95%. Useful views include the midesophageal long-axis, the midesophageal ascending aortic short-axis, and midesophageal aortic long-axis views. Unfortunately, a section of the aorta typically extending from the distal ascending aorta to the proximal arch is difficult to visualize with TEE due to the interposition of the air-filled left mainstem bronchus and trachea between it and the esophagus. The diagnostic hallmark of a dissection is the visualization of an intimal flap within the aorta separating a true lumen from a false lumen. It may be difficult to distinguish the true from the false lumen. However, the true lumen will usually appear smaller, has higher flow characteristics using CFD, and expands during systole. Additional findings may include visualization of aortic insufficiency, the presence of a pericardial effusion, and aortic dilatation. TEE can also be used to diagnose proximal abdominal aortic dissections that occur below the diaphragm using the descending aortic short- or long-axis views.

BIBLIOGRAPHY

Arntfield R, et al. Focused transesophageal echocardiography by emergency physicians is feasible and clinically influential: observational results from a Novel Ultrasound Program. *J Emerg Med.* 2016;50(2):286–294.

Baumgartner H, et al. Echocardiographic assessment of valve stenosis: EAE/ASE recommendations for clinical practice. *J Am Soc Echocardiogr.* 2009;22(1):1–23; quiz 101-2.

Bonow RO, et al. ACC/AHA 2006 guidelines for the management of patients with valvular heart disease: a report of the American College of Cardiology/American Heart Association Task Force on Practice Guidelines (writing committee to revise the 1998 Guidelines for the Management of Patients with Valvular Heart Disease): developed in collaboration with the Society of Cardiovascular Anesthesiologists: endorsed by the Society for Cardiovascular Angiography and Interventions and the Society of Thoracic Surgeons. *Circulation.* 2006;114(5):e84–e231.

Cheung AT, et al. Echocardiographic and hemodynamic indexes of left ventricular preload in patients with normal and abnormal ventricular function. *Anesthesiology.* 1994;81(2):376–387.

Colreavy FB, et al. Transesophageal echocardiography in critically ill patients. *Crit Care Med.* 2002;30(5):989–996.

Heidenreich PA, et al. Transesophageal echocardiography predicts mortality in critically ill patients with unexplained hypotension. *J Am Coll Cardiol.* 1995;26(1):152–158.

Hilberath JN, et al. Safety of transesophageal echocardiography. *J Am Soc Echocardiogr.* 2010;23(11):1115–1127; quiz 1220-1.

Hofer CK, et al. Therapeutic impact of intra-operative transoesophageal echocardiography during noncardiac surgery. *Anaesthesia.* 2004;59(1):3–9.

Khoury AF, et al. Transesophageal echocardiography in critically ill patients: feasibility, safety, and impact on management. *Am Heart J.* 1994;127(5):1363–1371.

Marijon E, et al. Prevalence of rheumatic heart disease detected by echocardiographic screening. *N Engl J Med.* 2007;357(5):470–476.

Markin NW, et al. A review of 364 perioperative rescue echocardiograms: findings of an anesthesiologist-staffed perioperative echocardiography service. *J Cardiothorac Vasc Anesth.* 2015;29(1):82–88.

Mayo PH, Narasimhan M, Koenig S. Critical care transesophageal echocardiography. *Chest.* 2015;148(5):1323–1332.

Pruszczyk P, et al. Noninvasive diagnosis of suspected severe pulmonary embolism: transesophageal echocardiography vs spiral CT. *Chest.* 1997;112(3):722–728.

Pruszczyk P, et al. Transoesophageal echocardiography for definitive diagnosis of haemodynamically significant pulmonary embolism. *Eur Heart J.* 1995;16(4):534–538.

Reeves ST, et al. Basic perioperative transesophageal echocardiography examination: a consensus statement of the American Society of Echocardiography and the Society of Cardiovascular Anesthesiologists. *J Am Soc Echocardiogr.* 2013;26(5):443–456.

Reichert CL, et al. Prognostic value of biventricular function in hypotensive patients after cardiac surgery as assessed by transesophageal echocardiography. *J Cardiothorac Vasc Anesth.* 1992;6(4):429–432.

Rudski LG, et al. Guidelines for the echocardiographic assessment of the right heart in adults: a report from the American Society of Echocardiography endorsed by the European Association of Echocardiography, a registered branch of the European Society of Cardiology, and the Canadian Society of Echocardiography. *J Am Soc Echocardiogr.* 2010;23(7):685–713; quiz 786-8.

Shanewise JS, et al. ASE/SCA guidelines for performing a comprehensive intraoperative multiplane transesophageal echocardiography examination: recommendations of the American Society of Echocardiography Council for Intraoperative Echocardiography and the Society of Cardiovascular Anesthesiologists Task Force for Certification in Perioperative Transesophageal Echocardiography. *Anesth Analg.* 1999;89(4):870–884.

Shiga T, et al. Diagnostic accuracy of transesophageal echocardiography, helical computed tomography, and magnetic resonance imaging for suspected thoracic aortic dissection: systematic review and meta-analysis. *Arch Intern Med.* 2006;166(13):1350–1356.

Shillcutt SK, et al. Use of rapid "rescue" perioperative echocardiography to improve outcomes after hemodynamic instability in noncardiac surgical patients. *J Cardiothorac Vasc Anesth.* 2012;26(3):362–370.

Takenaka K, et al. A simple Doppler echocardiographic method for estimating severity of aortic regurgitation. *Am J Cardiol.* 1986;57(15):1340–1343.

Vieillard-Baron A, et al. Transesophageal echocardiography for the diagnosis of pulmonary embolism with acute cor pulmonale: a comparison with radiological procedures. *Intensive Care Med.* 1998;24(5):429–433.

Wunderlich NC, Beigel R, Siegel RJ. Management of mitral stenosis using 2D and 3D echo-Doppler imaging. *JACC Cardiovasc Imaging.* 2013;6(11):1191–1205.

Zarauza J, et al. An integrated approach to the quantification of aortic regurgitation by Doppler echocardiography. *Am Heart J.* 1998;136(6):1030–1041.

Zoghbi WA, et al. Recommendations for noninvasive evaluation of native valvular regurgitation: a report from the American Society of Echocardiography developed in collaboration with the Society for Cardiovascular Magnetic Resonance. *J Am Soc Echocardiogr.* 2017;30(4):303–371.

12

Approach to the Patient with Shortness of Breath

Rachel Liu, Cristiana Baloescu

INTRODUCTION

Patients presenting with undifferentiated shortness of breath can be challenging because their presentations can have many potential etiologies: pulmonary, cardiac, mixed cardiopulmonary, gastrointestinal, neurologic, or other noncardiopulmonary reasons. It is important to evaluate all organ systems potentially involved using a standardized, structured fashion to reach helpful conclusions rapidly at the bedside.

Preceding chapters have explored and discussed organ-based evaluations utilizing ultrasound. This chapter will focus on integrating those applications into combined algorithmic approaches to undifferentiated shortness of breath.

Ultrasound protocols have been described for evaluation of a variety of symptoms and diagnostic concerns. Perhaps the most well-known is the focused assessment with sonography for trauma (FAST) examination looking for free fluid in the setting of trauma, which was expanded to the eFAST examination to assess for traumatic pneumothorax. Other well-known protocols that include assessments for dyspnea include the focused assessment with sonography for HIV-associated tuberculosis (FASH) and the rapid ultrasound in shock (RUSH) examination for hypotension.

Examples of specific algorithms for the ultrasound evaluation of undifferentiated dyspnea include the bedside lung ultrasound in emergency (BLUE) protocol and the rapid assessment of dyspnea with ultrasound (RADiUS) protocol. The BLUE protocol evaluates the lungs only and is useful for the diagnosis of pneumothorax, pulmonary edema, pulmonary consolidation, and pleural effusions. The RADiUS protocol includes echocardiographic and inferior vena cava (IVC) evaluation, in addition to the pulmonary examination. A fluid administration limited by lung sonography (FALLS) protocol combines cardiac and lung views to sequentially rule out obstructive and cardiogenic shock while expediting diagnosis of distributive (usually septic) shock and monitoring for development of pulmonary edema as a result of fluid resuscitation.

Most algorithms combine the cardiac examination (including the IVC) with a thoracic examination, culminating in a "focused chest" assessment, as many life-threatening etiologies of dyspnea have cardiopulmonary origins. This approach is similar to the methods for evaluation of undifferentiated chest pain and hypotension described in other chapters.

TECHNIQUE

The sequence for obtaining views varies, depending on the pretest probability of certain diagnoses obtained from the history and physical examination. Many sonologists choose to start with echocardiographic views, as the heart is essential.

Cardiac

The "5Es" approach is a problem-driven algorithm. The assessment for pathology is largely qualitative.

- Effusion—Is there an effusion? Is there pericardial tamponade?

- Parasternal long or short axis, apical four-chamber, or subxiphoid views
- Ejection (fraction)
  1. Is the left ventricular function normal or depressed? Is congestive heart failure a reason for dyspnea?
     - Parasternal long or short axis, apical four-chamber or subxiphoid views
  2. Is there acute focal wall motion abnormality, indicating acute myocardial infarction with dyspnea as a symptom equivalent?
     - Parasternal short axis, complemented by parasternal long axis or apical four-chamber view
- Equality—Is the right ventricle enlarged? Is there acute right heart strain from obstructive pathology such as a large pulmonary?
  - Parasternal long or short-axis, apical four-chamber views
- Exit—Is there thoracic aortic dilation? Is an aortic catastrophe causing the shortness of breath?
  - Parasternal long-axis view specifically measuring the aortic outflow tract (AOT)
- Entrance—What is the volume status (preload) entering the heart? Plethora and collapsibility of the IVC contribute to the interpretation of wall motion abnormalities and obstructive pathologies. Is hypovolemia causing shortness of breath?
  - Subxiphoid long-axis view reviewing IVC distensibility and respirophasic variations

If possible, obtain at least two views to confirm findings. Patient acuity, mobility, body habitus, and time constraints are all factors that may limit the number of views that can be obtained.

Lung

- Pleura—Is there a pneumothorax?
  - Sagittal view obtained in the second intercostal space
  - Review for pleural sliding; M-mode or power Doppler may be used for assistance
- Parenchyma
  - Is there pulmonary edema?
    - Sagittal view obtained in the second intercostal space
    - Review for B-lines
  - Is there pleural effusion or consolidation?

- Coronal view obtained in the right and left upper quadrant flanks evaluating the pleural space above the diaphragm
- Review the pleural space for presence of pleural effusion or consolidation from pneumonia or masses
- The "spine sign" is a clue to thoracic pathology

An algorithmic approach has been shown to narrow differential diagnoses and increase diagnostic confidence and accuracy in the setting of dyspnea, chest pain, or symptomatic hypotension. Fig. 12.1 presents the potential views to be interrogated as part of this algorithmic approach.

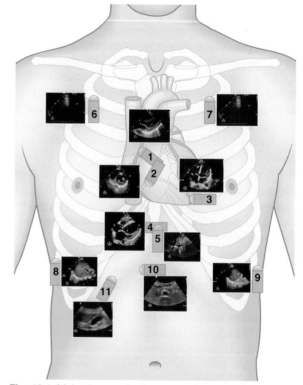

Fig. 12.1 Main views to be interrogated as part of a dyspnea evaluation algorithm: *1,* Parasternal long-axis view. *2,* Parasternal short-axis view. *3,* Apical four-chamber view. *4,* Subxiphoid view. *5,* IVC view. *6,* Sagittal right lung view, second intercostal space. *7,* Sagittal left lung view, second intercostal space. *8,* Coronal view, right upper quadrant. *9,* Coronal view, left upper quadrant *10,* Transverse view of abdominal aorta *11,* View of the gallbladder (Drawing based on Häggström M. Wikimedia Commons. Surface Anatomy of the Heart. https://commons.wikimedia.org/wiki/Category:Human_thorax#/media/File:Surface_anatomy_of_the_heart.png. Accessed April 9, 2019.)

EXAMPLES AND CASES

The following cases exemplify the use of an ultrasound protocol such as the one we propose, as well as examples of the pathology ultrasound can help uncover.

Case 1. Pericardial Effusion with Tamponade

A 54-year-old female with history of colon cancer metastatic to the lung, on chemotherapy, presents to the emergency department for dyspnea. She describes gradually worsening nonproductive cough and shortness of breath over the past week and noted worsening abdominal swelling and abdominal pain with nausea. She denies fever. Her physical examination is notable for tachycardia, lack of fever, and distended and tender abdomen.

Differential diagnosis in this case is broad and includes worsening metastatic disease, pleural effusion, pneumonia with or without empyema, acute coronary syndrome, small bowel obstruction, and pericardial effusion. Given the vague symptoms and large differential diagnosis, ultrasound would be helpful in excluding some etiologies on the differential and help the provider reach a diagnosis.

Utilizing the algorithmic approach as described earlier, the provider obtained point-of-care ultrasound (POCUS) images to aid with diagnosis. Fig. 12.2 shows the parasternal long-axis view with a large pericardial effusion and right ventricular collapse (better noted in cine-loop format, Video 12.1). Ultrasound of the lungs indicated an absence of B-lines and pleural effusions (Figs. 12.3–12.6),

arguing against a pulmonary cause for the patient's symptoms. The IVC is seen to be plethoric and noncollapsible, further supporting the diagnosis of tamponade (Fig. 12.7, better noted in cine-loop format, Video 12.2). The patient was taken to the catheterization laboratory for a pericardial drain placement.

Case 2. Pulmonary Embolus

A 75-year-old female presented to the emergency department with syncope. She was found to be febrile and hypotensive on arrival, and bedside laboratory testing revealed a lactic acid of 5. She had an indwelling Foley catheter placed for workup of vaginal bleeding a week prior.

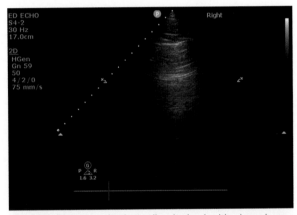

Fig. 12.3 Right anterior lung clip obtained with phased array probe showing absence of B-lines.

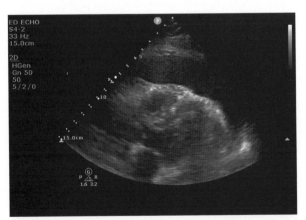

Fig. 12.2 Parasternal long-axis view with a large pericardial effusion and right ventricular collapse (better noted in cine-loop format, see Video 12.1).

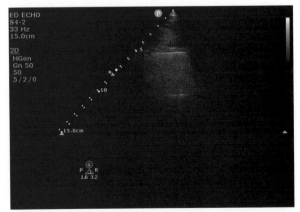

Fig. 12.4 Left anterior lung clip obtained with phased array probe showing absence of B-lines.

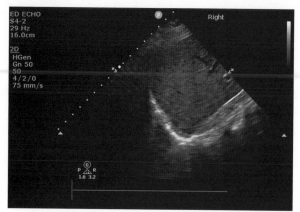

Fig. 12.5 Right lung base with no pleural effusion.

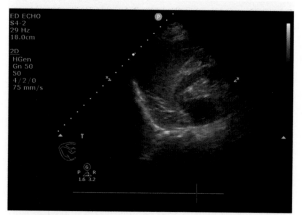

Fig. 12.6 Left lung base with no pleural effusion.

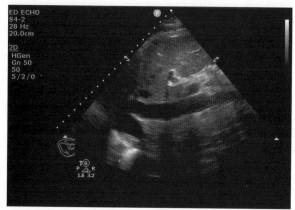

Fig. 12.7 Sagittal view of the inferior vena cava showing a plethoric and noncollapsible vessel (better noted in cine-loop format, see Video 12.2).

Differential diagnosis included sepsis from presumed urinary tract infection.

The patient did not improve with usual sepsis care. Despite fluid resuscitation and broad-spectrum antibiotics, she remained hypotensive. Providers performed point-of-care ultrasound.

The apical four-chamber view showed right ventricular enlargement and a mobile clot through the tricuspid valve, consistent with a clot in transit (Fig. 12.8 and Video 12.3). This clot can also be seen in the right atrium in the subxiphoid view in Fig. 12.9 and Video 12.4. The IVC, as seen in Fig. 12.10 and Video 12.5, is plethoric and noncollapsible. While undergoing computed tomography to evaluate for pulmonary embolus, the patient lost

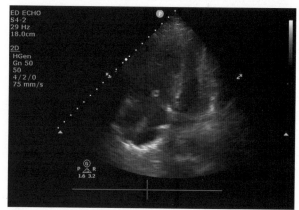

Fig. 12.8 Apical four-chamber view of the heart with right ventricular enlargement and mobile clot through the tricuspid valve (better noted in cine-loop format, see Video 12.3).

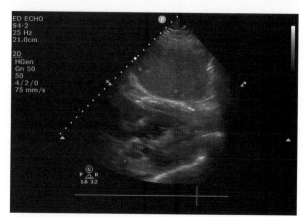

Fig. 12.9 Subxiphoid view with clot apparent in the right atrium (also noted in cine-loop format, see Video 12.4).

pulses and suffered a cardiac arrest. Fig. 12.11 shows a parasternal long-axis view of the heart during the code. Absence of cardiac activity can be seen better in cine-loop format in Video 12.6. Lung views from the patient (Figs. 12.12–12.15) show no pathology to explain the patient's symptoms. In conclusion, the point-of-care ultrasound showed a right ventricular thrombus in transit between the right atrium and right ventricle, together with a dilated right ventricle, consistent with acute pulmonary embolus and obstructive shock physiology. The cause of the cardiac arrest was most likely the breaking off of the clot in the right atrium/ventricle. This was in contrast to the initial impression of urinary tract infection causing sepsis.

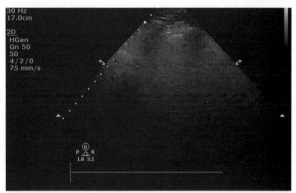

Fig. 12.12 Right anterior lung clip obtained with phased array probe showing absence of B-lines.

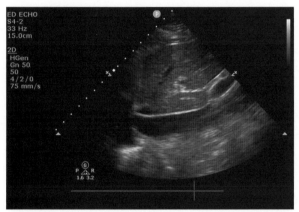

Fig. 12.10 Sagittal view of the IVC shows a plethoric vessel, which does not collapse with respiration (better noted in cine-loop format, see Video 12.5).

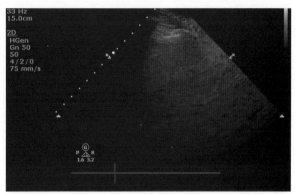

Fig. 12.13 Left anterior lung clip obtained with phased array probe showing absence of B-lines.

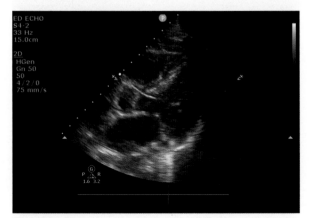

Fig. 12.11 Parasternal long-axis view of the heart during the code (Video 12.6).

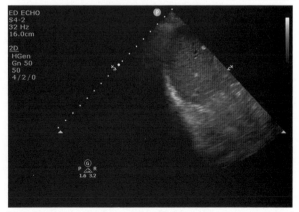

Fig. 12.14 Coronal view of the right lung base with no pleural effusion.

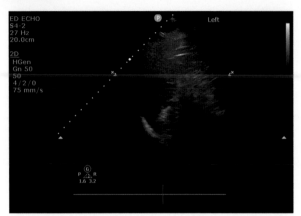

Fig. 12.15 Coronal view of the left lung base with no pleural effusion.

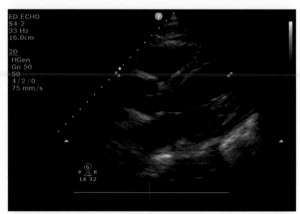

Fig. 12.16 Parasternal long-axis view of the heart (also see in cine-loop format, Video 12.7).

Case 3. Pneumonia

A 40-year-old female with nonsquamous cell lung cancer, known right lung necrotic mass, currently on chemotherapy, presented to the emergency department with worsening dyspnea, nonproductive cough, and subjective fevers for 2 days but worse since her bronchoscopy on the morning of the day of presentation. On examination, she was noted to be hypoxic to 90% on room air, hypotensive to 90/50 mm Hg, with diminished right-sided breath sounds.

The differential diagnosis in this case is broad, including pneumonia, pulmonary embolus, worsening tumor burden, pleural effusion, and empyema.

Using the algorithm described earlier, the providers were able to narrow this differential diagnosis. A parasternal long-axis view, as seen in Fig. 12.16, demonstrated no pericardial effusion, normal ejection fraction (better evaluated in cine-loop format, Video 12.7), no right ventricular enlargement to suggest right heart strain, and no aortic root dilation. A short-axis view at the level of the papillary muscles also demonstrated normal ejection fraction (Fig. 12.17 and Video 12.8). The patient had no evidence of alveolar interstitial syndrome in anterior lung fields (Figs. 12.18 and 12.19). The right lung base did show a spine sign, hepatization of lung, and air bronchograms, consistent with a unilateral infiltrative process (Figs. 12.20 and 12.21, Video 12.9). The diameter of the IVC was small, and the IVC was fully collapsible, further supporting an infectious cause of the symptoms (Fig. 12.22, Video 12.10). In this case,

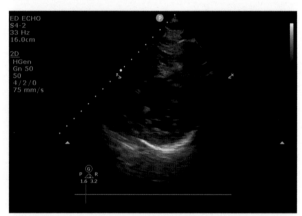

Fig. 12.17 Parasternal short-axis view of the heart at the level of the papillary muscles (also see in cine-loop format, Video 12.8).

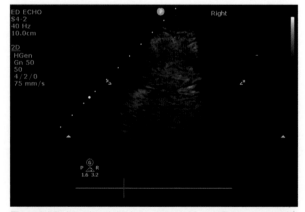

Fig. 12.18 Anterior right lung view with no B-lines and with pleural sliding.

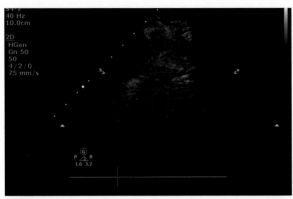

Fig. 12.19 Anterior left lung view with no B-lines and with pleural sliding.

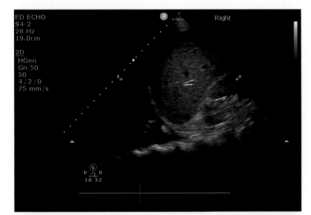

Fig. 12.20 Coronal view of the right lung base with spine sign, hepatization of lung, and air bronchograms, consistent with an infiltrative process.

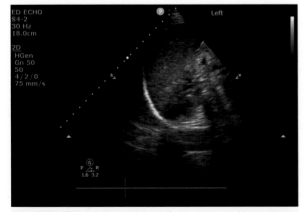

Fig. 12.21 Coronal view of the left lung base with no pleural effusion and no consolidation.

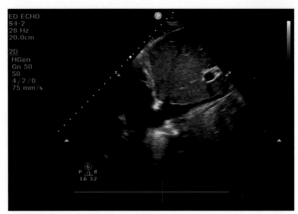

Fig. 12.22 Sagittal view of the IVC showing a flat vessel (also see in cine-loop format, Video 12.10).

point-of-care ultrasound revealed the diagnosis of a right-sided pneumonia causing the patient's symptoms, as evidenced by the right-sided consolidation with air bronchograms and absence of other pathologies.

Case 4. Pulmonary Edema from Congestive Heart Failure

A 60-year-old female with a history of untreated hypertension comes to the emergency department complaining of shortness of breath worse on exertion and at night. She denies any leg swelling, has had no recent travel, no fever, and no cough, but had some upper respiratory symptoms several weeks prior. She is afebrile, mildly hypoxic to 92% on room air, tachycardic with a heart rate of 105, tachypneic with respiratory rate of 24, and hypertensive with a blood pressure of 154/80 mm Hg.

Point-of-care ultrasound is performed, and a parasternal long-axis view demonstrates a severely depressed ejection fraction (Fig. 12.23 and Video 12.11), also noted on the parasternal short-axis view (Fig. 12.24 and Video 12.12). There are bilateral B-lines indicating alveolar interstitial syndrome (Fig. 12.25 and 12.26) and bilateral pleural effusions (Figs. 12.27 and 12.28). The patient's IVC is plethoric and poorly collapsible, and the liver shows hepatic vein dilation as well, indicating fluid overload (Fig. 12.29, better seen in cine-loop format, Video 12.13). The constellation of depressed ejection fraction, plethoric IVC, bilateral B-lines, and bilateral pleural effusions suggests fluid overload and heart failure as the cause of the patient's symptoms.

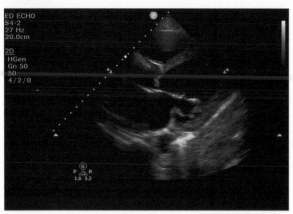

Fig. 12.23 Parasternal long-axis view demonstrating severely depressed ejection fraction (in cine-loop format, see Video 12.11).

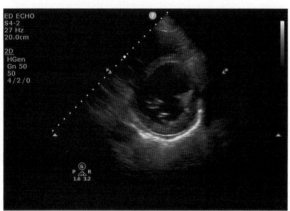

Fig. 12.24 Parasternal short-axis view at the level of the papillary muscles, with severely depressed ejection fraction (in cine-loop format, see Video 12.12).

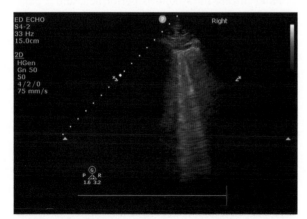

Fig. 12.25 Right anterior lung ultrasound with B-lines.

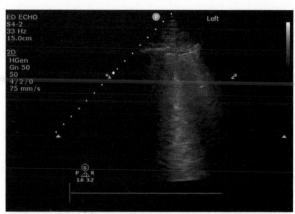

Fig. 12.26 Left anterior lung ultrasound with B-lines.

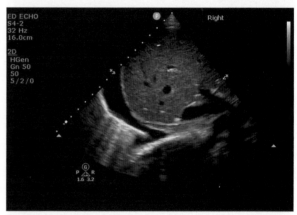

Fig. 12.27 Right coronal upper quadrant view demonstrating a spine sign and a right-sided pleural effusion.

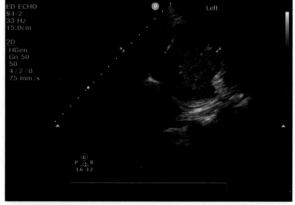

Fig. 12.28 Left coronal upper quadrant view demonstrating a left-sided pleural effusion.

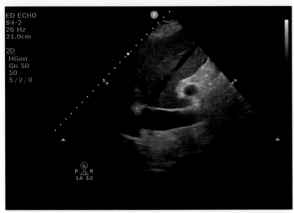

Fig. 12.29 Sagittal view of the IVC with plethoric IVC and dilation of the hepatic veins (Video 12.13 shows this in cine-loop format).

PEARLS AND LIMITATIONS

Flexibility in the order of areas examined with ultrasound is necessary, especially when evaluating a critically ill patient when time to diagnosis is important. It is reasonable to look first in the areas that can yield the most helpful information can take this out.

Limitations are expected when evaluating patients in an emergent setting. There are limitations in the time available for the ultrasound examination. Examinations may not be optimized due to lack of patient cooperation on examination in the setting of respiratory distress or pain, limitation in mobility, and competing simultaneous tests and procedures. Sometimes there are conflicting findings in the patient's presentation due to its complexity and the patient's illness, and ultrasound findings may point to competing or overlapping pathologies.

Point-of-care ultrasound should be integrated into a robust clinical evaluation of the patient.

BIBLIOGRAPHY

Ahn JH, et al. SEARCH 8Es: a novel point of care ultrasound protocol for patients with chest pain, dyspnea or symptomatic hypotension in the emergency department. *PLoS One.* 2017;12:1–13.

Grace, S. et al. Ovid: A prospective study of surgeon-performed ultrasound as the primary adjuvant modality for injured patient assessment? 2014;39:1–8.

Guttikonda SNR, Vadapalli K. Approach to undifferentiated dyspnea in emergency department: aids in rapid clinical decision-making. *Int. J. Emerg. Med.* 2018;11(1):21.

Hall MK, et al. The "5Es" of emergency physician-performed focused cardiac ultrasound: a protocol for rapid identification of effusion, ejection, equality, exit, and entrance. *Acad. Emerg. Med.* 2015;22:583–593.

Heller T, Wallrauch C, Goblirsch S, Brunetti E. Focused assessment with sonography for HIV-associated tuberculosis (FASH): a short protocol and a pictorial review. *Crit. Ultrasound J.* 2012;4:21.

Kirkpatrick AW, et al. Hand-held thoracic sonography for detecting post-traumatic pneumothoraces: the extended focused assessment with sonography for trauma (eFAST). *J Trauma - Inj Infect Crit Care.* 2004;57:288–295.

Lichtenstein DA. BLUE-protocol and FALLS-protocol: two applications of lung ultrasound in the critically ill. *Chest.* 2015;147:1659–1670.

Lichtenstein DA, Mezière GA. Relevance of lung ultrasound in the diagnosis of acute respiratory failure the BLUE protocol. *Chest.* 2008;134:117–125.

Manson W, Hafez NM. The rapid assessment of dyspnea with ultrasound: RADiUS. *Ultrasound Clin.* 2011;6:261–276.

Perera P, Mailhot T, Riley D, Mandavia D. The RUSH exam 2012: rapid ultrasound in shock in the evaluation of the critically ill patient. *Ultrasound Clin.* 2012;7:255–278.

Seif D, Perera P, Mailhot T, Riley D, Mandavia D. Bedside ultrasound in resuscitation and the rapid ultrasound in shock protocol. *Crit. Care Res. Pract.* 2012.

13

Approach to the Patient with Chest Pain

Rachel Liu, Cristiana Baloescu

INTRODUCTION

Undifferentiated chest pain presents a diagnostic dilemma because there are many potential causes, with some etiologies being imminently life threatening. These diagnoses often cannot be determined by history or physical examination alone. Patients may be hypotensive or deteriorate quickly, requiring emergent procedures. For these reasons, point-of-care ultrasound (POCUS) is used to evaluate chest pain.

The most urgent systems to evaluate are cardiac, aortic, and pulmonary, which can be performed together using a "focused chest" algorithm. Multiple algorithms exist, including a 5Es approach to review cardiac pathology, the SEARCH 8Es approach to assess the lung and heart, and a modified rapid ultrasound for shock and hypotension (RUSH) examination. Different algorithms prioritize ultrasound views in different orders. We recommend starting with the view most likely to yield a diagnosis based on initial history and physical.

TECHNIQUE

Because the heart is an essential organ upon which life depends, echocardiographic views are often obtained first to evaluate for life-threatening and immediately reversible causes.

Cardiac

The 5Es approach is a problem-driven algorithm. The assessment for pathology is largely qualitative.

- Effusion—Is there a pericardial effusion? Is there cardiac tamponade?
  - Parasternal long or short axis, apical four-chamber, or subxiphoid views
- Ejection (fraction)
  1. Is the left ventricular function preserved or depressed?
     - Parasternal long or short axis, apical four-chamber, or subxiphoid views
  2. Is there acute focal wall motion abnormality indicating acute myocardial infarction?
     - Mainly parasternal short axis, complemented by parasternal long axis or apical four-chamber view
- Equality—Is the right ventricle (RV) enlarged compared with the left ventricle indicating an acute obstructive process such as pulmonary embolus (PE)?
  - Parasternal long or short axis, apical four-chamber views
- Exit—Is there thoracic aortic dilation or dissection?
  - Parasternal long-axis (PSLA) view specifically measuring the aortic outflow tract (AOT)
  - The PSLA view should be performed at a depth great enough to visualize and measure the descending thoracic aorta in the same view
- Entrance—What is the volume status (preload) entering the heart? Is there hypervolemia or obstruction to blood flow?
  - Subxiphoid long-axis view reviewing inferior vena cava (IVC) distensibility and respirophasic variations

If possible, obtain at least two views to confirm findings. Patient acuity, mobility, body habitus, and time constraints are all factors that may limit the number of views that can be obtained.

Although valve assessment has not been incorporated into routine algorithms for chest pain echocardiographic assessment, concern for a new murmur or entities such as critical aortic stenosis should prompt valvular evaluation.

Pulmonary

- Is there a pneumothorax?
  - Sagittal view obtained in the second intercostal space
  - Review for lack of pleural sliding: M-mode or power Doppler may be used for assistance
- Is there significant pulmonary edema (chest pain from cardiac demand)?
  - Sagittal view obtained in the second intercostal space
  - Review for B-lines, which are vertically extending reverberation artifacts through the whole depth of field
- Is there pleural effusion or consolidation (chest pain from pleurisy)?
  - Coronal view obtained in the right and left upper quadrant flanks cephalad enough to see the pleural space above the diaphragm
  - Review the pleural space for the presence of pleural effusion (hypoechoic) or consolidations from pneumonia or masses (with hepatization containing air bronchograms)
  - In the presence of pathology, a "spine sign" will be seen, with the thoracic spine visualized extending cephalad past the diaphragm

Other lung views may be obtained if time is not limited.

Other Applications to Consider

If no reasons for chest pain etiology are found using echocardiographic and thoracic views, other etiologies can be considered.

- Is there a deep vein thrombosis (DVT)?
  - If a DVT is found, it may mean that chest pain can still be caused by a PE that is not extensive enough to cause evidence for RV enlargement or strain on echocardiography evaluation
  - Evaluate the saphenofemoral junction, common femoral vein, and popliteal vein to its trifurcation
- Does the patient have symptomatic cholelithiasis or cholecystitis causing chest pain that radiated from the epigastric region or right upper quadrant?

- Evaluate the gallbladder for presence of stone, thickened gallbladder wall, and pericholecystic fluid

The Views of This Algorithm

An algorithmic approach has been shown to narrow the differential diagnoses and increase diagnostic confidence and accuracy in the setting of dyspnea, chest pain, or symptomatic hypotension (Fig. 13.1).

EXAMPLES AND CASES

The following cases exemplify the use of an ultrasound protocol, such as the one we propose, as well

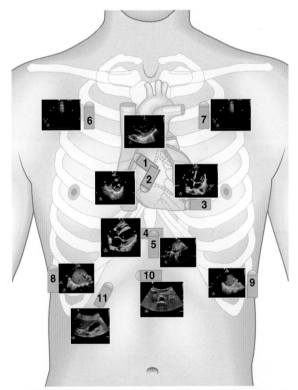

Fig. 13.1 Main views to be interrogated as part of a chest pain algorithm: (1) parasternal long-axis view; (2) parasternal short-axis view; (3) apical four-chamber view; (4) subxiphoid view; (5) IVC view; (6) sagittal right lung view, second intercostal space; (7) sagittal left lung view, second intercostal space; (8) coronal view, right upper quadrant; (9) coronal view, left upper quadrant; (10) transverse abdominal aorta in the epigastric area; and (11) subcostal view, with a longitudinal view of the gallbladder.

as examples of the pathology ultrasound can help uncover.

Case 1. Regional Wall Motion Abnormality

A 67-year-old male with a history of hypercholesterolemia on medications, prior negative stress test several years ago, and no diagnosed coronary artery disease presents to the emergency department with chest pain that started 3 hours prior. It is described as tight, nonradiating, and associated with nausea and diaphoresis. It improved with nitroglycerin administered in the ambulance. Electrocardiogram (EKG) showed J-point elevations in V1 and V2 without reciprocal changes, T wave, or ST-segment abnormalities.

Given the concerning patient history and nondiagnostic EKG, a point-of-care ultrasound was performed, clips of which are provided in Figs. 13.2 to 13.8 and Videos 13.1 to 13.7.

Ultrasound evaluation detected a posterior wall motion abnormality in the parasternal long- and short-axis views. An apical four-chamber view was not

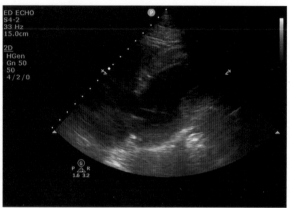

Fig. 13.2 Parasternal long-axis view of the heart; clip shows wall motion abnormality of the posterior wall of the left ventricle, not visible on static screenshot (see Video 13.1).

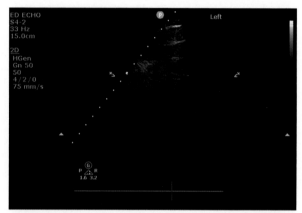

Fig. 13.4 Imaging of the left anterior lung with no B-lines and sliding noted; see Video 13.3.

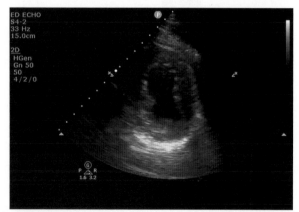

Fig. 13.3 Parasternal short-axis view of the heart; clip shows wall motion abnormality of the posterior wall of the left ventricle, not visible on static screenshot (see Video 13.2).

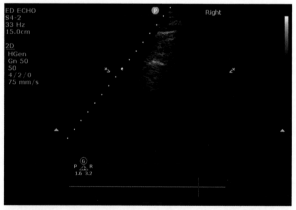

Fig. 13.5 Imaging of the right anterior lung with no B-lines and sliding noted (see Video 13.4).

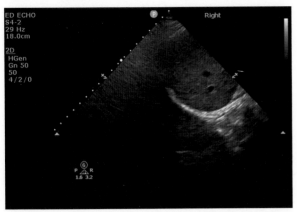

Fig. 13.6 Coronal view at the level of the diaphragm showing no right pleural effusion (see Video 13.5).

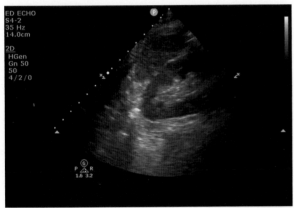

Fig. 13.7 Coronal view at the level of the diaphragm showing no left pleural effusion (see Video 13.6).

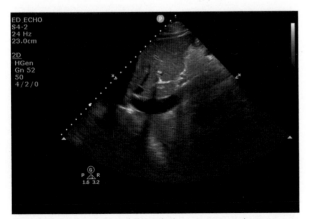

Fig. 13.8 Sagittal view of the inferior vena cava shows a normal-size vessel with respiratory variation (see Video 13.7).

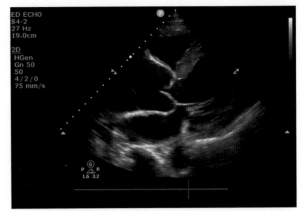

Fig. 13.9 Parasternal long-axis view showing a dilated aortic root and a subtle dissection flap (hyperechoic line best seen originating at the midpoint of the inferior wall of the ascending thoracic aorta). Cine-loop available in Video 13.8.

recorded for this patient. Evaluation also showed the presence of lung sliding, absence of B-lines, absence of pleural effusions, and a normal-sized, collapsible IVC. The combination of findings argued against pneumothorax, pneumonia, pericardial effusion, and dissection. The study revealed a focal wall motion abnormality consistent with acute coronary syndrome.

Case 2. Aortic Dissection

A 50-year-old male smoker with no significant medical problems was mowing the lawn and developed substernal chest pain, described as pressure with a dull component between the shoulder blades. Vital signs were normal, except for hypertension to 159/77 mm Hg. EKG was normal, and troponin negative. A point-of-care ultrasound was performed to elucidate the etiology of the chest pain, clips of which are provided in Figs. 13.9 to 13.14 and Videos 13.8 to 13.13.

Evaluation of the heart (Fig. 13.9) shows no pericardial effusion, and Video 13.8 demonstrates normal ejection fraction. The aortic root is enlarged, and a dissection flap is visible as a hyperechoic line inside the AOT. A portion of the descending thoracic aorta is visible inferior to the pericardium and is normal in caliber.

The apical five-chamber view in Fig. 13.10 and Video 13.9 shows another view of the enlarged AOT.

The rest of the clips show normal lungs, with slide sign present and no alveolar interstitial syndrome or pleural effusions.

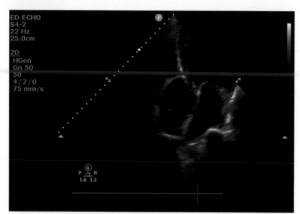

Fig. 13.10 Apical five-chamber view with a dilated aortic root visible to the left of the inferior part of the image, adjacent to the left atrium. The dilated aortic root is obscuring the right atrium in this screenshot. A dissection flap is also visible Findings can be better viewed in cine-loop format (Video 13.9).

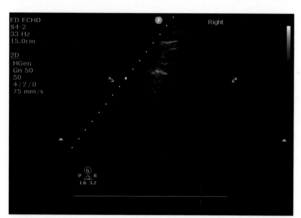

Fig. 13.11 Right anterior lung with no B-lines and no evidence of pneumothorax.

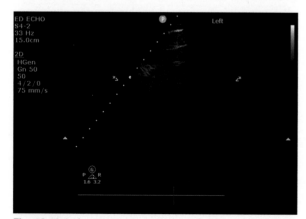

Fig. 13.12 Left anterior lung with no B-lines and no evidence of pneumothorax.

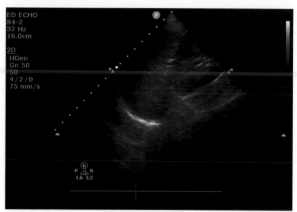

Fig. 13.13 Coronal view at the level of the right diaphragm showing no pleural effusion.

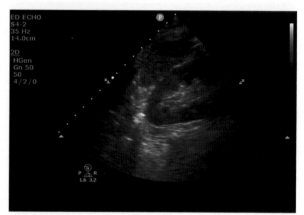

Fig. 13.14 Coronal view at the level of the left diaphragm showing no pleural effusion.

The ultrasound in this case identified thoracic aortic dissection that required emergent surgical management.

Case 3. Pneumothorax

A 50-year-old male with history of chronic obstructive pulmonary disease, systolic heart failure, and recent pneumonia on home oral antibiotics presents to the emergency department with shortness of breath. He is hypoxic to 89% on room air, but other vitals are normal. There is mild wheezing on examination, but the patient is not in distress and has good respiratory effort.

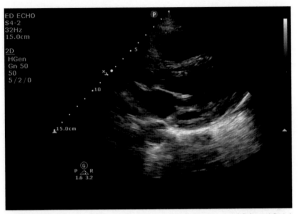

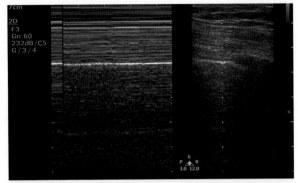

Fig. 13.17 This is an M-mode tracing of the right anterior lung showing sliding.

Fig. 13.15 Normal parasternal long-axis view; see Video 13.14 for cine-loop format.

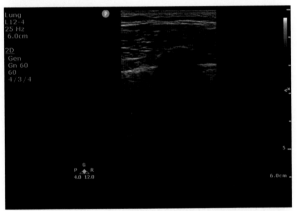

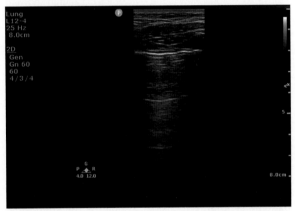

Fig. 13.16 Anterior lung view with linear probe showing presence of lung sliding on the right side.

Fig. 13.18 Anterior lung view with linear probe showing the presence of lung sliding on the left side.

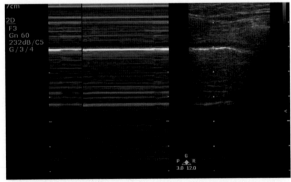

Using the algorithm described earlier, the providers obtain the clips shown in Figs. 13.15 to 13.21 and Videos 13.14 to 13.16.

Fig. 13.15 is indicative of a normal parasternal long view. There is no effusion, the ejection fraction is normal, the RV is not dilated, and the aortic root is normal in size.

Evaluation of the bilateral anterior lung views on M-mode (see Figs. 13.17–13.19) shows the difference between sliding (see Fig. 13.17) and no sliding (see Fig. 13.19). The patient has absent lung sliding on the left side. Clinical synthesis is required to interpret this finding, as loss of lung sliding is not diagnostic of pneumothorax but rather is diagnostic of the loss of the normal pleural interface.

Further interrogation of the lower lung fields shows no evidence of pneumonia or pleural effusion (Fig. 13.20 and 13.21). Ultimately, this patient was diagnosed with a pneumothorax.

Fig. 13.19 This is an M-mode tracing of the left anterior lung showing lack of sliding.

PEARLS AND LIMITATIONS

Flexibility in the order of areas examined with ultrasound is necessary, especially when evaluating a critically ill patient, where speed is of the essence.

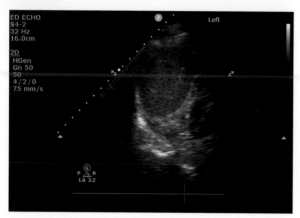

Fig. 13.20 Coronal view at the level of the diaphragm showing no pleural effusion.

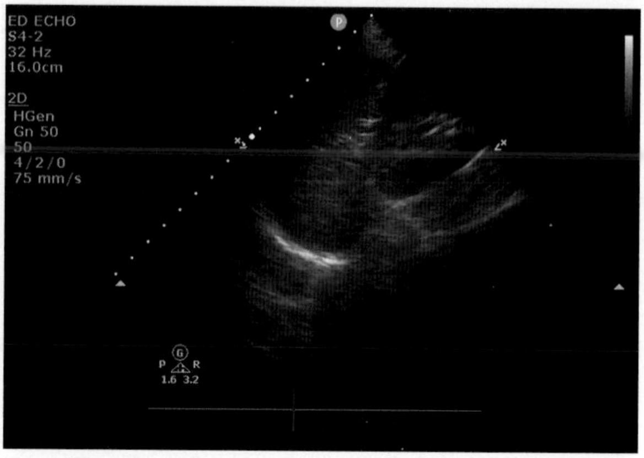

Fig. 13.21 Coronal view at the level of the diaphragm showing no pleural effusion.

The descending thoracic aorta can be visualized in cross-section inferior to the heart in the PSLA view. This is an opportunity to evaluate for dilation and presence of a dissection flap in that specific part of the thoracic aorta. It is an area easily overlooked and thus a pitfall of which to be aware.

High abdominal pain can present as chest pain. If the algorithm does not present any explanations for the patient's symptoms, consider evaluating the abdominal structures as well.

There are expected limitations when evaluating patients in an emergent setting in terms of time available for the ultrasound examination, inability to optimize views due to lack of patient cooperation on examination in the setting of respiratory distress and pain, or due to the need for intravenous line placement or other simultaneous tests and procedures.

Sometimes patients present with symptoms caused by overlapping pathologies, such as heart failure with pulmonary edema, chronic obstructive pulmonary disease with chronically enlarged RV, and pneumonia. This can generate complex ultrasound findings, or even ultrasound findings pointing to competing diagnoses, and requires careful clinical consideration.

BIBLIOGRAPHY

Ahn JH, et al. SEARCH 8Es: a novel point of care ultrasound protocol for patients with chest pain, dyspnea or symptomatic hypotension in the emergency department. *PLoS One.* 2017;12:1–13.

Hall MK, et al. The "5Es" of emergency physician-performed focused cardiac ultrasound: a protocol for rapid identification of effusion, ejection, equality, exit, and entrance. *Acad Emerg Med.* 2015;22:583–593.

Perera P, Mailhot T, Riley D, Mandavia D. The RUSH exam 2012: rapid ultrasound in shock in the evaluation of the critically ill patient. *Ultrasound Clin.* 2012;7:255–278.

Seif D, Perera P, Mailhot T, Riley D, Mandavia D. Bedside ultrasound in resuscitation and the rapid ultrasound in shock protocol. *Crit Care Res Pract.* 2012.

14

Ultrasound-Guided Resuscitation

Bjork Olafsdottir-Gardali, John S. Rose

USE OF ULTRASOUND IN THE UNDIFFERENTIATED HYPOTENSIVE PATIENT

Care of the undifferentiated hypotensive patient is a challenge for clinicians, and identifying life-threatening conditions that are readily reversible is a priority. Point-of-care ultrasound (POCUS) has had a prominent role over the past 20 years in the care of these patients. Focus on conditions that require emergent intervention, such as pneumothorax, intraabdominal hemorrhage, and pericardial effusion, has been an important addition to resuscitation practice.

The first description of a POCUS examination for the undifferentiated hypotensive patient was described by Rose et al. This examination protocol involves a focused three-view assessment evaluating for abdominal free fluid, pericardial fluid and cardiac activity, and abdominal aortic aneurysm. Subsequent protocols include additional views. The rapid ultrasound for shock and hypotension (RUSH) examination introduced a multipoint ultrasound (US) examination that includes detailed evaluation of the chest and abdomen to assess for causes of shock. Several other protocols have also emerged with varying numbers of US views. Regardless of the specific protocol involved, each of these protocols focuses on the use of US to rapidly identify etiologies of hypotension, with particular attention to conditions that require emergent intervention. Whether the shock is due to a cardiogenic etiology, an obstructive etiology, hypovolemia, or a distributive cause, an organized scanning protocol will narrow the differential diagnosis. The progress and sophistication in POCUS examinations allow detailed evaluation of the hypotensive patient.

The Heart

A focused cardiac US is central to all of the described protocols for US evaluation of the hypotensive patient. The techniques to perform focused echocardiography are explained in the echocardiography chapters.

The initial phase of resuscitation requires estimation of cardiac function, particularly left ventricular ejection fraction. Qualitatively evaluating ejection fraction is straightforward for sonographers of all skill levels. Categorization of the ejection fraction is trifold: preserved, moderately depressed, or severely depressed. This rapid estimate guides the resuscitation and determines whether the etiology of the hypotension is primarily cardiogenic.

Further interrogation of the heart is performed, depending on the clinical scenario. US is the modality of choice to identify pericardial fluid. This is best evaluated with a substernal or parasternal view. Sonographic characteristics of cardiac tamponade, characterized by right ventricular collapse and alteration of the intraventricular septum, are assessed on the focused cardiac examination. Evaluation of the aortic root is performed when there is suspicion for aortic dissection. With a parasternal long-axis view, an aortic root measurement (no greater than 3.5 cm) can be rapidly evaluated. Other signs of aortic root dissection include pericardial effusion and aortic valve insufficiency. However, these may not be present. Evaluation of the right heart for right heart strain is an important addition to the cardiac examination when massive pulmonary embolus is in the differential diagnosis. This is best assessed with the apical four-chamber view.

The Lungs

The addition of lung US has been an important addition to the POCUS evaluation of the hypotensive patient. The full description of this protocol is outlined in the pulmonary chapters. Originally described by Lichtenstein, the rapid pulmonary assessment provides several important data elements in differentiating types of shock.

Clinicians generally focus on two aspects of pulmonary US in the evaluation of the hypotensive patient. First is the identification of a pneumothorax. US accurately identifies pneumothoraxes. The determination of whether the pneumothorax is causing hypotension via a tension phenomenon is a clinical decision. The second is the identification of interstitial fluid. A rapid scan of the lungs to determine whether there is interstitial fluid consistent with pulmonary edema versus the absence of interstitial fluid may help the clinician determine whether there is a cardiogenic etiology for the hypotension. The presence of interstitial fluid also guides the fluid resuscitation. Patients with hypotension and pulmonary edema have more complex resuscitation algorithms, whether the primary source of hypotension is cardiogenic or not.

The Abdomen

Protocols evaluating for causes of hypotension include abdominal views. Of prime importance is the evaluation for free (intraperitoneal) fluid within the abdominal cavity. It is important to determine if a patient presenting with hypotension has free peritoneal fluid. The etiology of the free fluid requires clinical synthesis of the case. Providers will consider trauma, ruptured ectopic pregnancy, aortic catastrophe, and other less common etiologies. Importantly, US cannot differentiate the type of fluid in the abdomen. This must be considered in evaluating the examination. Given the time-dependent nature of intraperitoneal bleeding, excluding the presence of peritoneal free fluid is of critical importance. Protocols differ as to the number of peritoneal views that are

required and may include the right upper quadrant, left upper quadrant, and pelvic views or a single right upper quadrant view. It is important to consider the clinical context of the hypotensive patient. A single right upper quadrant view has been shown to have a very high sensitivity when performed on a hypotensive trauma patient. In addition, the right upper quadrant view is the technically easiest view to reliably obtain. For this reason, this view should be emphasized during the initial US scan of the abdomen in the hypotensive patient.

After a scan for peritoneal free fluid, attention is turned to the vessels of the abdomen. Evaluation of the inferior vena cava (IVC) is an important component of the evaluation of the undifferentiated hypotensive patient. The IVC diameter has been used as a surrogate for intravascular volume status in patients. It is surmised that rapid determination of the IVC diameter, as well as IVC collapsibility, determines the patient's intravascular volume status. This may help guide fluid resuscitation. The current published validity of this practice is mixed, however. Many factors affect the IVC diameter and collapsibility in addition to intravascular volume status. The IVC diameter is increased by elevated right-sided heart pressure, as seen in cardiac tamponade, pulmonary embolus, and heart failure. The diameter and collapsibility are changed with positive pressure ventilation. Although the IVC assessment has many factors that affect its accuracy, it remains a common component of intravascular volume assessment.

The abdominal aorta is interrogated in patients who present a concern for aortic catastrophe. Upon discovery of an abdominal aortic aneurysm, the clinician must decide based on clinical context if the aneurysm has ruptured, causing hypotension. As the aorta is retroperitoneal, one does not expect intraperitoneal free fluid with a ruptured abdominal aortic aneurysm. Size of the aneurysm and the context of the hypotension will contribute to the likelihood of the diagnosis. The presence of an abdominal aortic aneurysm may be the only evidence to suggest a ruptured aortic aneurysm as the cause of hypotension.

Some have described the addition of the femoral vessels to detect deep venous thrombosis as a component of the hypotensive protocol as surrogate markers for pulmonary embolus. In a critically ill patient, this examination may not contribute to narrowing the differential in an emergent fashion.

PUTTING IT ALL TOGETHER

Literature on the practice of undifferentiated hypotensive protocols is limited. A study by Jones et al. demonstrated that the use of a focused protocol of US to evaluate a hypotensive patient narrows the differential during the initial resuscitative phase. During emergency resuscitation, many important practices are utilized to exclude readily reversible causes of hypotension. The practice of POCUS evaluation of the hypotensive patient provides important data to rapidly determine the cause of the hypotension. Practitioners of POCUS must practice a clinically focused US evaluation of a hypotensive patient, rather than merely performing the prescribed views of any specific protocol. Rapidly identifying uncommon but reversible etiologies is paramount when dealing with the critically ill hypotensive patient (Table 14.1).

ULTRASOUND DURING CARDIAC ARREST

Use of US during cardiac arrest is an increasingly common practice. Empirically, it makes sense that viewing the heart directly would have an impact on resuscitative outcomes. In addition, it seems logical to conclude that US would guide the decision to continue or terminate resuscitation. However, data supporting these practices are inconclusive.

The use of US in the resuscitation of patients with cardiac arrest, both out-of-hospital and in-hospital, has been evaluated by a few small studies. A recent meta-analysis examined whether US predicts survival to hospital discharge. Conclusions from this meta-analysis support that the lack of organized cardiac activity is associated with a very poor prognosis. A more recent study evaluated the inter-rater heterogeneity of determining the definition of organized cardiac activity. With US, the heart may manifest variable degrees of motion. The lack of clarity in this definition impedes a clear interpretation of the current literature. Clinicians using US are commonly faced with a heart having some variable degrees of disorganized movement during electrical activity versus the complete absence of any cardiac activity. The current literature does not provide clear guidance on how to utilize the information gleaned on cardiac US in cardiopulmonary resuscitation (CPR). In addition, it has been questioned whether the routine use of US is helpful during resuscitation. Several studies illustrated that the use of US decreases the CPR fraction time (the proportion of time of active CPR over the total resuscitation time) and causes longer interruptions in CPR. There is preliminary work to evaluate the usefulness of transesophageal echocardiogram in cardiac arrest, with the intention of avoiding the interruption of chest compressions. The concept is early in development and has yet to be fully evaluated. Given that US typically delays chest compressions and lacks evidence of outcome benefit, the American Heart Association Committee on Cardiac Care does not currently support the routine use of US in cardiac arrest.

It should be noted that almost all CPR research using US currently is based upon adult data only. There are no published prospective trials on use in pediatric cardiac arrest resuscitation. Some observational reports suggest that US may help in the pulse check of pediatric patients and the evaluation of asystole. The American Heart Association guidelines that most recently addressed US in pediatric cardiac arrest state that there is insufficient evidence to recommend for or against US in pediatric resuscitation.

To date, there is no published protocol that incorporates US into CPR in an evidence-based fashion. Some important recent work suggests that US may be helpful in some specific types of cardiac arrests, such as pulseless electrical activity, and to identify organized cardiac activity when no palpable pulse is present. It is unclear, however, whether US offers any additional relevant information for the termination of resuscitation over already existing guidelines. Given this, the recommendations are to minimize any interruption of CPR when using US and apply US in a directed fashion when searching for acutely reversible conditions, if suspected.

TABLE 14.1   Summary of the Major Ultrasound Protocols for Medical Shock Assessment

Protocol	ACES	EGLS	Elmer/Noble	FALLS	Fate	POCUS	RUSH: Pump Tank Pipes	Trinity	UHP
Cardiac	1	2	1	3	1	3	1	1	3
IVC (inferior vena cava)	2	3	2	4		4	2		
Fast A/P FAST	4		3			1	3	3	1
Aorta	3					5	7	2	2
Lungs PTX (pneumothoax)		1	4	2		2	6		
Lungs effusion	5				2		4		
Lungs edema		4	5	1		6	5		
DVT (deep venous thrombosis)						7	8		
Ectopic pregnancy						8			

Numbers indicate examination sequences for each protocol.
(Modified from Seif D, Perera P, Mailot T et al. Bedside ultrasound in resuscitation and the rapid ultrasound in shock protocol. *Crit Care Res Pract.* 2012;2012:503254.)

BIBLIOGRAPHY

Aagaard R, et al. Timing of focused cardiac ultrasound during advanced life support - A prospective clinical study. *Resuscitation*. 2018;124:126–131.

Ahn JH, et al. SEARCH 8Es: a novel point of care ultrasound protocol for patients with chest pain, dyspnea or symptomatic hypotension in the emergency department. *PLoS One*. 2017;12(3):e0174581.

April MD, Long B. Does spontaneous cardiac motion, identified with point-of-care echocardiography during cardiac arrest, predict survival? *Ann Emerg Med*. 2018;71(2):208–210.

Atkinson P, et al. International Federation for Emergency Medicine Consensus Statement: sonography in hypotension and cardiac arrest (SHoC): an international consensus on the use of point of care ultrasound for undifferentiated hypotension and during cardiac arrest. *CJEM*. 2017;19(6):459–470.

Atkinson PR, et al. Abdominal and Cardiac Evaluation with Sonography in Shock (ACES): an approach by emergency physicians for the use of ultrasound in patients with undifferentiated hypotension. *Emerg Med J*. 2009;26(2):87–91.

Blaivas M, Fox JC. Outcome in cardiac arrest patients found to have cardiac standstill on the bedside emergency department echocardiogram. *Acad Emerg Med*. 2001;8(6):616–621.

Clattenburg EJ, et al. Point-of-care ultrasound use in patients with cardiac arrest is associated prolonged cardiopulmonary resuscitation pauses: a prospective cohort study. *Resuscitation*. 2018;122:65–68.

Costantino TG, et al. Accuracy of emergency medicine ultrasound in the evaluation of abdominal aortic aneurysm. *J Emerg Med*. 2005;29(4):455–460.

Fair J, et al. Transesophageal echocardiography: guidelines for point-of-care applications in cardiac arrest resuscitation. *Ann Emerg Med*. 2018;71(2):201–207.

Fojtik JP, Costantino TG, Dean AJ. The diagnosis of aortic dissection by emergency medicine ultrasound. *J Emerg Med*. 2007;32(2):191–196.

Gaspari R, et al. Emergency department point-of-care ultrasound in out-of-hospital and in-ED cardiac arrest. *Resuscitation*. 2016;109:33–39.

Ghane MR, et al. Accuracy of rapid ultrasound in shock (RUSH) exam for diagnosis of shock in critically ill patients. *Trauma Mon*. 2015;20(1):e20095.

Gui J, et al. Is the collapsibility index of the inferior vena cava an accurate predictor for the early detection of intravascular volume change? *Shock*. 2018;49(1):29–32.

Huis In 't Veld MA, et al. Ultrasound use during cardiopulmonary resuscitation is associated with delays in chest compressions. *Resuscitation*. 2017;119:95–98.

Jones AE, et al. Randomized, controlled trial of immediate versus delayed goal-directed ultrasound to identify the cause of nontraumatic hypotension in emergency department patients. *Crit Care Med*. 2004;32(8):1703–1708.

Kleinman ME, et al. Part 14: pediatric advanced life support: 2010 American Heart Association Guidelines for Cardiopulmonary Resuscitation and Emergency Cardiovascular Care. *Circulation*. 2010;122(18 suppl 3):S876–S908.

Knudtson JL, et al. Surgeon-performed ultrasound for pneumothorax in the trauma suite. *J Trauma*. 2004;56(3):527–530.

Kuhn M, et al. Emergency department ultrasound scanning for abdominal aortic aneurysm: accessible, accurate, and advantageous. *Ann Emerg Med*. 2000;36(3):219–223.

Labovitz AJ, et al. Focused cardiac ultrasound in the emergent setting: a consensus statement of the American Society of Echocardiography and American College of Emergency Physicians. *J Am Soc Echocardiogr*. 2010;23(12):12251230.

Lichtenstein D. Lung ultrasound in acute respiratory failure an introduction to the BLUE-protocol. *Minerva Anestesiol*. 2009;75(5):313–317.

Lichtenstein. BLUE-protocol and FALLS-protocol: two applications of lung ultrasound in the critically ill. *Chest*. 2015;147(6):1659–1670.

Lichtenstein, Meziere GA. Relevance of lung ultrasound in the diagnosis of acute respiratory failure: the BLUE protocol. *Chest*. 2008;134(1):117–125.

Link MS, et al. Part 7: Adult Advanced Cardiovascular Life Support: 2015 American Heart Association Guidelines Update for Cardiopulmonary Resuscitation and Emergency Cardiovascular Care. *Circulation*. 2015;132(18 suppl 2):S444–S464.

Long E, et al. Does respiratory variation of inferior vena cava diameter predict fluid responsiveness in spontaneously ventilating children with sepsis. *Emerg Med Australas*. 2018.

Ma OJ, et al. Evaluation of hemoperitoneum using a single-vs multiple-view ultrasonographic examination. *Acad Emerg Med*. 1995;2(7):581–586.

Mandavia DP, et al. Bedside echocardiography by emergency physicians. *Ann Emerg Med*. 2001;38(4):377–382.

Mayron R, et al. Echocardiography performed by emergency physicians: impact on diagnosis and therapy. *Ann Emerg Med*. 1988;17(2):150–154.

Milne J, et al. Sonography in hypotension and cardiac arrest (SHoC): rates of abnormal findings in undifferentiated hypotension and during cardiac arrest as a basis for consensus on a hierarchical point of care ultrasound protocol. *Cureus*. 2016;8(4):e564.

Molokoane-Mokgoro K, Goldstein LN, Wells M. Ultrasound evaluation of the respiratory changes of the inferior vena cava and axillary vein diameter at rest and during positive pressure ventilation in spontaneously breathing healthy volunteers. *Emerg Med J*. 2018;35(5):297–302.

Ng NYY, et al. Evaluation for occult sepsis incorporating NIRS and emergency sonography. *Am J Emerg Med.* 2018.

Niendorff DF, et al. Rapid cardiac ultrasound of inpatients suffering PEA arrest performed by nonexpert sonographers. *Resuscitation.* 2005;67(1):81–87.

Orso D, et al. Accuracy of ultrasonographic measurements of inferior vena cava to determine fluid responsiveness: a systematic review and meta-analysis. *J Intensive Care Med.* 2018. https://doi.org/10.1177/0885066617752308.

Perera P, et al. The RUSH exam: rapid ultrasound in shock in the evaluation of the critically lll. *Emerg Med Clin North Am.* 2010;28(1):29–56. vii.

Perkins AM, Liteplo A, Noble VE. Ultrasound diagnosis of type a aortic dissection. *J Emerg Med.* 2010;38(4):490–493.

Rose JS, et al. The UHP ultrasound protocol: a novel ultrasound approach to the empiric evaluation of the undifferentiated hypotensive patient. *Am J Emerg Med.* 2001;19(4):299–302.

Salen P, et al. Does the presence or absence of sonographically identified cardiac activity predict resuscitation outcomes of cardiac arrest patients? *Am J Emerg Med.* 2005;23(4):459–462.

Schmidt GA. POINT: should acute fluid resuscitation be guided primarily by inferior vena cava ultrasound for patients in shock? *Yes. Chest.* 2017;151(3):531–532.

Sekiguchi H, et al. Focused cardiac ultrasound in the early resuscitation of severe sepsis and septic shock: a prospective pilot study. *J Anesth.* 2017;31(4):487–493.

Steffen K, et al. Return of viable cardiac function after sonographic cardiac standstill in pediatric cardiac arrest. *Pediatr Emerg Care.* 2017;33(1):58–59.

Tayal VS, Graf CD, Gibbs MA. Prospective study of accuracy and outcome of emergency ultrasound for abdominal aortic aneurysm over two years. *Acad Emerg Med.* 2003;10(8):867–871.

Tsung JW, Blaivas M. Feasibility of correlating the pulse check with focused point-of-care echocardiography during pediatric cardiac arrest: a case series. *Resuscitation.* 2008;77(2):264–269.

Volpicelli G. Usefulness of emergency ultrasound in nontraumatic cardiac arrest. *Am J Emerg Med.* 2011;29(2):216–223.

Wilkerson RG, Stone MB. Sensitivity of bedside ultrasound and supine anteroposterior chest radiographs for the identification of pneumothorax after blunt trauma. *Acad Emerg Med.* 2010;17(1):11–17.

Wu C, et al. The predictive value of bedside ultrasound to restore spontaneous circulation in patients with pulseless electrical activity: a systematic review and meta-analysis. *PLoS One.* 2018;13(1):e0191636.

Wu J, et al. Evaluation of the fluid responsiveness in patients with septic shock by ultrasound plus the passive leg raising test. *J Surg Res.* 2018;224:207–214.

SECTION 4

Focused Assessment with Sonography in Trauma

15

FAST of the Abdomen – Beyond the Basics: False Positives, Limitations, and Approach to the Unstable Patient

John R. Richards, John P. McGahan

INTRODUCTION

The development of focused assessment with sonography for trauma (FAST) over 30 years ago enabled clinicians to rapidly screen for injury at the bedside of patients, especially those hemodynamically unstable for transport to the computed tomography (CT) suite. The identification of free fluid within the peritoneal cavity, pericardium, and pleural spaces can be accomplished with point-of-care ultrasound (US) immediately upon patient arrival to the hospital. Other applications of FAST include detection of solid organ injury, pneumothorax, fractures, and serial examinations, as well as use in prehospital transport and multiple casualty settings as a triage tool. Before FAST, invasive procedures such as diagnostic peritoneal lavage and exploratory laparotomy were commonly utilized to diagnose intraabdominal injury (IAI). Today the FAST examination has evolved into a more comprehensive study of the abdomen, heart, chest, and inferior vena cava, and many variations in technique, protocols, and interpretation exist.

US was first utilized for the examination of trauma patients in the 1970s in Europe. It was not widely adopted in North America until the 1990s, during which time the FAST acronym was defined as "focused abdominal sonography for trauma." As FAST evolved into a more comprehensive examination, the acronym was changed to "focused assessment with sonography for trauma." Since then, FAST has become the common initial screening modality in trauma centers worldwide, and it is included in the Advanced Trauma Life Support (ATLS) program for evaluation of the hypotensive trauma patient. A unique aspect of FAST is that it is routinely utilized by radiologists, emergency physicians, surgeons, and paramedics with variable training and experience. Over time, a new role for FAST has evolved, in which its use in the evaluation of unstable, hypotensive trauma patients is emphasized. The most effective use of FAST has been rapid triage of hemodynamically unstable trauma patients to definitive intervention.

In the mid-2000s, the addition of US evaluation of the thorax to detect pneumothorax to the traditional FAST examination resulted in a new acronym, "e-FAST," or extended FAST. Several other protocols have been developed for evaluation of shock, respiratory distress, and cardiac arrest, some of which feature echocardiography. The number of different protocols for evaluation of the critically injured or ill patient is a source of confusion, especially as even more protocols are developed with creative acronyms and abbreviations. In this chapter we will focus on the abdominal portion of the overall FAST examination, as point-of-care evaluation of the heart and lungs is covered in separate chapters.

ULTRASOUND TECHNIQUE

The original FAST scan included views of the right upper quadrant, which included the perihepatic area and hepatorenal recess (Morison's pouch), of the left upper quadrant encompassing the perisplenic view, the suprapubic view (pouch of Douglas), and later a subxiphoid pericardial view (Fig. 15.1). The preferred initial site for detection of free fluid with FAST is the right upper quadrant view using a lower-frequency (3.5–5 MHz) curved array transducer. The liver serves as an acoustic window during insonation of the hepatorenal space and liver parenchyma. In the left upper quadrant view, the spleen is the target during examination of the splenorenal fossa and perisplenic area. Cephalad scanning enables visualization of the left pleural space. Moving the probe caudally brings the inferior pole of the left kidney and paracolic gutter into view. The perisplenic area may be inadequately scanned due to difficult physical access. Rolling the patient to the right side and/or having the patient take a deep breath is helpful in evaluating this area, as small amounts of free fluid may collect superiorly to the spleen. The suprapubic view enables visualization of the most dependent space in the peritoneal cavity. The transducer is placed above the pubic symphysis in a sagittal plane and swept side to side, then rotated transversely and repeated. Reverse Trendelenburg positioning may enhance the detection of free fluid in the pelvis. The visualization of small amounts of free fluid in the pelvis is aided by the presence of a full bladder. When free fluid is present, it is most frequently located posterior or superior to the bladder and/or the uterus. Free fluid in the pelvis can be missed when a Foley catheter is placed to empty the

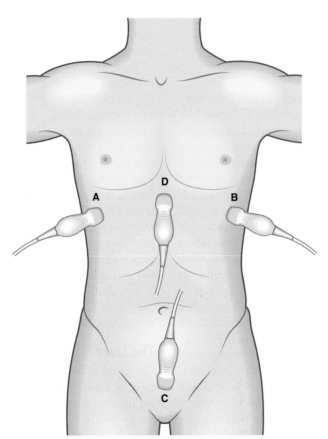

Fig. 15.1 Probe placement. The original FAST scan included views of the (A) right upper quadrant, which included the perihepatic area and hepatorenal recess (Morison's pouch); (B) left upper quadrant encompassing the perisplenic view; (C) the suprapubic view (pouch of Douglas); and, later, (D) a subxiphoid pericardial view.

bladder, as the acoustic window for examining the pelvis is removed, limiting the sonographer's ability to discern small amounts of pelvic fluid. Bowel gas, subcutaneous emphysema, and obesity represent common obstacles to full sonographic visualization.

The volume of free fluid necessary to enable detection with FAST is a well-known limitation. In one early study, the mean minimum detectable free-fluid volume in 100 patients undergoing diagnostic peritoneal lavage was 619 mL in the right upper quadrant view. Trendelenburg positioning may improve visualization of free fluid in the splenorenal and hepatorenal interface. FAST performed in the Trendelenburg position enables detection of smaller amounts of hepatorenal free fluid than supine. Even smaller volumes of free fluid are required for detection in the pelvic views of FAST, with median minimal volume of fluid of 100 mL. Scoring systems have been described in the past, and the common theme among these studies is the larger the amount and number of sites of free fluid, the greater the likelihood of injury or need for surgical intervention.

Hemoperitoneum

Free fluid detected by US is assumed to be hemoperitoneum, which usually appears anechoic or hypoechoic compared with adjacent solid organs. During prolonged periods, this hemorrhage may organize into clots and become more echogenic-appearing on US. In the absence of injury or other pathology, free fluid should not be found within the peritoneal cavity on US, with the exception of the suprapubic view: only small amounts of rectouterine (pouch of Douglas) free fluid in women of childbearing age should be detectable. These small free-fluid collections of up to 50 mL in the pouch of Douglas are considered physiologic, and amounts exceeding 50 mL should be regarded as pathologic in the setting of trauma. As the initial FAST represents a "snapshot" in time, serial examinations performed on stable blunt trauma patients may be useful (Fig. 15.2). Examination after stabilization gives the sonographer more time for a comprehensive scan. With active intraperitoneal hemorrhage, the amount of free fluid should theoretically increase with time. Serial FAST examinations have been reported to decrease the false-negative rate by up to 50% and may be a logical alternative for stable trauma patients, patients with a sudden change in hemodynamic status or physical examination, and pregnant patients to mitigate radiation exposure.

False Negatives and Positives

The sensitivity of FAST ranges from 69% to 98% and specificity from 95% to 100% for detection of hemoperitoneum. The initial studies of FAST reporting high sensitivity compared FAST findings with patient outcome and not CT. Later studies comparing FAST with CT results showed lower sensitivity, largely due to the fact that CT detected isolated solid organ injuries without the presence of hemoperitoneum. Since then, more recent critical evaluations of FAST have appeared, highlighting its high false-negative rate in stable trauma patients. In hemodynamically stable patients, a negative FAST without follow-up CT may miss an IAI. Thus the potential for underdiagnoses of IAI with FAST is now well recognized. Clinical suspicion, mechanism of injury, and change in clinical examination or hemodynamic status should always be included in deciding upon further diagnostic testing in patients with negative initial FAST. For patients with negative FAST, observation, serial FAST, CT, or contrast-enhanced US may be chosen.

False-positive scans may result from detection of ascites, peritoneal dialysate, ventriculoperitoneal shunt outflow, polycystic ovarian disease, and ovarian cyst rupture. Massive intravascular volume resuscitation may result in a false-positive FAST examination from intravascular to intraperitoneal fluid transudation. Although free fluid detected by FAST in trauma patients is assumed to be hemoperitoneum, it can also represent injury-related urine, bile, and bowel contents. Patients with delayed presentation after trauma may have hemoperitoneum containing clots, which can have mixed echogenicity and be missed or misinterpreted. Perinephric fat, which widens the hepatorenal and splenorenal interface, may be misinterpreted as free fluid or subcapsular hematoma, also known as the *"double-line"* sign. Comparison views of each kidney may be helpful in these cases.

The Liver

Detection of liver injury, even in the absence of free fluid, is possible with point-of-care US. Although not included in the FAST protocol, careful insonation of the normally homogenous liver parenchyma for any irregularities may detect injuries such as lacerations, contusions, and hematomas. Ultrasound has been shown to have very high sensitivity for detection of grades III and higher liver injury. For parenchymal

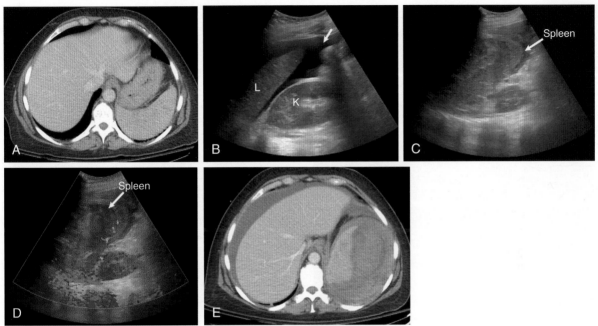

Fig. 15.2 Serial FAST in a 44-year-old man with blunt abdominal trauma from a motor vehicle accident with abdominal pain. (A) Initial CT scan was interpreted as normal. Slight inhomogeneity of the spleen was thought to be due to normal enhancement of splenic pulp. (B) Nine hours later, the patient developed hypotension, and a bedside FAST examination was performed, which demonstrated free fluid in the upper abdomen (*arrow*) and pelvis. *K*, Kidney; *L*, liver. (C) Real-time images showed marked heterogeneity to the spleen. (D) Color flow demonstrated a fairly avascular appearance of the spleen. (E) Patient was resuscitated and underwent CT, during which a large spleen laceration with subcapsular hematoma and free fluid was detected. Patient was rushed to the operating room for successful emergency splenectomy. (From Richards JR, McGahan JP. Focused assessment with sonography in trauma (FAST) in 2017: what radiologists can learn. *Radiology*. 2017;283:30–48. Copyright: Radiological Society of North America [2017].)

injuries detected with US, three distinct patterns are identified. The most common sonographic pattern is a discrete hyperechoic area visualized within the hepatic architecture, followed by a diffuse hyperechoic pattern (Fig. 15.3). The least common pattern is a discrete hypoechoic focus. Hepatic injuries may be difficult to detect when the liver capsule remains intact. The liver has a greater volume than the spleen; thus small intraparenchymal lesions may be missed with the rapid FAST technique.

The Spleen

Rapid identification of spleen injuries is important due to the highly vascular nature of this organ and the potential for extensive and life-threatening intraperitoneal hemorrhage. The majority of spleen injuries have associated hemoperitoneum. However, if the capsule of the spleen remains intact after trauma, hemoperitoneum may not be detected. In these situations several distinct patterns of parenchymal appearance have been identified on US for spleen injuries. The most common sonographic patterns are diffuse heterogeneous (both hyperechoic and hypoechoic), discrete hyperechoic, discrete hypoechoic, and perisplenic crescent (Figs. 15.4–15.6). More recently, contrast-enhanced US has been shown to be more sensitive in detecting spleen and other solid organ injuries compared with conventional sonography.

The Kidneys

The kidneys are retroperitoneal structures, and unless significant trauma occurs directly to the kidney, it is unlikely that free fluid would be observed in the abdomen. In one study of isolated renal injury, free fluid was

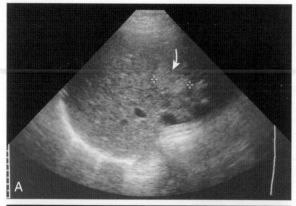

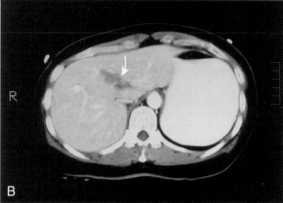

Fig. 15.3 A 46-year-old female pedestrian was struck by an automobile. (A) The sonogram demonstrates a discrete hyperechoic lesion (*arrow with markers*) and subhepatic free fluid. (B) The corresponding CT scan shows a laceration of the left lobe of the liver (*arrow*). (From Richards JR, McGahan JP, Pali MJ, Bohnen PA. Sonographic detection of blunt hepatic trauma: hemoperitoneum and parenchymal patterns of injury. *J Trauma.* 1999;47:1092–1097. copyright: Lippincott Williams & Wilkins [1999].)

detected in only 7 of 20 patients. The majority of renal injuries occurs with concomitant other major organ injuries, such as splenic rupture, liver laceration, or tears of the bowel or mesentery that require operative repair. However, careful interrogation of the renal parenchyma may reveal hyperechoic, hypoechoic, and mixed abnormalities representing lacerations, contusion, and hematomas (Figs. 15.7–15.10). Such findings, especially when hematuria is concurrently detected, should prompt further imaging with CT. The most common pitfall on US is interpretation of perinephric fat, which widens the hepatorenal and splenorenal interface. Perinephric fat may be misinterpreted as free fluid or subcapsular

hematoma, also known as the *"double-line" sign*. Comparison views of each kidney may be helpful in these cases.

The Uterus and Pregnancy

Blunt and penetrating trauma is the leading cause of nonobstetric maternal mortality, affecting up to 7% of pregnancies. It is an important cause of fetal loss, and most obstetric complications from trauma occur in the third trimester. For pregnant trauma patients, US is advantageous, in that there is no contrast material or radiation exposure to the mother or fetus. In addition to the rapid assessment for free fluid, US can assess for fetal heart motion, fetal activity, amniotic fluid volume, approximate gestational age, and placenta. A small number of studies have shown FAST in pregnant patients with blunt abdominal trauma to have similar sensitivity and specificity to nonpregnant patients. Examination of the placenta is very important, as abruption may have a variety of appearances, such as thickened or avascular regions without accompanying free fluid in the pelvis. Fetal cardiac activity should always be checked with M-mode US, and the fetus should be examined for other injuries sustained during impact to the maternal abdomen. The gravid uterus may distort the usual sonographic landmarks in the suprapubic view. Thus evaluation of the pouch of Douglas for hemoperitoneum in this patient subgroup requires careful technique and some experience. Distinguishing between intrauterine and extrauterine fluid can be challenging. Free intraperitoneal fluid may result from hemorrhage due to solid-organ IAI, amniotic fluid from uterine rupture, or both. For patients with negative or equivocal FAST examinations, continuous cardiotocographic monitoring should commence as early as possible to screen for placental abruption.

The ability to detect free fluid in the pregnant patient may differ for different stages of pregnancy. For instance, there is a higher rate of detection of free fluid in the first and second trimesters of pregnancy compared with the third trimester of pregnancy. However, there is a higher rate of false-positive detection of free fluid in the first trimester compared with the second or third trimester. This may be secondary to "physiologic" free fluid often seen in the first trimester of pregnancy. Patients in whom free pelvic fluid is detected in the first trimester of pregnancy without significant trauma should undergo continuous monitoring or follow-up

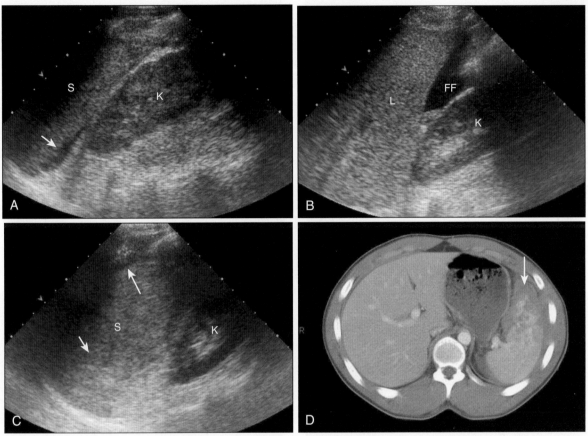

Fig. 15.4 Blunt abdominal trauma after a snowboarding accident in a 19-year-old man. The patient was treated nonsurgically and was discharged later without complications. (A) Sagittal sonogram of the splenorenal interface showing free fluid (*arrow*). *K,* Kidney; *S,* spleen. (B) Transverse sonogram of the right upper quadrant showing free fluid (*FF*) in the Morison's pouch. *L,* liver. (C) Another sagittal view of the left upper quadrant showing inhomogeneous splenic parenchyma with a hyperechoic focus (*short arrow*) and subcapsular fluid (*long arrow*). (D) Computed tomogram showing splenic rupture with perisplenic free fluid (*arrow*). (From Richards JR, McGahan PJ, Jewell MG, Fukushima LC, McGahan JP. Sonographic patterns of intraperitoneal hemorrhage associated with blunt splenic injury. *J Ultrasound Med.* 2004;23:387–394. Copyright: John Wiley & Sons [2004].)

US. There is even greater difficulty detecting IAI with FAST in the late second or third trimester of pregnancy. Placental abruption may have devastating consequences for both the fetus and mother but may be a difficult sonographic diagnosis. The normal placenta usually has a fairly homogeneous appearance until the late third trimester (Fig. 15.11), when placental calcifications may occur. During abruption of the placenta, there may be subtle sonographic changes, such as a more heterogeneous appearance. Placental thickening may also be observed (Fig. 15.12). It is important, if possible, to compare the emergency point-of-care US examination with any prior obstetrical US images to evaluate for any change in the appearance of the placenta. The anterior placenta is more prone to injury from direct impact to the anterior abdominal wall. In rare circumstances low-dose CT may be needed to diagnose placental injury when significant trauma occurs. Careful US examination may also detect rare fetal injuries (Fig. 15.13). In any pregnant patient with trauma fetal monitoring, an M-mode US should always be performed.

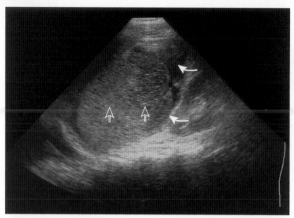

Fig. 15.5 Longitudinal ultrasound of the left upper quadrant demonstrates subtle, diffuse, disorganized appearance of the spleen, with an echogenic cephalad portion (*large open arrow*) and hypoechoic caudal portion (*small open arrow*). Focal echogenic areas are also noted within the hypoechoic crescent surrounding the spleen (*curved arrow*). (From Richards JR, McGahan JP, Jones CD, Zhan S, Gerscovich EO. Ultrasound detection of blunt splenic injury. *Injury*. 2001;32:95–103. Copyright: Elsevier [2001].)

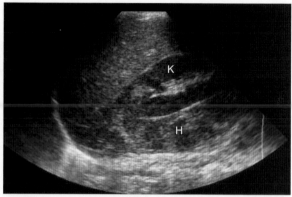

Fig. 15.7 Hematoma posterior to the kidney. Longitudinal ultrasonogram demonstrates hematoma (*H*) posterior to the kidney (*K*) causing anterior displacement of the kidney. (From McGahan JP, Richards JR, Jones CD, Gerscovich EO. Use of ultrasonography in the patient with acute renal trauma. *J Ultrasound Med*. 1999;18:207–213. Copyright: John Wiley & Sons [1999].)

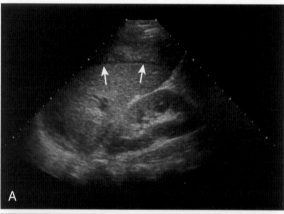

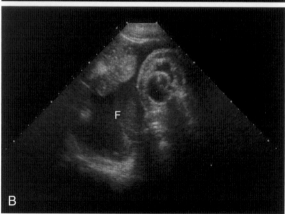

Fig. 15.6 (A) Longitudinal ultrasound of the left upper quadrant demonstrates a hypoechoic crescent (*arrows*) surrounding the spleen. (B) Longitudinal ultrasound of the pelvis reveals free fluid (*F*) as less echogenic than the perisplenic crescent. (From Richards JR, McGahan JP, Jones CD, Zhan S, Gerscovich EO. Ultrasound detection of blunt splenic injury. *Injury*. 2001;32:95–103. Copyright: Elsevier [2001].)

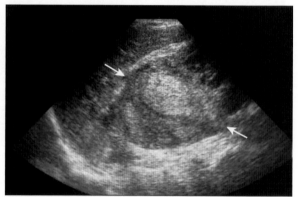

Fig. 15.8 Grade III renal injury. Longitudinal ultrasonogram demonstrates mixed isoechoic and hyperechoic patterns in the enlarged renal fossa (*arrows*), which at nephrectomy was found to show renal parenchymal fragmentation with active hemorrhage. (From McGahan JP, Richards JR, Jones CD, Gerscovich EO. Use of ultrasonography in the patient with acute renal trauma. *J Ultrasound Med*. 1999;18:207–213. Copyright: John Wiley & Sons [1999].)

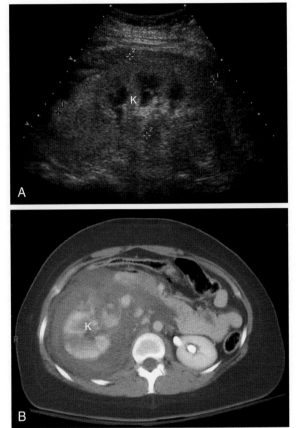

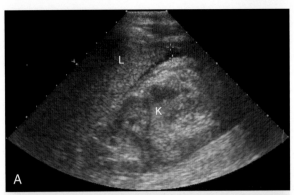

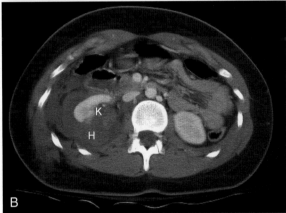

Fig. 15.9 A 24-year-old male involved in a motorcycle crash who sustained a grade III renal laceration requiring nephrectomy. (A) Transverse ultrasonogram of the right kidney (*K*) reveals distorted parenchyma with mixed echogenicity and no clearly visualized renal capsule. There is a surrounding hematoma noted as well. (B) CT demonstrates kidney (*K*) disruption and a large surrounding hematoma. (From McGahan PJ, Richards JR, Bair AE, Rose JS. Ultrasound detection of blunt urological trauma: a 6-year study. *Injury.* 2005;36:762–770. Copyright: Elsevier [2005].)

Fig. 15.10 A 17-year-old female in a high-speed motor vehicle crash with subsequent grade III renal laceration requiring nephrectomy. (A) Longitudinal ultrasonogram of the right upper quadrant demonstrates disorganized architecture of the kidney (*K*) with mixed echogenicity. The renal capsule is not clearly defined. There is hypoechoic free fluid in Morison's pouch (*markers*). *L*, liver. (B) CT demonstrates the lacerated kidney (*K*) with surrounding hematoma and areas of active hemorrhage (*H*). (From McGahan PJ, Richards JR, Bair AE, Rose JS. Ultrasound detection of blunt urological trauma: a 6-year study. *Injury.* 2005;36:762–770. Copyright: Elsevier [2005].)

Bowel and Mesentery

Early detection of bowel and mesenteric injuries with FAST is notoriously difficult, as volume of hemorrhage and/or extravagated bowel contents is usually minimal just after the time of injury. Loops of fluid-filled bowel should not be confused with free intraperitoneal fluid, and these loops can usually be distinguished from free fluid because they are round and have peristalsis (Fig. 15.14). Additionally, pneumoperitoneum from bowel perforation can mimic air within small and large bowel loops on US, or appear as echogenic lines, bands, or spots with posterior reverberation artifacts.

Free air shifts to the least dependent areas of the peritoneal cavity with change in patient position and is referred to as the *shifting phenomenon.* Ultrasound can detect pneumoperitoneum: when both free fluid and air are present in the peritoneal cavity, the "peritoneal stripe sign" may be visualized with US. Nondependent air may appear as a thickened, echogenic peritoneal stripe with or without reverberation artifacts. The additional view of the "interloop" space, a triangular hypoechoic area between loops of bowel, was shown to improve the sensitivity of FAST in both primary and secondary examinations.

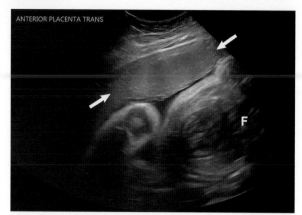

Fig. 15.11 Normal anterior placenta. Real-time ultrasound examination of third-trimester pregnancy demonstrating fetal parts (*F*) and the anterior placenta (*arrows*). Note the homogeneous appearance to the placenta.

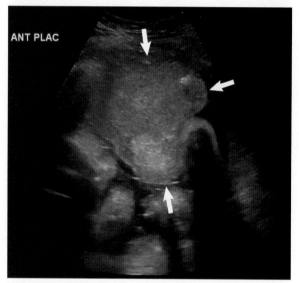

Fig. 15.12 Placental abruption. Real-time ultrasound examination of third-trimester pregnancy after maternal abdominal trauma demonstrates very thickened and heterogeneous appearance to the placenta (*arrows*).

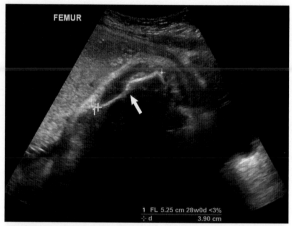

Fig. 15.13 Fractured femur (*arrow*) of the fetus. Real-time ultrasound examination demonstrates "step-off" of the midshaft of the femur representing in utero femoral fracture from trauma. (From Richards JR, McGahan JP. Focused assessment with sonography in trauma (FAST) in 2017: what radiologists can learn. *Radiology*. 2017;283:30–48. Copyright: Radiological Society of North America [2017].)

CONCLUSION

Since its early inception, the use of FAST to detect IAI initially focused on the detection of free fluid. At present, FAST has been expanded to include further interrogation of the heart, lungs, and inferior vena cava (e-FAST). During FAST, it has been shown that intraparenchymal abnormalities may be detected and may be important clues to the presence of IAI, especially in the absence of free fluid. These solid-organ findings, including the uterus, should prompt the clinician to seek further diagnostic testing so that these injuries are not missed. Serial US examinations, contrast-enhanced US, CT, and magnetic resonance imaging (MRI) are possible options to supplement FAST. Additionally, it is important for clinicians utilizing FAST to understand its limitations, especially in stable adult patients with low-impact blunt trauma and in pediatric patients.

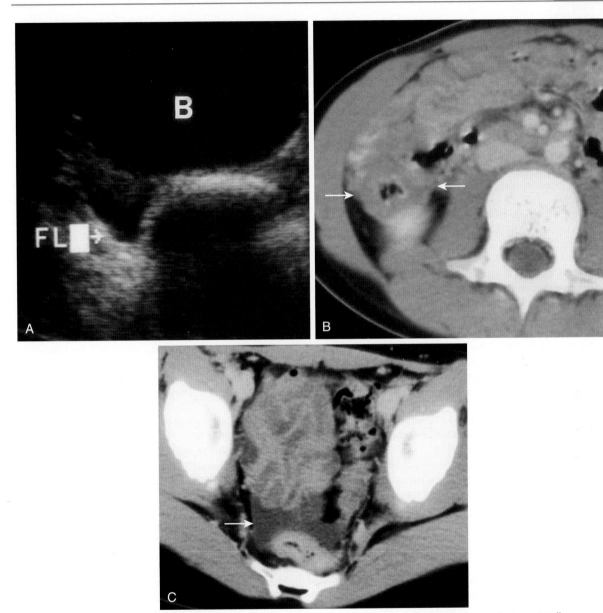

Fig. 15.14 Ascending colon laceration. (A) Transverse ultrasound scan of the pelvis demonstrates a small amount of free fluid posterior to the bladder. *B*, Bladder; *FL*, fluid. (B) CT abdominal scan demonstrates thickening of the lower ascending colon (*arrows*). (C) CT scan of the pelvis demonstrates fluid posterior to the bladder (*arrow*), with loops of bowel anteriorly. (From Richards JR, McGahan JP, Simpson JL, Tabar P. Bowel and mesenteric injury: evaluation with emergency abdominal US. *Radiology.* 1999;211:399–403. Copyright: Radiological Society of North America [1999].)

BIBLIOGRAPHY

Abrams BJ, Sukumvanich P, Seibel R, Moscati R, Jehle D. Ultrasound for the detection of intraperitoneal fluid: the role of Trendelenburg positioning. *Am J Emerg Med.* 1999;17(2):117–120.

Asrani A. Sonographic diagnosis of pneumoperitoneum using the "enhancement of the peritoneal stripe sign." A prospective study. *Emerg Radiol.* 2007;14(1):29–39.

Blackbourne LH, Soffer D, McKenney M, et al. Secondary ultrasound examination increases the sensitivity of the FAST exam in blunt trauma. *J Trauma.* 2004;57(5):934–938.

Boulanger BR, Kearney PA, Brenneman FD, Tsuei B, Ochoa J. Utilization of FAST (Focused Assessment with Sonography for Trauma) in 1999: results of a survey of North American trauma centers. *Am Surg.* 2000;66(11):1049–1055.

Braccini G, Lamacchia M, Boraschi P, et al. Ultrasound versus plain film in the detection of pneumoperitoneum. *Abdom Imaging.* 1996;21(5):404–412.

Branney SW, Wolfe RE, Moore EE, et al. Quantitative sensitivity of ultrasound in detecting free intraperitoneal fluid. *J Trauma.* 1995;39(2):375–380.

Brown MA, Sirlin CB, Farahmand N, Hoyt DB, Casola G. Screening sonography in pregnant patients with blunt abdominal trauma. *J Ultrasound Med.* 2005;24(2):175–181.

Carter JW, Falco MH, Chopko MS, Flynn Jr WJ, Wiles III CE, Guo WA. Do we really rely on FAST for decision-making in the management of blunt abdominal trauma? *Injury.* 2015;46(5):817–821.

Chiu WC, Cushing BM, Rodriguez A, et al. Abdominal injuries without hemoperitoneum: a potential limitation of focused abdominal sonography for trauma (FAST). *J Trauma.* 1997;42(4):617–623.

Huang MS, Liu M, Wu JK, Shih HC, Ko TJ, Lee CH. Ultrasonography for the evaluation of hemoperitoneum during resuscitation: a simple scoring system. *J Trauma.* 1994;36(2):173–177.

Jehle D, Guarino J, Karamanoukian H. Emergency department ultrasound in the evaluation of blunt abdominal trauma. *Am J Emerg Med.* 1993;11(4):342–346.

Jehle D, Stiller G, Wagner D. Sensitivity in detecting free intraperitoneal fluid with the pelvic views of the FAST exam. *Am J Emerg Med.* 2003;21(6):476–478.

Kornezos I, Chatziioannou A, Kokkonouzis I, et al. Findings and limitations of focused ultrasound as a possible screening test in stable adult patients with blunt abdominal trauma: a Greek study. *Eur Radiol.* 2010;20:234–238.

McGahan JP, Horton S, Gerscovich EO, et al. Appearance of solid organ injury with contrast-enhanced sonography in blunt abdominal trauma: preliminary experience. *AJR Am J Roentgenol.* 2006;187(3):658–666.

McGahan JP, Phillips HE, Reid MH, Oi RH. Sonographic spectrum of retroplacental hemorrhage. *Radiology.* 1982;142:481–485.

McGahan JP, Richards JR, Gillen M. The focused abdominal sonography for trauma scan: pearls and pitfalls. *J Ultrasound Med.* 2002;21(7):789–800.

McGahan JP, Richards JR, Jones CD, Gerscovich EO. Use of sonography in the patient with acute renal trauma. *J Ultrasound Med.* 1999;18(3):207–213.

McGahan JP, Rose J, Coates TL, Wisner DH, Newberry P. Use of sonography in the patient with acute abdominal trauma. *J Ultrasound Med.* 1997;16(10):653–664.

McKenney KL, McKenney MG, Cohn SM, et al. Hemoperitoneum score helps determine need for therapeutic laparotomy. *J Trauma.* 2001;50(4):650–654.

Melniker LA, Leibner E, McKenney MG, Lopez P, Briggs WM, Mancuso CA. Randomized controlled clinical trial of point-of-care, limited ultrasonography for trauma in the emergency department: the first sonography outcomes assessment program trial. *Ann Emerg Med.* 2006;48(3):227–235.

Muradali D, Wilson S, Burns PN, Shapiro H, Hope-Simpson D. A specific sign of pneumoperitoneum on sonography: enhancement of the peritoneal stripe. *AJR Am J Roentgenol.* 1999;173(5):1257–1262.

Nunes LW, Simmons S, Hallowell MJ, Kinback R, Trooskin S, Kozar R. Diagnostic performance of trauma US in identifying abdominal or pelvic free fluid and serious abdominal or pelvic injury. *Acad Radiol.* 2001;8(2):128–136.

Ollerton JE, Sugrue M, Balogh Z, D'Amours SK, Giles A, Wyllie P. Prospective study to evaluate the influence of FAST on trauma patient management. *J Trauma.* 2006;60(4):785–791.

Ormsby EL, Geng J, McGahan JP, Richards JR. Pelvic free fluid: clinical importance for reproductive age women with blunt abdominal trauma. *Ultrasound Obstet Gynecol.* 2005;26(3):271–278.

Pearl WS, Todd KH. Sonography for the initial evaluation of blunt abdominal trauma: a review of prospective trials. *Ann Emerg Med.* 1996;27(3):353–361.

Richards JR, McGahan JP. Focused assessment with sonography in trauma (FAST) in 2017: what radiologists can learn. *Radiology.* 2017;283:30–48.

Richards JR, McGahan JP, Jones CD, Zhan S, Gerscovich E. Ultrasound detection of blunt splenic injury. *Injury.* 2001;32(2):95–103.

Richards JR, McGahan JP, Pali MJ, Bohnen PA. Sonographic detection of blunt hepatic trauma: hemoperitoneum and parenchymal patterns of injury. *J Trauma.* 1999;47(6):1092–1097.

Richards JR, McGahan JP, Simpson JL, Tabar P. Bowel and mesenteric injury: evaluation with emergency abdominal US. *Radiology.* 1999;211(2):399–403.

Richards JR, Ormsby EL, Romo MV, Gillen MA, McGahan JP. Blunt abdominal injury in the pregnant patient: detection with US. *Radiology.* 2004;233(2):463–470.

Röthlin MA, Näf R, Amgwerd M, Candinas D, Frick T, Trentz O. Ultrasound in blunt abdominal and thoracic trauma. *J Trauma.* 1993;34(4):488–495.

Rozycki GS, Ochsner MG, Schmidt JA, et al. A prospective study of surgeon-performed ultrasound as the primary adjuvant modality for injured patient assessment. *J Trauma.* 1995;39(3):492–498.

Sato M, Yoshii H. Reevaluation of ultrasonography for solid-organ injury in blunt abdominal trauma. *J Ultrasound Med.* 2004;23(12):1583–1596.

Scalea TM, Rodriguez A, Chiu WC, et al. Focused assessment with sonography for trauma (FAST): results from an international consensus conference. *J Trauma.* 1999;46(3):466–472.

Shanmuganathan K, Mirvis SE, Sherbourne CD, Chiu WC, Rodriguez A. Hemoperitoneum as the sole indicator of abdominal visceral injuries: a potential limitation of screening abdominal US for trauma. *Radiology.* 1999;212(2):423–430.

Sierzenski PR, Schofer JM, Bauman MJ, Nomura JT. The double-line sign: a false positive finding on the focused assessment with sonography for trauma (FAST) examination. *J Emerg Med.* 2011;40(2):188–189.

Sirlin CB, Casola G, Brown MA, et al. US of blunt abdominal trauma: importance of free pelvic fluid in women of reproductive age. *Radiology.* 2001;219(1):229–235.

Sirlin CB, Casola G, Brown MA, Patel N, Bendavid EJ, Hoyt DB. Quantification of fluid on screening ultrasonography for blunt abdominal trauma: a simple scoring system to predict severity of injury. *J Ultrasound Med.* 2001;20(4):359–364.

Slutzman JE, Arvold LA, Rempell JS, Stone MB, Kimberly HH. Positive FAST without hemoperitoneum due to fluid resuscitation in blunt trauma. *J Emerg Med.* 2014;47(4):427–429.

vanSonnenberg E, Simeone JF, Mueller PR, Wittenberg J, Hall DA, Ferrucci Jr JT. Sonographic appearance of hematoma in liver, spleen, and kidney: a clinical, pathologic, and animal study. *Radiology.* 1983;147(2):507–510.

Abdomen Ultrasound

16

Liver and Spleen

John P. McGahan, Deborah J. Rubens

THE LIVER

Normal Liver

Normal Anatomy. The cephalad portion of the liver is bounded by the diaphragm. The caudal extent of the liver is in close proximity to the stomach, the duodenum, and the large bowel and lies just cephalad to the pancreas. Using the Couinaud classification of liver anatomy, the liver is divided into eight segments. Segment 1 is the caudate lobe. The caudate's boundary is the inferior vena cava (IVC) posteriorly and the portal vein and the echogenic fissure of the ligamentum venosum more anteriorly. The main lobar fissure, which extends from the gallbladder to the middle hepatic vein, divides the right from the left lobe of the liver (Fig. 16.1). Knowledge of the location of the main lobar fissure is useful to locate the gallbladder, especially if the gallbladder is contracted or is full of stones. The gallbladder lies in the caudal extent of the main lobar fissure. The left lobe contains segments 2, 3, and 4A and 4B; the right lobe contains segments 5, 6, 7, and 8. The ligamentum teres is an easily identifiable landmark, which is the fibrous remnant of the umbilical vein. It separates segment 3 and segment 4B of the left lobe. The left hepatic vein can be thought of as the more cephalad extension of the ligamentum teres and divides segment 2 and segment 4A of the left lobe of the liver. The right hepatic vein divides the more posterior segments 6/7 from the more anterior segments 5/8 of the right lobe (Figs. 16.1 and 16.2).

The common hepatic artery usually arises from the celiac artery and passes as the proper hepatic artery anterior to the portal vein. Common hepatic artery variants include the right hepatic artery arising from the superior mesenteric artery and passing posterior to the portal vein as a replaced right hepatic artery. There are a number of variants of the origin and branches of the hepatic artery, including a replaced or accessory left hepatic artery. Most of these variants are not easily visualized with ultrasound (US).

Ultrasound Findings/Technique. When scanning the liver, multiple transverse and longitudinal scans are obtained with the patient supine. Usually the liver is scanned with a curved array transducer with center frequency from 3 to 5 MHz. Higher-frequency linear array transducers may be used to examine the liver surface to assess for cirrhotic nodules.

The subcostal approach may be used for visualization of the right lobe, especially if the patient can hold a deep inspiration. Portions of the right lobe of the liver will require the patient to be placed in the right anterior oblique position. Using this technique, it is important to place the transducer parallel to the intercostal space. If this is not done, there will be acoustic shadowing from adjacent ribs, which prevents good visualization of the liver. The transducer often must be angled in a cephalad direction to scan the majority of the right lobe of the liver. Scanning performed intercostally may be helpful to identify the subdiaphragmatic portion of the liver, such as segments 7 and 8. Unfortunately, it may be difficult to visualize all portions of the right lobe of the liver because of the shadowing by the lung. This is why scanning in the intercostal space with the

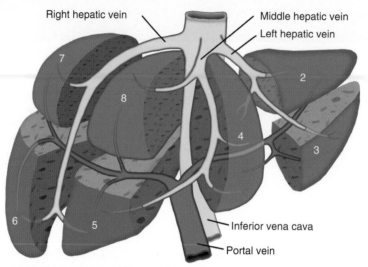

Fig. 16.1 Segmental anatomy of the liver. The drawing shows a segmental anatomy of the liver with the middle hepatic vein dividing the right lobe of the liver (segments 5–8) from the left lobe of lobe liver (segments 2–4). The right hepatic vein divides segments 5 and 8 from segments 6 and 7, with a left hepatic vein dividing segments 2 and 3 from segment 4. Portal veins then divide the other segments of the liver. (From McGahan J. *General and Vascular Ultrasound: Case Review*. 3rd ed. Philadelphia, PA: Elsevier; 2016:294, Fig. S38-3.)

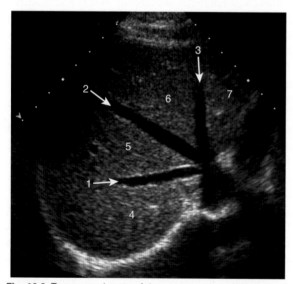

Fig. 16.2 Transverse image of the upper portion of the liver. (*1*, right hepatic vein; *2*, middle hepatic vein; *3*, left hepatic vein. Segments of the liver include *4*, segment 7; *5*, segment 8; *6*, segment 4A; *7*, segment 2.) (From McGahan J. *General and Vascular Ultrasound: Case Review*. 3rd ed. Philadelphia, PA: Elsevier; 2016:279, Fig. S22-2.)

right side of the abdomen elevated is important. The left lobe can be scanned using an anterior subxiphoid approach.

Normally, the liver appears as a homogeneous structure, with echogenicity slightly greater than or equal to the kidney. This internal comparison is important, as with increasing hepatic steatosis there will be increasing echogenicity of the liver. The homogeneous echogenicity is only interrupted by the portal triads and the hepatic veins. The size of the liver is variable, with the length of the right lobe of the liver varying between 13 and 17 cm. Liver volume is not usually calculated, and there is considerable variability in the size of the right and left lobes of the liver.

Color Doppler ultrasound is important to use to identify the portal vein and its normal direction of hepatopetal flow (toward the liver). In patients with cirrhosis, the portal vein can increase in size. Eventually there can be hepatofugal (reversed) flow in the portal vein. Color flow may be helpful to identify any thrombus in the portal vein. Pulsed Doppler ultrasound is used to identify the direction of flow in the portal vein. Color flow in the hepatic veins is easily obtained and is helpful to exclude occlusion of the hepatic veins. Pulse Doppler may be used to identify

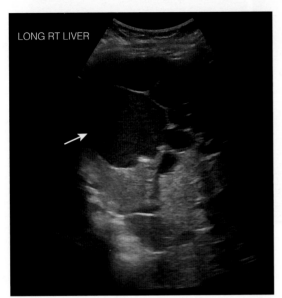

LONG RT LIVER

Fig. 16.3 Hemorrhagic cyst and polycystic liver disease. Ultrasound image through the liver demonstrates multiple small cysts within the liver, as well as a larger cyst with increased echoes (*arrow*) with good through transmission corresponding to a hemorrhagic cyst within the liver.

the normal triphasic hepatic waveform. The IVC can be identified posterior to the liver and heading anteriorly to the right atrium. The hepatic artery can be seen with color and noting its arterial waveform with pulsed Doppler.

Liver: Etiologies of Right Upper Quadrant Pain

Hepatic Cysts. A hepatic cyst is rarely the etiology of right upper quadrant (RUQ) pain, unless it is large enough to distort the liver capsule or it has hemorrhaged internally. Cysts are anechoic with smooth walls with good through transmission. Cysts with avascular septations or debris are called *complex cysts*. Upper abdominal pain may occur with hemorrhage into a hepatic cyst. Cysts with internal hemorrhage may become echogenic, appear more complex, or have a fluid/blood interface (Fig. 16.3). Although a complex cyst may be due to hemorrhage, the differential for a complex hepatic cyst is fairly broad (Fig. 16.4). The differential can include anything from a postoperative or posttransplant hematoma to postoperative seroma or biloma (Fig. 16.5). Historical information is important in narrowing the ultrasound differential. Rarer causes of more complex hepatic cysts are listed in Table 16.1. If

a complex cyst is encountered, computed tomography (CT) or magnetic resonance imaging (MRI) may be useful for better characterization.

Abscess. Bacterial liver abscesses are an etiology of acute abdominal pain. Bacterial abscesses are usually hypoechoic but may be isoechoic or echogenic (Videos 16.1–16.3). They may have thick or poorly defined walls (Figs. 16.6 and 16.7). They may be difficult to diagnose on ultrasound. Therefore the clinical presentation is helpful. Again, CT or MRI may be needed to better characterize an hepatic abscess. Liver abscesses may be secondary to infection from adjacent structures, such gallbladder perforation into the liver from acute cholecystitis (Fig. 16.8, Video 16.4). An hepatic abscess may also occur from hematogenous spread due to acute diverticulitis or appendicitis. It is important to realize that although abscesses often appear complex with thick internal separations, they may also appear solid and could be confused with a solid mass (see Figs. 16.6 and 16.7).

Amebic abscesses are usually round or oval, with a lack of a significant echogenic wall. They are less echogenic than normal liver and are more homogeneous compared with bacterial abscesses. They often have clearly defined margins. History of travel to an endemic area is helpful as an important clue in narrowing the differential.

Echinococcal abscesses are endemic in some geographic locations. *Echinococcus granulosus* may affect the liver, lung, kidneys, spleen, and other organs. In the liver they have external cysts called *ectocysts* and internal cysts called *endocysts*. The liver may form a fibrous reaction around the cyst called a *pericyst*. This infection has a variety of appearances within the liver, including a simple cyst, multiple cysts that are encapsulated, a cyst with smaller daughter cysts, or a cyst with internal debris, to name a few. They may be confused with a simple or a more complex hepatic cyst with hemorrhage.

Fungal abscesses are rare. They often occur in immunocompromised patients. History is important. The offending organism is often *Candida*. These lesions are usually multiple and small. They may have a target appearance with a more central echogenicity surrounded by a hypoechoic halo.

Hepatic Tumors. Rarely hepatic tumors can cause acute pain. In most situations acute pain only occurs when

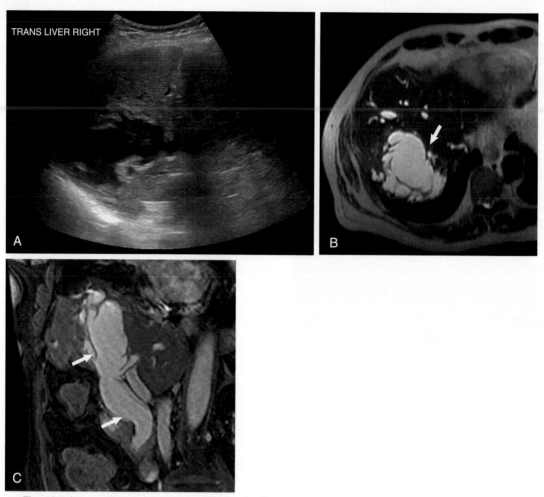

Fig. 16.4 Intrapapillary mucinous neoplasm of the liver. (A) Transverse ultrasound of the upper abdomen demonstrates a poorly marginated cyst with internal echoes. (B) Corresponding T2-weighted MRI demonstrates this multiseptated cyst (*arrow*). (C) This coronal T2-weighted MRI better demonstrates the communication between the multiseptated cyst and the common bile duct of this intrapapillary mucinous neoplasm (*arrows*) of the biliary tract.

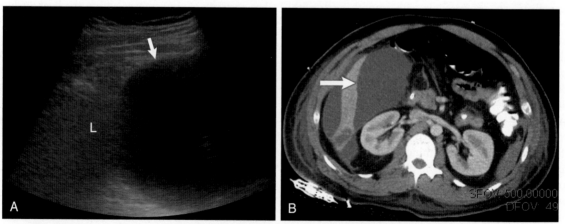

Fig. 16.5 Biloma. (A) Longitudinal scan of the liver (*L*) demonstrates a large fluid collection (*arrow*) in this postoperative patient with prior abdominal trauma. (B) Corresponding CT scan demonstrating large biloma (*arrow*).

TABLE 16.1	Potential Differential of a Complex Hepatic Cyst
Hemorrhagic cyst	Pseudoaneurysms (use color flow)
Infected cyst	Polycystic renal disease (multiple hepatic cysts)
Biloma	Multiple hepatic cysts
Abscess	Mucinous (cystic) biliary tumor
Echinococcal cyst	
Necrotic hepatic tumor	

these tumors are large enough to distort the liver capsule or when the tumor ruptures. Hepatic hemangiomas are the most common benign primary hepatic tumors. They are usually echogenic and well marginated, with little color flow. They have a characteristic outer-to-central fill-in on contrast-enhanced ultrasound, CT, or MRI. They are usually discovered incidentally but may be the cause of abdominal discomfort if large enough.

Hepatic adenomas are associated with use of birth control pills and have a propensity for bleeding.

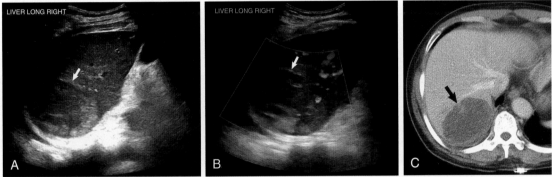

Fig. 16.6 Liver abscess: *K. pneumoniae*. (A) Transverse ultrasound of the upper abdomen demonstrates an isoechoic or slightly hypoechoic mass (*arrow*) in the right lobe of the liver, which represented a bacterial liver abscess. (Note small right pleural effusion). (B) Color Doppler ultrasound demonstrates very little color flow noted within this abscess (*arrow*). (C) CT scan with contrast of the upper abdomen demonstrates a well-demarcated, low-density mass (*arrow*), which was later drained percutaneously with the specimen cultured that revealed an abscess due to *K. pneumoniae*.

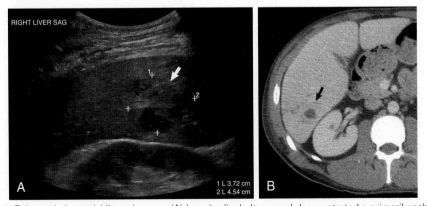

Fig. 16.7 Echogenic bacterial liver abscess. (A) Longitudinal ultrasound demonstrated a primarily echogenic mass (*calipers* and *arrow*). There is a small cystic component noted posteriorly. (B) Contrast-enhanced CT scan demonstrated the majority of the abscess (*arrow*) was not easily identified except for the cystic component of the mass.

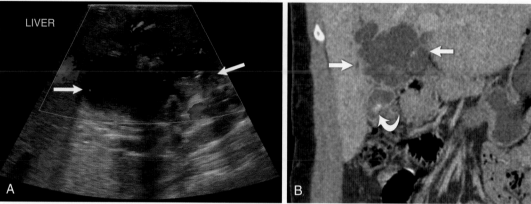

Fig. 16.8 Liver abscess secondary to perforated gallbladder. (A) Transverse ultrasound through the caudal aspect of the right lobe of the liver demonstrates thick-walled, poorly demarcated fluid collection (*arrows*), which corresponded to a liver abscess from a perforated gallbladder. (B) Coronal CT scan demonstrates the liver abscess (*arrows*) and part of the gallbladder with a radiopaque stone (*curved arrow*).

Hepatic malignances include liver metastases and primary malignancy such as hepatocellular carcinoma (HCC) or cholangiocarcinoma. Metastatic liver tumors, as with HCC may have a variety of appearances. Metastases often have an echogenic center with a surrounding hypoechoic halo appearing as a "target" sign on sonography. Discrete hypoechoic lesions is another common pattern. There is usually a history of a primary malignancy. HCC usually occurs in patients with cirrhosis or hepatitis B. Both metastatic liver disease and primary HCC may cause discomfort, due to size or intratumoral hemorrhage.

Trauma. Acute trauma will cause acute RUQ pain from injury to the liver, gallbladder, or other organs. This is discussed in Chapter 15, on ultrasound in trauma.

Chronic Liver Disease

Cirrhosis/Ascites. Patients with chronic liver disease may present with abdominal pain and discomfort. Chronic liver disease may develop into cirrhosis. Etiologies of cirrhosis can include hepatitis, hepatic steatosis, alcohol, or any other of a number of etiologies. Patients with cirrhosis have hepatic findings, including a coarsened liver texture, surface nodularity, and a shrunken liver (Fig. 16.9). However, these patients may present with discomfort due to the sequela of portal hypertension. Cirrhosis causes an increased pressure gradient between the IVC and the portal vein. The portal vein enlarges and may develop slow flow or reversal

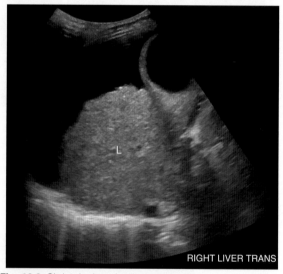

Fig. 16.9 Cirrhosis. Longitudinal ultrasound demonstrated the echogenic liver (*L*), which is surrounded by ascites. Note the dilated gallbladder anteriorly.

of flow, with eventual development of portosystemic collaterals, splenomegaly, and ascites. Ascites is a common etiology of patient discomfort and may require multiple paracentesis for management. The technique for ultrasound-guided paracentesis is presented in Chapter 29. Other complications of portal hypertension include portal vein or hepatic vein thrombus or obstruction. Briefly, a thrombus may be echogenic, isoechoic, or hypoechoic on grayscale sonography. As such, either

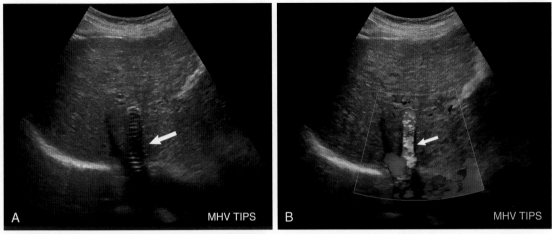

Fig. 16.10 Normal TIPS. (A) Real-time ultrasound examination demonstrates the appearance of a TIPS (*arrow*). (B) This same image with color flow demonstrates color aliasing within the TIPS (*arrow*).

color Doppler or pulsed Doppler will be needed to detect the thrombus or occlusion. The color and pulsed Doppler findings of portal venous occlusion is not discussed in full detail in this emergency ultrasound text.

Transjugular Intrahepatic Portosystemic Shunt. Patients with portal hypertension may require a portocaval shunt. This includes placement of a stent from the hepatic vein, usually the right hepatic vein, into the portal vein. This is called a *transjugular intrahepatic portosystemic shunt* (*TIPS*). These patients may present in an emergent situation acutely or at a later date due to TIPS malfunction. These patients may develop liver failure and require liver transplant. Acute problems with a TIPS may be either nonvascular or vascular. Common nonvascular problems with a TIPS occur usually immediately after shunt placement and are commonly fluid collections such as hematoma or, less frequently, a biloma.

TIPS malfunction is a vascular complication due to stent stenosis or occlusion. Malfunction can occur acutely or chronically, resulting in recurrences of ascites. These malfunctions may be secondary to narrowing or occlusion of the TIPS. A TIPS may be seen with grayscale ultrasound but is better identified using color or power Doppler ultrasound (Fig. 16.10). The IVC and the portal vein must also be studied. When evaluating for TIPS malfunction, pulsed Doppler ultrasound of the portal vein; the IVC; and the proximal, mid, and

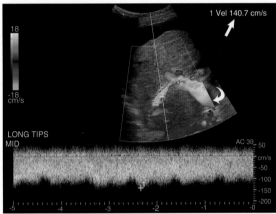

Fig. 16.11 Doppler of normal TIPS. Color flow imaging demonstrates flow within the portal vein (*curved arrow*). Also, the Doppler cursor is placed within the TIPS. Velocities within the TIPS are measured at 140 cm/sec (*arrow*), which is within normal limits.

distal TIPS is needed for complete hemodynamic evaluation. Typically, angle-corrected velocities in the TIPS are from 90 to 190 cm/sec (Fig. 16.11). Any value out of this range may indicate TIPS malfunction. Typical post-TIPS velocities in the portal vein are usually above 40 cm/sec. Decreasing velocity in the portal vein may indicate TIPS malfunction. When the TIPS is functioning normally, the blood flow in the main portal vein is toward the liver, whereas the blood flow from the left and right portal vein should be toward the stunt. If the flow in the right and left portal vein is toward the liver,

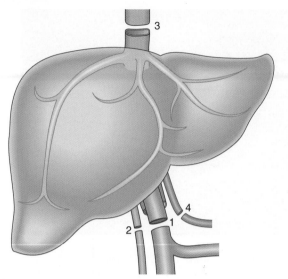

Fig. 16.12 Liver transplant anatomy. There are four separate surgical anastomosis sites with orthotopic liver transplant. The surgical anastomosis sites include the portal vein *(1)*, the common bile duct *(2)*, the inferior vena cava *(3)*, and the hepatic artery *(4)*.

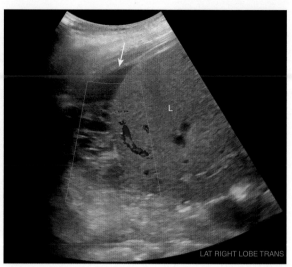

Fig. 16.13 Resolving hematoma posttransplant. Several days after liver transplant this complex fluid collection is noted (*arrow*), which corresponded to resolving hematoma. *L*, Liver.

this can indicate TIPS malfunction. Changes in velocities within any portion of the shunt or reversal of flow in the right or left portal vein are indicative of TIPS malfunction.

Liver Transplants. Patients with end-stage liver disease may require liver transplant. Detailed explanation of the technique of liver transplant is beyond the scope of this text. In essence, four connections between the donor liver and the recipient must be made. This includes the IVC (with the hepatic vein), the portal vein, the hepatic artery, and the common bile duct (Fig. 16.12). Complications may occur with any of these anastomoses. In the acute phase, complications may be nonvascular, such as a hematoma or a biloma (Figs. 16.5 and 16.13). Vascular complications can occur both acutely and chronically. The most common and difficult hepatic transplant complications include hepatic artery stenosis or thrombosis and bile duct stricture or leak. The portal vein or the IVC anastomosis less commonly malfunctions. Hepatic artery thrombosis and stenosis are especially critical to detect because the bile ducts are exclusively supplied by the hepatic artery. If the hepatic artery becomes occluded, this can result in biliary necrosis (Fig. 16.14). Biliary necrosis is a devastating

event due to recurrent biliary abscess formation. These require multiple drainages, and in some cases, the patient requires retransplantation. Doppler ultrasound of the proper hepatic artery and the more distal parenchymal arteries is helpful to evaluate for possible hepatic artery stenosis. The resistive index (RI) in the hepatic artery is calculated automatically by most ultrasound units. The RI is the peak systolic velocity minus the end diastolic velocity divided by the peak systolic velocity (Fig. 16.15). Normally, if the RI in the right and left hepatic artery is less than 0.4 and 0.5, respectively, this is suspicious for stenosis. Another helpful sign of hepatic artery stenosis is a delayed and decreased upstroke of the hepatic artery. This is called the *tardus parvus waveform of the artery* (see Fig. 16.14). These Doppler indices are explained in more detail in Chapter 19, on renal ultrasound.

THE SPLEEN

Normal Spleen

Normal Anatomy. The spleen is a predominantly intraperitoneal organ that is bounded by the diaphragm posteriorly, laterally, and superiorly. The retroperitoneal portion of the spleen is in continuity with the left kidney, the splenic flexure of the colon, the tail of the pancreas, and portions of the stomach. Accessory spleens, appearing as small homogeneous nodules in the left upper quadrant (LUQ), are common (Fig. 16.16).

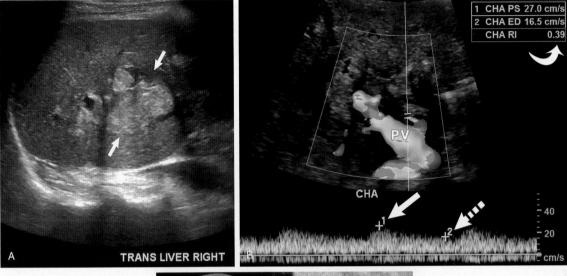

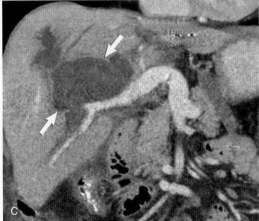

Fig. 16.14 Biliary necrosis secondary to hepatic artery thrombosis. The patient ultimately required retransplantation. (A) Transverse ultrasound shows a hyperechoic lobulated mass (*arrows*) centrally in the right lobe, corresponding to an area of hepatic necrosis. (B) Color and spectral Doppler image of the common hepatic artery. Note the Doppler tracing, which shows the tardus parvus waveform. The peak systolic velocity (*arrow*) and the end diastolic velocity (*broken arrow*) were measured and show an RI of 0.39 (*curved arrow*). These findings are concerning for hepatic artery stenosis or thrombosis. (C) Coronal CT performed 1 day later confirms massive biliary necrosis (*arrows*) superior to the portal vein.

Ultrasound Findings/Technique. The spleen may be imaged using an intercostal approach with the patient supine. Alternatively, the spleen may be examined using a subcostal approach with the left side of the abdomen elevated. If this technique is used, having the patient take a deep inspiration may aid in better visualization of the spleen. However, if there is significant overlapping lung, an expiratory view can also be used. The splenic artery and vein are best identified with color Doppler ultrasound.

The splenic parenchyma is homogeneous, with echogenicity greater than that of the adjacent left kidney. It is usually more echogenic than the liver, but this ratio may reverse if there is significant hepatic steatosis.

Various methods have been used to determine splenomegaly, including the use of splenic volume, splenic volume index, or splenic index. The normal upper limit of splenic length is 13 cm, and the width is usually less than or equal to 6 cm. However, in day-to-day practice, the splenic length alone is sufficient and a longitudinal diameter greater than 13 cm indicates splenomegaly (Fig. 16.17).

Left Upper Quadrant Pain: Etiologies. Etiologies of LUQ pain are listed in Table 16.2. Many of these causes of pain are less serious, such as constipation or dyspepsia.

More serious conditions resulting in LUQ pain are related to the gastrointestinal tract and require investigation with CT or other diagnostic tests. Pancreatic etiologies of LUQ pain can include pancreatitis, which is discussed in Chapter 18 on the pancreas. LUQ pain due to renal colic or hydronephrosis is discussed in Chapter 19, on the kidney.

The spleen is often the forgotten organ in the abdomen, as it is an uncommon cause of left upper abdominal pain. Traumatic splenic injury is the most common etiology of LUQ pain and will be further discussed in Chapter 15, on trauma. The spleen may be the cause of pain when it is associated with a large mass or if there is generalized splenomegaly, including infarction and/or rupture. Etiologies of splenomegaly include portal

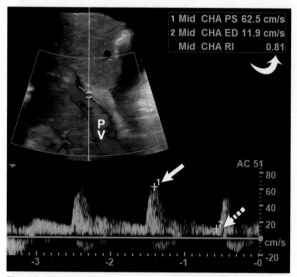

Fig. 16.15 Hepatic artery Doppler can be used for a variety of purposes, including helping to predict hepatic artery stenosis. This is done by noting an RI that is less than 0.5. The RI is automatically calculated by placing the caliber on the peak systole (*arrow*) and end diastole (*broken arrow*). In this case, the RI is 0.81 (*curved arrow*). *PV*, Portal vein.

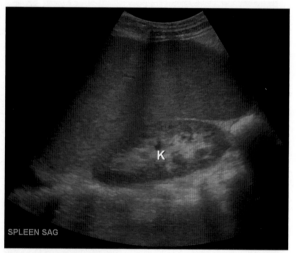

Fig. 16.17 Splenomegaly. Longitudinal real-time ultrasound exam demonstrating the left kidney (*K*) measuring approximately 11 cm in length. Note the anterior located spleen, which is nearly twice as long as the adjacent kidney, representing splenomegaly.

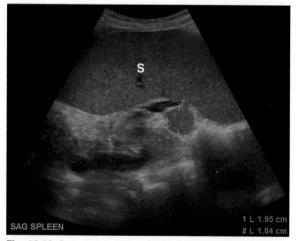

Fig. 16.16 Accessory spleen. Coronal ultrasound demonstrating the spleen (*S*) and a small nodule (*calipers*). This nodule is adjacent to the spleen, representing an accessory spleen.

TABLE 16.2 **Potential Etiologies of Left Upper Quadrant Pain**
I. *More Benign*
Dyspepsia
Constipation
II. *Gastrointestinal*
Gastroenteritis
Diverticulitis
Inflammatory Bowel Disease
Irritable Bowel Disease
III. Renal Colic/Hydronephrosis
IV. Pancreatitis
V. Splenic Etiologies (see discussion)

hypertension from cirrhosis, infections, hematologic disorders, infiltrative disease, collagen vascular disease, or neoplasm. Anemia, thrombocytopenia, and myelodysplasia cause diffuse splenic enlargement. Inflammatory splenic enlargement may occur with viral, bacterial, parasitic, or fungal infections. Whereas viral infections such as mononucleosis cause homogeneous enlargement, fungal infections such as *Candida*, *Aspergillosis*, or *Cryptococcus* often demonstrate multiple solid hypoechoic or target lesions throughout the spleen (Fig. 16.18). These are similar to the appearance of the same infection within the liver. Rarely, bacterial abscesses may occur within the spleen, also similar in appearance to bacterial hepatic abscesses.

These patients often present with fever and LUQ pain related to the cause of the abscess, which can include adjacent pancreatitis or diverticulitis. Focal masses within the spleen may be cystic or solid and are rarely the cause of pain, unless there is associated splenomegaly or rupture (Fig. 16.19). True cysts within the spleen are rare. Splenic cysts are usually posttraumatic pseudocysts. They have the typical ultrasound features of cysts; however, the wall may contain calcification (Fig. 16.20). Pancreatitis may extend to the spleen through the retroperitoneum and present with pancreatic pseudocysts. Cystic malignancies, other cystic tumors, or cystic infections in the spleen are rare. Hydatid cysts are an important consideration when encountering a splenic cyst in a person at risk for echinococcosis. Of the solid lesions, hemangiomas are the most common primary tumors of the spleen and are usually homogeneously echogenic. Splenic metastases are uncommon in the absence of other metastatic disease in the abdomen. The exception to this is lymphoma, which is the most common primary splenic malignancy. Lymphoma may present with homogeneous splenic enlargement, or the spleen may contain multiple hypoechoic nodules (Fig. 16.19). Angiosarcoma is a rare but aggressive, highly vascular, primary malignant splenic tumor, which may present with pain and splenic enlargement. If a complex cyst or splenic mass is identified by sonography, CT correlation may be needed.

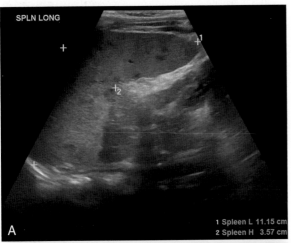
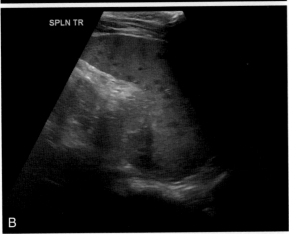

Fig. 16.18 Splenic microabscesses. (A and B) Transverse and longitudinal ultrasound of the spleen demonstrating multiple hypoechoic structures throughout the spleen, which correspond to microabscesses due to candidiasis.

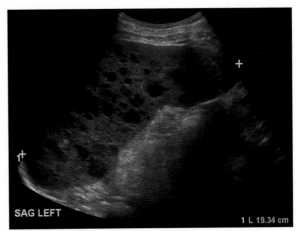

Fig. 16.19 Splenic lymphoma. Longitudinal ultrasound demonstrating multiple hypoechoic masses with splenomegaly secondary to splenic involvement due to lymphomas.

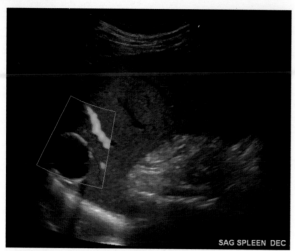

SAG SPLEEN DEC

Fig. 16.20 Splenic pseudocyst. Longitudinal power Doppler ultrasound of the spleen demonstrates an avascular cyst with an echogenic rim, stable for 3 years, consistent with a posttraumatic pseudocyst. The spleen is mildly enlarged as a sequela of prior portal hypertension.

BIBLIOGRAPHY

Hui JY, Yang MK, Cho DH, et al. Pyogenic liver abscesses caused by *Klebsiella pneumoniae*: US appearance and aspiration findings. *Radiolog.* 2007;242:769–776.

Kishina M, Koda M, Tokunaga S, et al. Usefulness of contrast-enhanced ultrasound with sonazoid for evaluating liver abscess in comparison with conventional B-mode ultrasound. *Hepatol Res.* 2015;45:337–342.

Labib PL, Aroori S, Bowles M, Stell D, Briggs C. Differentiating simple hepatic cysts from mucinous cystic neoplasms: radiological features, cyst fluid tumour marker analysis and multidisciplinary team outcomes. *Dig Surg.* 2017;34:36–42.

Pakala T, Molina M, Wu GY. Hepatic echinococcal cysts: a review. *J Clin Transl Hepatol.* 2016;4:39–46.

Ralls PW, Colletti PM, Quinn MF, Halls J. Sonographic findings in hepatic amebic abscess. *Radiolog.* 1982;145:123–126.

Sun K, Zhu W, Luo Y, Li Y, Zhou X. Transient segmental enhancement of pyogenic liver abscess: a comparison between contrast-enhanced ultrasound and computed tomography. *J Comput Assist Tomogr.* 2018;42:133–138.

Wang X, Cai YQ, Chen YH, Liu XB. Biliary tract intraductal papillary mucinous neoplasm: report of 19 cases. *World J Gastroenterol.* 2015;21:4261–4267.

Gallbladder and Biliary

John P. McGahan

THE GALLBLADDER

Normal Anatomy

The normal anatomy of the gallbladder, biliary tract, and surrounding organs is presented in Fig. 17.1. The gallbladder is connected via the cystic duct to the common hepatic duct, forming the common bile duct (CBD) that drains into the duodenum through the head of the pancreas. In most situations, the hepatic artery lies between the CBD and the more posteriorly located portal vein.

Ultrasound Techniques/Findings

Imaging of the gallbladder is performed using a low-frequency transducer, such as a curved array (typically 3–6 MHz frequency). It is best to visualize the gallbladder and CBD in a parasagittal, as well as transverse plane, in real time. Patients are often imaged in a supine position; however, turning the patient in a lateral decubitus or right anterior oblique position may improve visualization. Occasionally, placement of the probe in other positions, such as intercostal or through the right flank, may be helpful for gallbladder visualization. Careful and deliberate interrogation of the entire gallbladder is imperative, as stones may be impacted in the gallbladder neck or pass through the cystic duct into the CBD and cause biliary ductal obstruction. The examiner may find a sonographic Murphy's sign to be useful. A simple test is performed by placing the probe over the gallbladder to elicit pain. We find that placing the probe in different positions may be best to localize the true site of the pain. Thus probe pressure to the right of the gallbladder, over the gallbladder, and then over the mid-epigastric region may be used to best identify the true site of pain. A sonographic Murphy's sign is defined as the presence of maximum tenderness elicited by direct probe pressure over the sonographically located gallbladder. If analgesics have been administered, a Murphy's sign may be more difficult to elicit. On ultrasound we are evaluating the gallbladder primarily for stones, signs of inflammation of the gallbladder, and/or biliary obstruction. If the extrahepatic biliary ductal system appears dilated, then scanning through the liver as well as the head of the pancreas to evaluate the extrahepatic biliary system is important. It is important to document potential etiologies of biliary ductal obstruction such as choledocholithiasis and/or distal mass within the pancreas. When there is biliary ductal obstruction but no identifiable etiology on ultrasound, a computed tomography (CT) scan of the abdomen should be performed. Magnetic resonance imaging (MRI) may be useful to better identify etiologies of biliary obstruction such as choledocholithiasis.

Cholelithiasis and Mimics

Cholelithiasis. The principal imaging features that distinguish gallstones are mobility, echogenic focus, and acoustic shadowing (Fig. 17.2, Video 17.1 and Video 17.2). Multiple studies have shown sensitivities of ultrasound of approximately 95%, with even higher positive and negative predictive values. Gallstones may also demonstrate a "twinkle" artifact on color Doppler imaging (Fig. 17.3). When an echogenic focus is identified in the gallbladder, first shadowing should

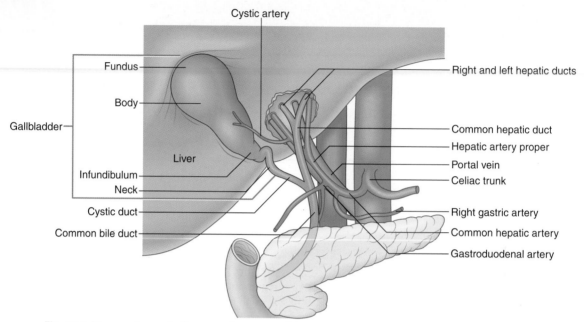

Fig. 17.1 Diagram demonstrating normal anatomy of the upper abdomen, including the relationship of the hepatic artery to the common bile duct and the biliary ductal system. (Redrawn with permission from Soni NJ. *Point of Care Ultrasound*. Philadelphia, PA: Elsevier; 2015:146, Fig. 19.2.)

be confirmed. This is followed by repositioning the patient to demonstrate stone mobility. This can include having the patient upright or standing. Stones lodged in the cystic duct may not move. Careful attention to surrounding structures is important, so as not to confuse an echogenic bowel (which can create a "dirty shadow") with gallstones (Fig. 17.4). This artifact can be differentiated from stones by scanning the patient in different positions and noting that the bowel is not within the gallbladder fossa, as well as noting peristalsis within the bowel (Video 17.3). Scanning in different planes or obliquely may be necessary to separate adjacent bowel from the gallbladder (see Fig. 17.4). A Refraction artifact, which is a mildly echogenic area in the region of the neck of the gallbladder that produces acoustic shadowing, can also be confused for gallstones. This edge artifact is due to refraction or from the multiple small valves of Heister within the cystic duct. Other nonmobile echogenicities within the gallbladder, which may be confused with cholelithiasis, are listed in Table 17.1.

The gallbladder is best examined when the patient is fasting. In emergent situations, the patient may not always be adequately prepped. Thus when the patient is not fasting, the gallbladder may be contracted. Even in these situations, gallstones may be identified. Also, the gallbladder may be in a permanent state of contraction in cases of chronic cholecystitis. In these situations the wall, echo, and shadow, or "WES," triad is observed. This corresponds to a visualization of the anterior gallbladder *wall*, with *echogenicity* representing the echogenic gallstones and posterior acoustic *shadowing* (Fig. 17.5, Videos 17.4–17.6). Again, this WES triad is fairly specific for chronic cholecystitis and cholelithiasis, but in patients with gallstones who are not fasting, their gallbladder may have a similar appearance. "Twinkle" artifact can also be seen in this entity (see Video 17.6). Patients with porcelain gallbladders will have an echogenic gallbladder wall with some shadowing. A porcelain gallbladder may predispose a patient to gallbladder cancer.

Cholelithiasis Mimic: Sludge. Tumefactive sludge is often an incidental finding when there is examination of the gallbladder in a patient with right upper quadrant pain. Tumefactive biliary sludge may mimic gallstones

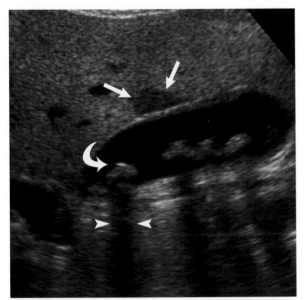

Fig. 17.2 Cholelithiasis/focal fatty sparing of the liver. Scans through the gallbladder demonstrated multiple echogenic foci (*curved arrow*) with acoustic shadowing (*arrowheads*), which are consistent with gallstones. In addition, there is a focal hypoechoic region noted anterior to the gallbladder (*arrows*), which represents an area of focal fatty sparing in a patient with diffuse fatty infiltration of the liver. (From McGahan J. *General and Vascular Ultrasound: Case Review.* 3rd ed. Philadelphia, PA: Elsevier; 2016:117, Fig. 57-1.)

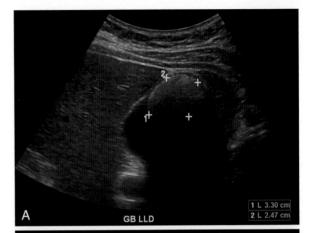

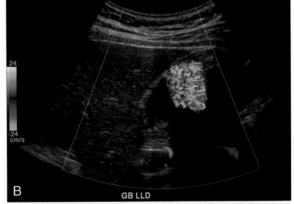

Fig. 17.3 Gallstone with "twinkle" artifact. (A) Large gallstone (*calipers*) in a contracted gallbladder. (B) Color Doppler demonstrates mosaic appearance to the color originating at the anterior surface of the gallbladder, representing the "twinkle" artifact.

or a mass. However, sludge will not shadow. Often this sludge may be mobile (Fig. 17.6). Thus with repositioning of the patient, sludge may move. Additionally, adding color or power Doppler to the evaluation should demonstrate lack of vascularity in the sludge. There can be an exception to the rule of no acoustic shadowing with sludge. If gallstones are surrounded by sludge, they may produce the "twinkle" artifact or shadowing. Other causes of gallbladder masses and mimics of cholelithiasis are listed in Table 17.2.

Gallbladder Masses: Polyps. Both benign and malignant gallbladder masses may be encountered when examining the gallbladder in the acute setting. This includes gallbladder polyps, cancer, or, rarely, metastasis (Fig. 17.7, Video 17.7). Most polyps are small and may resolve spontaneously. However, adenomatous polyps may be precancerous.

Gallbladder Cancer. Gallbladder cancer may be missed on routine ultrasound. This is probably due to the fact that

gallstones are often present in patients with gallbladder cancer, and any mass within the gallbladder may be obscured by the gallstones. Gallbladder carcinoma can be echogenic, isoechoic, or hypoechoic, and usually does have color Doppler flow. Gallbladder cancer may cause either diffuse or focal thickening of the gallbladder wall (Fig. 17.8). Primary gallbladder cancer may invade the adjacent liver. Various cancers, including melanoma and gastrointestinal (GI) cancers, may metastasize to the gallbladder and appear as a vascular gallbladder mass.

Adenomyomatosis. Adenomyomatosis is characterized by epithelial proliferation and mucosal diverticula called *Rokitansky–Aschoff sinuses.* The most common

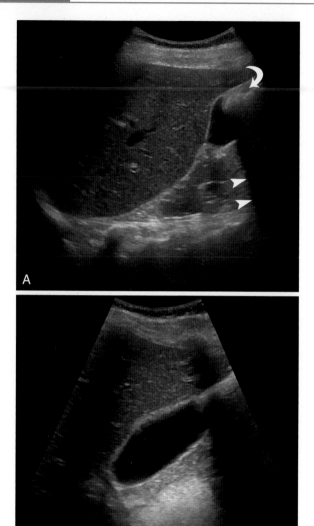

Fig. 17.4 Bowel mimicking gallstones. (A) This longitudinal scan of the liver and gallbladder demonstrates an echogenic focus (*curved arrow*) noted anteriorly within the gallbladder with distal acoustic shadowing (*arrows*). (B) Another scan, using different probe angulation, demonstrates the echogenic focus. This was bowel that moved, and there was no evidence of cholelithiasis.

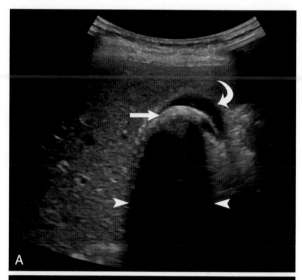

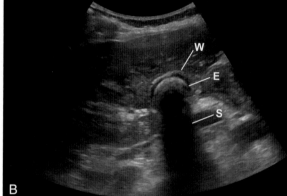

Fig. 17.5 Wall echo shadow (WES) triad. (A) Transverse image demonstrating anterior gallbladder wall (*curved arrow*) and partially collapsed gallbladder surrounding a large gallstone (*arrow*). Posterior to this there is an echogenic focus with acoustic shadowing (*arrow heads*) representing a large gallstone. There is still some fluid within the gallbladder. (B) In another patient, there is a near completely contracted gallbladder with anterior gallbladder wall (*W*) surrounding the gallstone as an echogenicity (*E*) and distal acoustic shadowing (*S*), giving the WES appearance.

TABLE 17.1 Nonmobile Echogenicities in the Gallbladder That May Shadow
• Stone lodged in the gallbladder neck
• Stone adherent to gallbladder wall
• Gallbladder fold
• Intramural gas secondary to emphysematous cholecystitis
• Adenomyomatosis with stone in Rokitansky–Aschoff sinus

form creates localized and confined wall thickening at the fundus of the gallbladder. This thickening can be so great, it appears as a mass and may be hard to distinguish from gallbladder cancer. There are other rare forms of segmental or diffuse adenomyomatosis. The pathognomonic finding of adenomyomatosis is the presence of hyperechoic foci, most commonly noted in the anterior wall of the gallbladder, which produces a

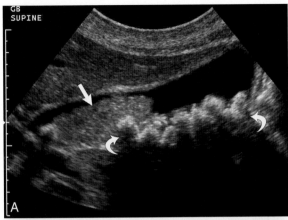

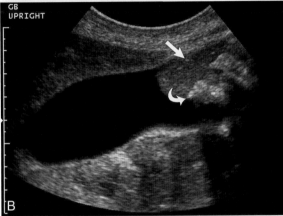

Fig. 17.6 Biliary sludge and cholelithiasis. (A) To the left side of the image there is an echogenic mass (*arrow*) without shadowing within the gallbladder lumen representing gallbladder sludge. To the right, there are multiple echogenic foci (*curved arrows*) with acoustic shadowing, representing gallstones. (B) When the patient is placed in an upright position, this mass (*arrow*) is mobile and falls to the dependent portion of the gallbladder. Note: Multiple echogenicities (*curved arrow*) within this echogenic sludge represent the gallstones.

comet tail artifact that decreases in width and amplitude more posteriorly (Fig. 17.9, Videos 17.8 and 17.9). This is thought to be secondary to cholesterol crystals within the Rokitansky–Aschoff sinuses in the gallbladder wall. Color Doppler will show a "twinkle artifact" in this entity (see Fig. 17.9), which is similar to the "twinkle" artifact seen with gallstones.

Acute Right Upper Quadrant Pain

The American College of Radiology has imaging criteria for patients with right upper quadrant pain who have fever, leukocytosis, and a clinical positive Murphy's sign, and recommends ultrasound as the first-line test in these situations (Table 17.3). Patients may present with acute or chronic pain in the right upper quadrant of the abdomen. The level and acuity of pain are secondary to the etiology of the pain. For instance, chronic pain may be secondary to chronic cholecystitis and cholelithiasis, whereas more acute pain may be secondary to acute cholecystitis, gallbladder perforation, or acute biliary obstruction. Abnormalities of the liver, biliary tract, pancreas, or kidney should be considered in the differential as listed in Table 17.4. In some situations, the etiology of the pain may not be discovered or may be secondary to etiologies that may require other imaging, such as CT.

Acute Calculus Cholecystitis. There are different etiologies for acute cholecystitis, but often there is an obstructing gallstone in the cystic duct. Sonographic findings that are nonspecific but may be suggestive of acute cholecystitis include the presence of gallstones; gallbladder sludge; gallbladder distention; and an asymmetrical, thickened gallbladder wall

TABLE 17.2 Cholelithiasis and Possible Mimics

Cause	Finding
Multiple stones	Echogenic layer with acoustic shadowing.
Sludge/sludgeball	Usually dependent, no color. Often mobile.
Stones and sludge	Stones surrounded by sludge (as above).
Blood	Dependent in gallbladder /or fills entire gallbladder. No shadowing.
Pus	Similar to blood, but with finding of acute cholecystitis.
Pseudo-sludge	A curvilinear echogenicity whose borders may project beyond the gallbladder and may disappear with different transducer orientations.
Parasites	Only in endemic areas or in patients from these areas.
Gallbladder polyps	Small masses with or without color flow.
Gallbladder cancer	Gallbladder mass with color flow and wall thickening, and often gallstones.

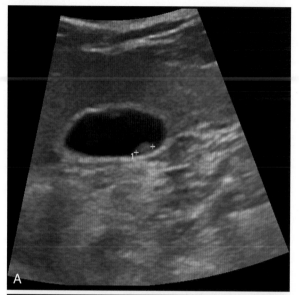

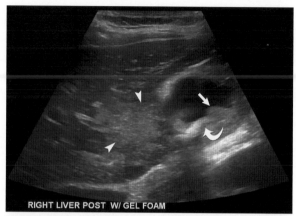

Fig. 17.8 Gallbladder carcinoma. Longitudinal scan of the gallbladder demonstrates a gallstone (*curved arrow*) with a nonmobile mass (*arrow*) in the gallbladder. There is also gallbladder wall thickening. An ill-defined mass (*arrowheads*) in the liver represents local invasion into the liver from the gallbladder adenocarcinoma.

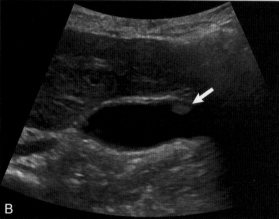

Fig. 17.7 Gallbladder polyps. (A) This image demonstrates an echogenic focus without shadowing (*calipers*) in the dependent portion of the gallbladder, representing a gallbladder polyp. If proper technique was not used, this could be misinterpreted as a gallstone. (B) In another patient, there is an anterior echogenic focus (*arrows*) without acoustic shadowing, representing a gallbladder polyp.

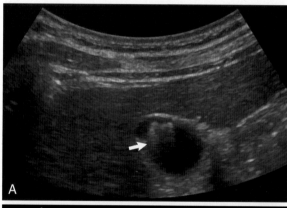

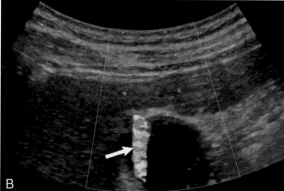

Fig. 17.9 Adenomyomatosis. (A) Transverse scan through the gallbladder demonstrates a few echogenic foci with "ring-down artifact" (*arrow*). Note this is different than in cholelithiasis, where there is acoustic shadowing. (B) In the same region there is "twinkle" artifact (*arrow*), which can be seen with both adenomyomatosis and cholelithiasis.

(Fig. 17.10, Video 17.10). Pericholecystic fluid is also another suggestive sign. Intraluminal membranes are suggestive of gangrenous cholecystitis. A sonographic positive Murphy's sign is defined as a presence of maximum tenderness elicited by direct pressure of the transducer over the sonographically located gallbladder. As noted previously, placing the ultrasound probe to the right of the gallbladder, then over the gallbladder, and then over the epigastrium will help localize the site of pain. This sign is often

TABLE 17.3   Imaging Criteria Patients with Fever, Elevated White Blood Cell Count, Positive Murphy's Sign

Radiologic Procedure	Rating	Comments	Relative Radiation Level
Ultrasound abdomen	9		◯
MRI abdomen without and with contrast	6	Based on ultrasound findings, this generally should follow an ultrasound of the right upper quadrant.	◯
Cholescintigraphy	6		☢ ☢
CT abdomen with contrast	6		☢ ☢ ☢
MRI abdomen without contrast	4		◯
CT abdomen without contrast	4		☢ ☢ ☢
CT abdomen without and with contrast	3		☢ ☢ ☢ ☢

Note: Rating scale: 1, 2, and 3 = usually not appropriate; 4, 5, and 6 = may be appropriate; 7, 8, and 9 = usually appropriate. (From Yarmish GM, Smith MP, Rosen MP, et al. ACR appropriateness criteria right upper quadrant pain. *J Am Coll Radiol.* 2014;11[3]:316–322.)

TABLE 17.4   Potential Etiologies of Right Upper Quadrant Pain, Including Those Due to Gallbladder Disease, Biliary Disease, or Disease in Surrounding Organs

- Cholelithiasis
- Acute calculus cholecystitis
- Acute acalculous cholecystitis
- Complications of acute cholecystitis
- Biliary obstruction
- Pancreatic mass (see Chapter 18)
- Pancreatitis (see Chapter 18)
- Hepatitis, hepatic abscess/mass (see Chapter 16)
- Pyelonephritis or renal obstruction (see Chapter 19)
- Renal colic/abscess (see Chapter 19)
- Gastroenteritis/colon disease
- Abdominal aortic aneurysm
- Right lower lobe pneumonia
- No identified etiology

present in patients with acute cholecystitis. The presence of cholelithiasis and a positive sonographic Murphy's sign had a high positive predictive value in the diagnosis of acute cholecystitis. However, administration of analgesia may reduce the reliability of this sign, and thus will reduce the sensitivity of ultrasound in diagnosing acute calculous cholecystitis. The presence of gallstones and a sonographic Murphy's sign are the most sensitive findings for acute cholecystitis. Gallbladder wall thickening and

pericholecystic fluid are considered important, but secondary, signs of acute cholecystitis. Some consider gallstones plus wall thickening to be sensitive in the diagnosis of acute cholecystitis.

Although a number of different ultrasound findings are suggestive of acute cholecystitis, gallbladder wall thickening is a nonspecific finding that can be seen in a number of different disease states (Table 17.5).

Other findings in acute cholecystitis include gallbladder distinction and sludge. Gallbladder sludge usually indicates the presence of gallbladder stasis, which can be identified in patients who are hospitalized. A distended gallbladder may be seen in the presence of acute cholecystitis but may be a normal finding or can be secondary to more distal biliary ductal obstruction. More recently, angle-corrected hepatic artery velocities over 100 cm/sec have been shown to be a useful sign in predicting acute cholecystitis. Unfortunately, elevated hepatic artery velocities can be seen in a number of conditions, including intrinsic liver disease. Thus all ancillary ultrasound findings, such as the presence of positive ultrasound Murphy's sign, wall thickening, or sludge, must be taken into the clinical context, as many of these findings may be secondary to a number of etiologies.

There are a number of different complications of acute cholecystitis, including emphysematous cholecystitis and gangrenous cholecystitis. Air may be

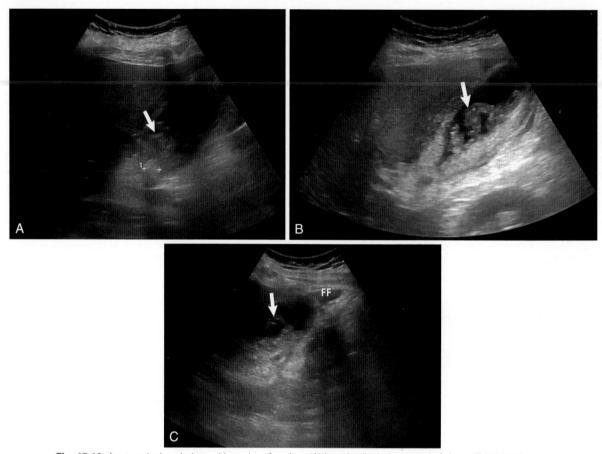

Fig. 17.10 Acute calculus cholecystitis and perforation. (A) Longitudinal ultrasound of the gallbladder demonstrates an echogenic focus with acoustic shadowing in the gallbladder (*calipers*). There is surrounding debris/biliary sludge (*arrow*). (B) Within the gallbladder itself, there are large amounts of debris and sludge (*arrow*), and the question of gangrenous cholecystitis was considered. There is gallbladder wall thickening. (C) There is also free fluid noted around the tip of the gallbladder (*FF*). There is sludge and debris in the gallbladder (*arrow*). This patient was noted to have acute calculus cholecystitis with perforation.

detected within the gallbladder or lumen and/or can be seen within the gallbladder wall, and often changes with position in these patients. Perforation of the gallbladder may occur, resulting in a pericholecystic abscess formation.

Acute Acalculous Cholecystitis. This is an extremely difficult diagnosis to make by ultrasound. Usually, these patients have had a prolonged intensive care stay or have been hospitalized for major surgery, trauma, or other severe illnesses. The exact etiology of acalculous cholecystitis is not known, but pathogenesis may be multifactorial and include

TABLE 17.5 **Causes of Gallbladder Wall Thickening**
• Acute cholecystitis
• Chronic cholecystitis
• Cirrhosis
• Hypoproteinemia
• Renal failure
• Congestive heart failure
• Acute viral hepatitis
• Pancreatitis
• Adenomyomatosis (focal)
• Gallbladder cancer (focal)
• Gallbladder wall varices

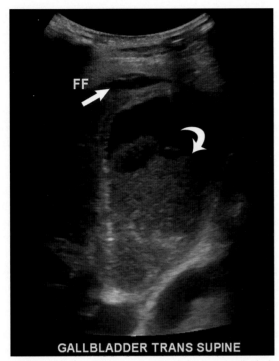

GALLBLADDER TRANS SUPINE

Fig. 17.11 Acute acalculous cholecystitis. Longitudinal ultrasounds of the gallbladder in an intensive care patient that demonstrate a distended gallbladder with sludge (*arrowhead*) in the dependent portion of the gallbladder. There was gallbladder wall thickening and a small amount of free fluid (*arrow*). This patient was shown to have acute acalculous cholecystitis.

TABLE 17.6	Causes of Enlarged Gallbladder
• Prolonged fasting
• Postsurgical
• Hyperalimentation
• Diabetes
• Acute cholecystitis
• Common bile duct obstruction

ischemia of the gallbladder, biliary stasis, and sepsis. As mentioned, this diagnosis is very difficult (Fig. 17.11). Gallbladder wall thickening may be present, but this is a nonspecific finding seen in patients with hypoalbuminemia, acute hepatitis, heart failure, or chronic liver disease (see Table 17.5). There may be focal or complex pericholecystic fluid collections, and some patients may have a very distended gallbladder. However, these findings are nonspecific as well (Table 17.6). A positive Murphy's sign by ultrasound may be unreliable in the hospitalized patient, as they are often heavily sedated, and thus eliciting pain may be difficult. Both gallbladder sludge and a distended gallbladder may be seen in these patients but are nonspecific findings (see Table 17.6). Thus the diagnosis of an acalculous cholecystitis may rest on the combined ultrasound findings and clinical picture in the patient, making this diagnosis difficult, if not elusive. Color flow Doppler

should be performed when looking at the gallbladder wall, as, rarely, varices within the gallbladder wall cause gallbladder wall thickening in patients with cirrhosis. These may be large or small cystic structures within or adjacent to the gallbladder wall that appear as irregular thickening. With color flow, these varices are seen as vascular channels.

Emphysematous Cholecystitis. Emphysematous cholecystitis is a rare entity. Its etiology is probably not secondary to cystic duct obstruction, but rather cystic arterial occlusion and/or gallbladder wall ischemia. Gallstones need not be present, but are present in 50% of the cases.

The sonographic findings include intramural gas in the gallbladder wall appearing echogenic with shadowing or ring-down artifact posteriorly. Intraluminal air will change position if the patient is turned, as the air may rise to a nondependent portion of the gallbladder. One pitfall is patients with biliary stents often have air within their gallbladder wall (Fig. 17.12, Video 17.11). Adenomyomatosis is another entity within the differential for intramural air. However, there will be only focal ring-down artifact, as discussed previously.

Gangrenous Cholecystitis. This is a difficult diagnosis to make by sonography. Gangrenous cholecystitis occurs often in the elderly diabetic patient. Most of these patients have cholelithiasis. Patients may be afebrile, and the white blood cell count may be normal. Unfortunately, once the gallbladder has become gangrenous, often it is denervated. Thus right upper quadrant pain and/or tenderness may be diminished, and a sonographic Murphy's sign may or may not be present. However, intraluminal membranes strongly suggest the diagnosis. There also may be an irregular, thickened gallbladder wall.

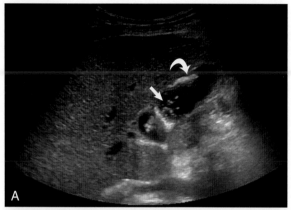

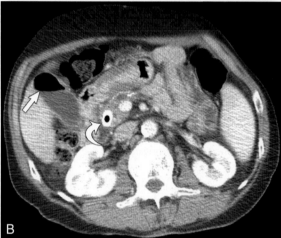

Fig. 17.12 Air within the gallbladder lumen. (A) Longitudinal ultrasound of the gallbladder demonstrates anterior echogenic linear focus with some shadowing (*curved arrow*). A similar echogenic focus along a septation within the gallbladder was seen. There are also multiple small echogenic foci (*arrow*) in the gallbladder lumen, which were observed to rise toward the nondependent portion of the gallbladder. All of this corresponded to air within the gallbladder lumen. (B) A CT scan of the abdomen demonstrates the patient had a biliary stent in place (*curved arrow*), and an air–fluid level was noted within the gallbladder (*arrow*).

Other Etiologies of Right Upper Quadrant Abdominal Pain

Liver: Abscess or Mass. Other etiologies of right upper quadrant pain may only be appreciated with careful scanning. Among these etiologies are hepatic infections. A patient with a hepatic abscess may present with sepsis, elevated white blood cell count, and abdominal pain. Patients with hepatic cysts or tumors may present with pain due to the mass effect. These cysts or masses may

have internal hemorrhage, which produces pain. Acute liver abnormalities are presented in more detail in Chapter 16, on liver disease.

Renal: Obstruction and Pyelonephritis. Renal abnormalities, such as pyelonephritis, may present with flank pain and hematuria. Patients may also have acute flank pain from renal colic due to renal stones or more distal obstruction. These are presented in more detail in Chapter 19, on renal disease.

Gastrointestinal. Upper GI abnormalities may be considered within the differential, but less commonly have ultrasound features. Patients with gastroenteritis, duodenitis, peptic ulcer disease, colitis, or colon cancer can present with upper abdominal pain. Many times patients with right upper quadrant pain have no ultrasound etiology for their pain. In these situations, other studies, such as CT, may be helpful.

Pancreas: Pancreatitis or Mass. Upper abdominal pain may be secondary to pancreatic abnormalities. These can include anything from pancreatitis to pancreatic masses, which cause biliary obstruction. Acute pancreatic disease is presented in more detail in Chapter 18, on the pancreas.

THE BILIARY SYSTEM

Normal Anatomy

The right and the left hepatic ducts join to form the common hepatic duct. This is located anterior to the portal vein. The cystic duct joins the common hepatic duct to create the CBD (see Fig. 17.1). However, it may be difficult to note the confluences of the cystic duct with the common hepatic duct, and thus the term *common duct* is often used to describe the common hepatic and/ or CBD. Usually, the CBD lies anterior to the hepatic artery, which lies anterior to the portal vein, forming the portal triad.

Ultrasound Findings

The intrahepatic bile ducts can be seen as they run parallel to the portal veins and hepatic arteries. Because of the relatively small size, normal intrahepatic bile ducts are very difficult to demonstrate. Close to the porta hepatis, rather small tubular structures representing bile ducts can be identified, usually anterior to the main right and left

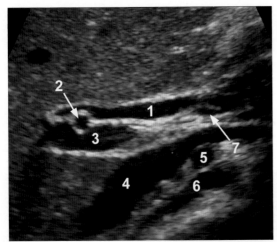

Fig. 17.13 Normal longitudinal scan of the common bile duct. Longitudinal image of the porta hepatis with the following structures labeled: *1*, common hepatic duct; *2*, right hepatic artery; *3*, portal vein; *4*, inferior vena cava; *5*, right renal artery; *6*, crus of the diaphragm; *7*, cystic duct. (From McGahan J. *General and Vascular Ultrasound: Case Review*. 3rd ed. Philadelphia, PA: Elsevier; 2016:45, Fig. 22-1.)

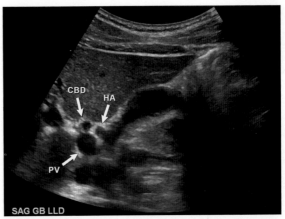

Fig. 17.14 Portal triad. "Mickey Mouse" parasagittal image demonstrates the more posteriorly located portal vein (*PV*) and the more anteriorly located common bile duct (*CBD*) (which is usually to the left) and the hepatic artery (*HA*) (which is usually to the right).

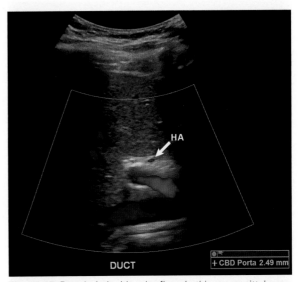

Fig. 17.15 Portal triad with color flow. In this parasagittal scan, color flow is utilized to demonstrate flow in the hepatic artery (*HA*), which is to the right, and the common bile duct (*calipers*), which is to the left. The portal vein is more posterior.

branches of the portal vein. The intrahepatic bile ducts are identified by scanning both in the transverse and parasagittal planes. Additionally, by slightly elevating the right side of the patient, longitudinal scanning can help identify the common duct. Usually, the CBD is anterior to the hepatic artery, and both are anterior to the main portal vein (Fig. 17.13). The gallbladder can be followed to a hyperechoic line, which is the main lobar fissure. The portal vein appears as a dot at the base, which has been called the *explanation point*. With probe angulation, the hepatic artery (to the right) and the CBD (to the left) lie above the portal vein and form the "Mickey Mouse" view (Fig. 17.14) of the portal triad. Color flow can be used to help distinguish the hepatic artery from the CBD (Fig. 17.15). Color flow is helpful to distinguish the portal vein from the bile ducts. However, in some situations where the hepatic artery originates from the superior mesenteric artery, as the replaced hepatic artery, the hepatic artery will lie posterior to the portal vein (Fig. 17.16).

Biliary Ductal Dilatation

There are a number of etiologies of biliary ductal dilatation (Table 17.7). Patients with biliary ductal disease may present with different symptoms depending on the etiology of the biliary ductal obstruction. Patients with pancreatic cancer or distal cholangiocarcinoma may present with painless jaundice. Patients who present with choledocholithiasis and cholecystitis may present with pain and jaundice. Patients with pain, fever, and elevated liver function tests may have cholangitis.

Normal versus Dilated Ducts. There are a number of different criteria for making the diagnosis of biliary ductal dilatation. Some of the sonographic features that are important are noting tubular structures adjacent to the intrahepatic portal veins larger than 2

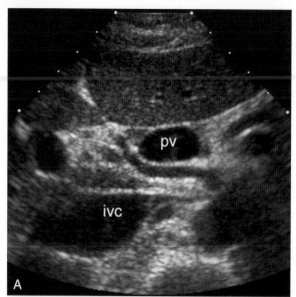

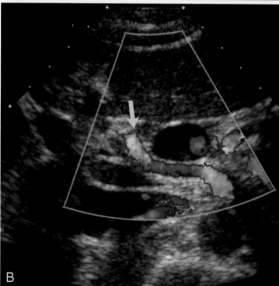

Fig. 17.16 Replaced hepatic artery. (A) In this transverse image of the upper abdomen, a tubular structure lies posterior to the portal vein (*pv*) and anterior to the inferior vena cava (*ivc*). (B) Color Doppler demonstrates this is a replaced hepatic artery (*arrow*) from the superior mesenteric artery that runs posterior, rather than anterior, to the portal vein. (From McGahan J. *General and Vascular Ultrasound: Case Review*. 3rd ed. Philadelphia, PA: Elsevier; 2016:21, Figs. 10-1 and 10-2.)

TABLE 17.7 **Causes of Biliary Ductal Dilatation**
• Postoperative stricture
• Pancreatic carcinoma
• Cholangiocarcinoma
• Metastatic disease
• Choledocholithiasis
• Pancreatitis
• Cholangitis (different etiologies)

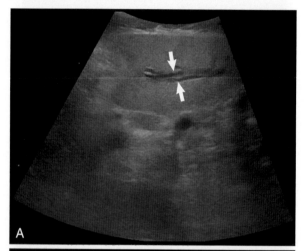

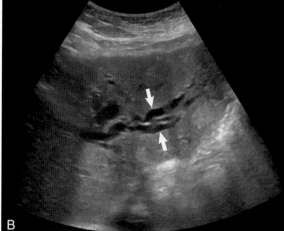

Fig. 17.17 Biliary ductal dilatation, mild to severe. (A) This transverse image through the left lobe of the liver demonstrates a "double duct" or "double barrel shotgun" sign with the portal vein and the slightly dilated bile duct seen together (*arrows*). Note the bile ducts are approximately the same size as the portal vein, indicating biliary ductal dilatation. (B) In another patient, transverse image through the left lobe of the liver, there is more severe biliary ductal dilatation that demonstrates the "double duct" or "double barrel shotgun" sign (*arrows*), which is more prominent, and indicates more severe biliary ductal dilatation.

mm in diameter or more than 40% the diameter of the adjacent portal vein (Fig. 17.17). The extrahepatic CBD measurements are usually less than 6 mm. Extrahepatic biliary ductal dilatation may be mild or severe (Fig. 17.18, Video 17.12). If severe, there is marked intrahepatic

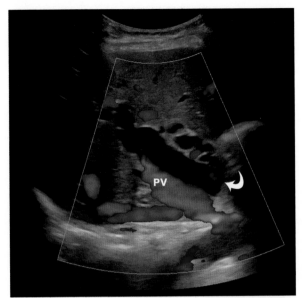

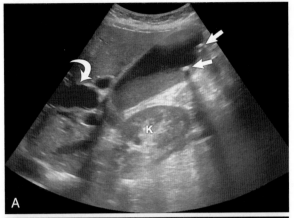

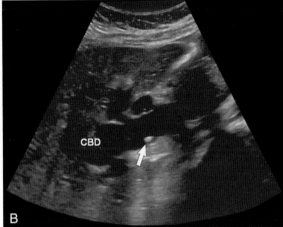

Fig. 17.18 Severe biliary ductal dilatation. (A) Examination of the porta hepatis, with color flow demonstrating the portal vein (*PV*) noted posteriorly and the markedly dilated common bile duct (*curved arrow*).

Fig. 17.19 Choledocholithiasis. (A) This longitudinal ultrasound shows the dilated common duct (*curved arrow*) and a gallbladder with sludge and gallstones (*arrows*) that cast an acoustic shadow (*K*, Kidney). (B) In this image there is a dilated common bile duct (*CBD*) with a single stone (*arrow*). Choledocholithiasis is very difficult to identify on ultrasound.

biliary ductal dilation, and often concomitant gallbladder enlargement or gallbladder sludge may be present (Fig. 17.19, Video 17.13). However, there has been considerable debate concerning the CBD measurement. In the elderly, it has been postulated that there is minimal increased size of the CBD with advancing age, especially after age 60. Also, it has been observed in some patients after cholecystectomy that the CBD may be enlarged. In some series the postcholecystectomy patients exceed the 6-mm cutoff more frequently than those without cholecystectomy. We have observed that there may be a prominent extrahepatic system without intrahepatic dilatation in postcholecystectomy patients. Thus one always must struggle between sensitivity and specificity in making the diagnosis of biliary ductal dilatation. Certainly in this situation, the clinical picture, including elevated hepatic/biliary laboratory values, is important. If there is ductal dilatation, then a precise etiology should be determined. Thus examination of the CBD in both the longitudinal and transverse planes may be helpful to exclude choledocholithiasis. Other etiologies of biliary ductal dilation include pancreatic etiologies, which are better discussed in Chapter 18, on the pancreas and may require a CT for diagnosis.

Pitfalls. In patients with biliary-enteric anastomosis, there may be dilatation of the biliary ductal system. In these patients, air from enteric reflux may cause shadowing in the periphery of the liver. In patients with severe cirrhosis and portal hypertension, there may be dilated hepatic arteries, which appear as dilated ducts. Additionally, when there is obstruction of the portal vein, multiple collateral veins appear as cavernous transformation of the portal vein. The veins appear as multiple vascular tubes in the porta hepatis. In both situations, color Doppler is useful to distinguish the dilated hepatic arteries and/or regions of cavernous transformation of the portal vein from dilated ducts. Finally, although biliary ductal dilatation is usually distal, it may occur focally within one branch of the biliary ductal system; thus both the right and the left lobe of the liver must be carefully scanned.

Causes of Biliary Ductal Dilatation

Choledocholithiasis. Choledocholithiasis is one etiology of biliary ductal dilatation. However, common duct stones are very difficult to identify on sonography. High-resolution ultrasound scanners improve resolution (see Fig. 17.19). Often, manual compression by the sonographer/sonologist is needed on both transverse and longitudinal scans to identify the more distal common duct. Stones appear as hyperechoic structures within the duct. Often, these stones will shadow, but the shadow may be difficult to produce. There are several pitfalls in identifying choledocholithiasis. Calcified arteries adjacent to the common duct may have an echogenic focus with shadowing. Pancreatic calcifications may be very echoic in the head of the pancreas. Even surgical clips after cholecystectomy may be close to the common duct and mimic stones. All these can serve as potential pitfalls in the diagnosis of choledocholithiasis. Finally, biliary sludge, which is similar to the sludge noted within the gallbladder, can be identified within the common duct and mimic a stone.

Mirizzi's Syndrome. A rare but correctable cause of extrahepatic biliary ductal obstruction is Mirizzi's syndrome (Fig. 17.20). In this syndrome, an impacted stone in the cystic duct causes partial mechanical obstruction of the common hepatic duct by the compression from the cystic duct stone. Thus the patient has a dilated common hepatic duct at that site. Sonographic features include a gallstone impacted in the distal cystic duct with dilatation in the biliary system, including the common hepatic duct.

Cholangiocarcinoma. Cholangiocarcinoma and adenocarcinoma of the pancreas are common causes of biliary ductal dilatation. In distal cholangiocarcinoma, the mass may not be easily identified with ultrasound and CT or MRI, with magnetic resonance cholangiopancreatography (MRCP) is needed. However, in pancreatic adenocarcinoma, a hypoechoic mass may be identified in the head of the pancreas. Usually CT or MRI is needed to evaluate the extent of the disease. Also, cholangiocarcinoma may not always occur distally but occur in the hilar region, or so-called *Klatskin's tumor,*

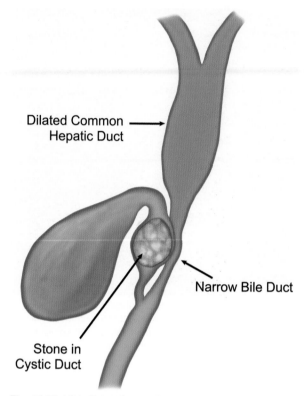

Fig. 17.20 Mirizzi's syndrome. Diagram of an impacted stone lodged in the cystic duct with surrounding edema that causes narrowing and obstruction of the common hepatic duct.

in which the patient may present with jaundice. Hilar masses will not dilate the extrahepatic biliary ductal system, but there will be dilatation at the junction of the right and left hepatic ducts as well as intrahepatic biliary system. A mass in this region may be difficult to identify with ultrasound.

Cholangitis. Recurrent pyogenic cholangitis is identified with both intrahepatic and extrahepatic biliary ductal dilatation with multiple soft, pigmented stones and purulent material. The gallbladder is often distended in these cases.

AIDS-related cholangitis may cause intrahepatic and extrahepatic biliary ductal dilatation. Usually, AIDS-related cholangitis is due to cryptosporidium or cytomegalovirus. This can result in a number of different sonographic findings, including distal biliary and/or intrahepatic ductal dilatation and strictures. There may also be gallbladder wall thickening in this entity.

Both acute bacterial cholangitis and primary sclerosing cholangitis may also produce intrahepatic biliary ductal dilatation. Close clinical correlation is needed in these cases.

Biloma. Biloma usually occurs as a complication of surgery or blunt and penetrating trauma and appears as a well-defined cystic structure noted in the right upper quadrant of the abdomen. The differential would include a hematoma or abscess, both of which usually have more internal echoes. Often CT is utilized as the next examination after ultrasound in these patients. A biloma may be confirmed by performing MRCP with a hepatobiliary agent such as Eovist. This agent is excreted into the biliary tract and will fill a biloma.

BIBLIOGRAPHY

Cartwright SL, Knudson MP. Diagnostic imaging of acute abdominal pain in adults. *Am Fam Physician.* 2015;91:452–459.

Chawla S, Trick WE, Gilkey S, Attar BM. Does cholecystectomy status influence the common bile duct diameter? a matched-pair analysis. *Dig Dis Sci.* 2010;55:1155–1160.

Chung CJ, Sivit CJ, Rakusan TA, Chandra RS, Ellaurie M. Hepatobiliary abnormalities on sonography in children with HIV infection. *J Ultrasound Med.* 1994;13:205–210.

Corwin MT, Siewert B, Sheiman RG, Kane RA. Incidentally detected gallbladder polyps: is follow-up necessary?-- Long-term clinical and US analysis of 346 patients. *Radiology.* 2011;258:277–282.

Fakhry J. Sonography of tumefactive biliary sludge. *AJR Am J Roentgenol.* 1982;139:717–719.

Graham MF, Cooperberg PL, Cohen MM, Burhenne HJ. The size of the normal common hepatic duct following cholecystectomy: an ultrasonographic study. *Radiology.* 1980;135:137–139.

Horrow MM, Horrow JC, Niakosari A, Kirby CL, Rosenberg HK. Is age associated with size of adult extrahepatic bile duct: sonographic study. *Radiology.* 2001;221:411–414.

Kim HC, Yang DM, Jin W, Ryu JK, Shin HC. Color doppler twinkling artifacts in various conditions during abdominal and pelvic sonography. *J Ultrasound Med.* 2010;29:621–632.

Kumar A, Senthil G, Prakash A, et al. Mirizzi's syndrome: lessons learnt from 169 patients at a single center. *Korean J Hepatobiliary Pancreat Surg.* 2016;20:17–22.

Laing FC, Jeffrey RB, Wing VW. Improved visualization of choledocholithiasis by sonography. *AJR Am J Roentgenol.* 1984;143:949–952.

Levy AD, Murakata LA, Abbott RM, Rohrmann Jr CA. From the archives of the AFIP. Benign tumors and tumorlike lesions of the gallbladder and extrahepatic bile ducts: radiologic-pathologic correlation. *Radiographics.* 2002;22:387–413.

Lim JH, Ko YT, Lee DH, Hong KS. Oriental cholangiohepatitis: sonographic findings in 48 cases. *AJR Am J Roentgenol.* 1990;155:511–514.

Loehfelm TW, Tse JR, Jeffrey RB, Kamaya A. The Utility of Hepatic Artery Velocity in Diagnosing Patients With Acute Cholecystitis. (NY): *Abdom Radiol.* 2017.

MacDonald FR, Cooperberg PL, Cohen MM. The WES triad -- a specific sonographic sign of gallstones in the contracted gallbladder. *Gastrointest Radiol.* 1981;6:39–41.

McArthur TA, Planz V, Fineberg NS, Tessler FN, Robbin ML, Lockhart ME. The common duct dilates after cholecystectomy and with advancing age: reality or myth? *J Ultrasound Med.* 2013;32:1385–1391.

Raghavendra BN, Subramanyam BR, Balthazar EJ, Horii SC, Megibow AJ, Hilton S. Sonography of adenomyomatosis of the gallbladder: radiologic-pathologic correlation. *Radiology.* 1983;146:747–752.

Ralls PW, Colletti PM, Lapin SA, et al. Real-time sonography in suspected acute cholecystitis. Prospective evaluation of primary and secondary signs. *Radiology.* 1985;155:767–771.

Ralls PW, Colletti PM, Quinn MF, Lapin SA, Morris UL, Halls J. Sonography in recurrent oriental pyogenic cholangitis. *AJR Am J Roentgenol.* 1981;136:1010–1012.

Teefey SA, Dahiya N, Middleton WD, et al. Acute cholecystitis: do sonographic findings and WBC count predict gangrenous changes? *AJR Am J Roentgenol.* 2013;200:363–369.

Yarmish GM, Smith MP, Rosen MP, et al. ACR appropriateness criteria right upper quadrant pain. *J Am Coll Radiol.* 2014;11:316–322.

18

Pancreas

John P. McGahan

NORMAL ANATOMY

The pancreas is mostly within the retroperitoneum in the anterior pararenal space. However, the tail of the pancreas is actually an intraperitoneal structure and in close relationship with the splenorenal ligament. To best understand the anatomy of the pancreas, an understanding of embryology is necessary. The pancreas develops from two pancreatic buds: the dorsal bud and the ventral bud. With development, the ventral bud of the pancreas rotates posterior to the duodenum and becomes the uncinate process. The dorsal bud comprises most of the pancreas. The main pancreatic duct usually enters with or in close proximity to the common bile duct into the duodenum at the major papilla, through the duct of Wirsung. The distal part of the dorsal pancreatic duct forms the duct of Santorini and can persist as an accessory pancreatic duct and enters the duodenum at the minor papilla. On occasion, the entire pancreatic duct enters the duodenum through the accessory duct of Santorini. When this anatomic variant is found with the ventral and dorsal pancreatic ducts not fusing, this is termed *pancreatic divisum*. This important to note, as this can be an etiology of acute and/or recurrent pancreatitis.

In most adults, the anterior/posterior dimension of the pancreas can vary from 2.0 to 3.0 cm in thickness. The head of the pancreas is anatomically in close approximation to the "C" loop of the duodenum. The splenic vein forms the posterior margin of the pancreas and joins the superior mesenteric vein in the region of the head or neck of the pancreas (Fig. 18.1). The uncinate process projects posteriorly from the pancreatic head. The neck is the thinnest portion of the pancreas and is the region between the body and the head, usually at the confluence of the splenic and superior mesentery vein. The superior mesenteric artery is noted posterior to the pancreas. It can be recognized by the mesenteric fat surrounding it.

ULTRASOUND TECHNIQUES/FINDINGS

The pancreas is usually fairly homogeneous in appearance. A scanning window is provided through the left lobe of the liver. Often, the partially collapsed stomach or pylorus of the stomach can be seen. The muscular wall of the stomach will be hypoechoic and can be confused with the pancreatic duct. The pancreas is often obscured by bowel gas, and as such moderate probe pressure is utilized. The body of the pancreas is the portion of the pancreas most commonly identified. Visualization of the head of the pancreas may be aided by using a right subcostal approach and angling the transducer medially. The tail of the pancreas is often difficult to identify but may be aided by having the patient drink de-gassed water. Within the head of the pancreas, the gastroduodenal artery is seen anteriorly, whereas the common bile duct is seen more posteriorly in the pancreatic head (Fig. 18.2). The pancreatic duct can be seen in normal patients. The superior mesenteric vein joins the splenic vein and is noted posterior to the pancreas. The superior mesenteric artery is seen as a rounded structure, which is recognized by the echogenic mesentery fat surrounding it (see Fig. 18.2).

The pancreas is just as or slightly more echogenic than the liver. With age, there can be a change in the size and echogenicity of the pancreas. If there is gradual atrophy of the pancreas, there may be fatty replacement of the pancreas with fibrosis and fat, which increases the echogenicity of the pancreas. Pancreatic atrophy may be better identified with computed tomography (CT). The pancreas may be seen not only with a transverse scan but also with a parasagittal scan. Depending on the parasagittal plane that is used, the liver and the stomach are visualized. Surrounding vascular structures help with the localization of the pancreas (Fig. 18.3).

ACUTE ABDOMINAL PAIN

Acute Pancreatitis

Patients with acute pancreatitis usually present with pain, vomiting, and abdominal tenderness. Laboratory findings include elevation of lipase and amylase. There are a variety of etiologies of acute pancreatitis. These are included in Table 18.1. Probably the most common etiology is gallstones in the common bile duct. Thus the gallbladder should be scanned for any evidence of cholelithiasis. Also, careful scanning of the common bile duct may identify choledocholithiasis. Choledocholithiasis is difficult to identify and is discussed in more detail in Chapter 17, on the gallbladder and biliary tract. Acute peripancreatic fluid collection may occur with either interstitial pancreatitis or in necrotizing pancreatitis. After 4 weeks the fluid collections in both entities have well-defined walls. In interstitial pancreatitis, the fluid collections are called *pseudocysts*, and in necrotizing pancreatitis, the fluid collections are called *walled-off necrosis*.

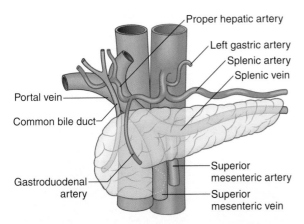

Fig. 18.1 Diagram of the pancreas showing its relationship with surrounding vascular structures. (From Hertzberg B. *Ultrasound, The Requisites*. 3rd ed. Philadelphia, PA: Elsevier; 2015: 180, Fig. 7-1.)

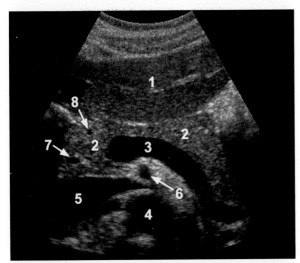

Fig. 18.2 Transverse image of the pancreas. Transverse image of the upper abdomen through the liver (*1*) demonstrates the pancreas (*2*). Within the head of the pancreas is the common bile duct (*7*) and the gastroduodenal artery (*8*). Also, the posterior boundary of the pancreas is the confluence of the splenic vein and the superior mesenteric vein (*3*). The superior mesenteric artery (*6*) lies anterior to the aorta (*4*). (*5*, IVC.) (From McGahan JP, Teefey SA, Needleman L. *General and Vascular Ultrasound*. 3rd ed. Philadelphia, PA: Elsevier; 2016: 45, Fig. 22-2.)

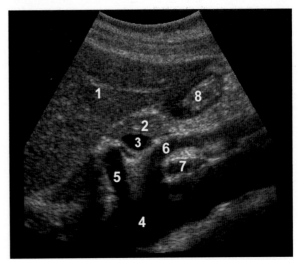

Fig. 18.3 Longitudinal view of the pancreas and upper abdomen. (*1*, liver; *2*, pancreas; *3*, splenic vein; *4*, aorta; *5*, celiac axis; *6*, superior mesenteric artery [SMA]; *7*, left renal vein; *8*, gastric antrum.) (From McGahan JP, Teefey SA, Needleman L. *General and Vascular Ultrasound*. 3rd ed. Philadelphia, PA: Elsevier, 2016: 45, Fig. 22-3.)

In mild acute pancreatitis, ultrasound appearance may be normal. However, subtle features can be identified with ultrasound in acute pancreatitis (Fig. 18.4). One of these features is enlargement of the pancreas. This is the most common feature identified with acute pancreatitis. Unfortunately, many times there is no prior ultrasound for comparison, and thus enlargement of the pancreas, unless it is focal, may be difficult to detect. The measurement of the anterior/posterior dimension of the pancreas varies between patients and location in the pancreas. Usually, the anterior/posterior measurement of the head is <3 cm, the body is <2.5 cm, and the tail is <2.0 cm. Usually, the enlargement is diffuse, but it may be focal. If focal, it often occurs in the head of the pancreas. This focal enlargement from pancreatitis may be difficult to differentiate from a pancreatic mass, such as pancreatic cancer.

The second finding of acute pancreatitis is decreased gland echogenicity. However, this is not always present. With acute pancreatitis, the pancreas appears hypoechoic or may have hypoechoic regions. Finally, the margins of the pancreas may be poorly defined. There can also be surrounding fluid collections. Fig. 18.4 shows a case of a patient who had a prior scan when there was no evidence of pancreatitis, followed by a scan when the patient had acute pancreatitis. In this case of acute pancreatitis, there are subtle findings of slightly decreased echogenicity and slightly increased thickness of the pancreas. There are also ill-defined pancreatic margins in this case. Fluid collections may appear in different areas around the pancreas with acute pancreatitis. If seen, they may be helpful to confirm the diagnosis. Approximately 40% of patients with acute pancreatitis develop fluid

collections. In acute interstitial pancreatitis, these fluid collections are homogeneous in terms of fluid density, whereas in acute necrotizing pancreatitis, these fluid collections are heterogeneous on ultrasound.

Subacute Pancreatitis (Pseudocysts)

Fluid collections occurring with interstitial pancreatitis that become encapsulated after 4 weeks from the onset of symptoms are called *pseudocysts*. Pseudocysts require this time to mature to a point where they can be drained surgically. Pseudocysts may be very small and seen as a cystic mass in or about the pancreas. If there is no other prior imaging, small pseudocysts and cystic tumors

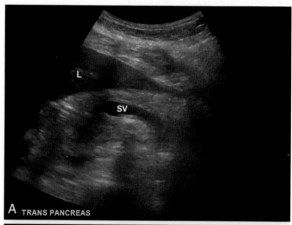

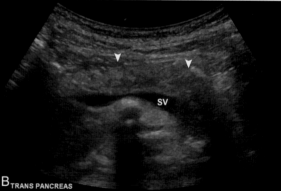

Fig. 18.4 Acute pancreatitis. (A) Ultrasound image of the upper abdomen demonstrates some increased echogenicity of the pancreas, probably reflecting some atrophy within the pancreas. *L,* Liver. Note the margins of the pancreas are very distinct. *SV,* Splenic vein. (B) Five days later the patient had a bout of acute pancreatitis with elevated lipase. On this scan note the pancreas (*arrowheads*) appears more hypoechoic and was slightly enlarged compared with earlier baseline images. *SV,* Splenic vein. The pancreatic margins are less distinct.

TABLE 18.1   **Causes of Acute Pancreatitis**

a. Choledocholithiasis
b. Alcohol
c. Medications
d. Infection (viral)
e. Pancreatic etiologies
　1. Annular pancreas
　2. Pancreatic divisum
f. Systemic processes
　1. Autoimmune
　2. Hypercalcemia
　3. Hyperlipidemia
g. Injury

of the pancreas may have a very similar appearance (Videos 18.1 and 18.2). Larger pseudocysts may develop after pancreatitis. These pseudocysts are encapsulated and anechoic with good through-transmission (Fig. 18.5). These are fairly easy to diagnose, as there usually has been an antecedent more-pronounced case of acute pancreatitis with resultant surrounding fluid collections that eventually develop into pseudocysts. These patients may present with pain or discomfort.

Patients who present after a bout of acute necrotizing pancreatitis can develop other fluid collections. In more severe pancreatitis, there may be regions of pancreatic necrosis. Fluid collections are more heterogeneous and have no definable wall. In time, these fluid collections may develop a well-defined wall but are very heterogeneous. This is called *walled-off necrosis* (Video 18.3). In pancreatic necrosis, there is nonenhancing pancreatic parenchyma, as seen on contrast-enhanced CT. Ultrasound can identify the sequalae of pancreatic necrosis, which is the development of walled-off, heterogeneous fluid collections (Fig. 18.6, Video 18.3). This is a very serious disease and can result in a fatal outcome.

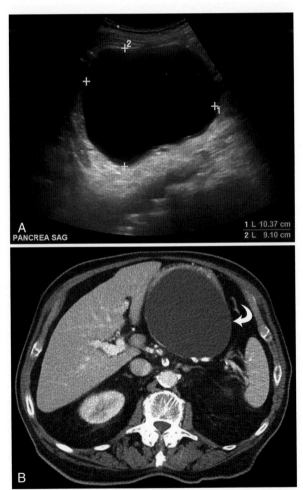

Fig. 18.5 Large pancreatic pseudocyst. (A) Parasagittal scan demonstrating large pseudocyst (*calipers*) noted within the body of the pancreas. Note the cyst is homogeneous. Cyst measured approximately 10 cm by 9 cm. (B) Corresponding CT scan demonstrating large pseudocyst (*curved arrow*) originating from the pancreas, which displaced the stomach anteriorly.

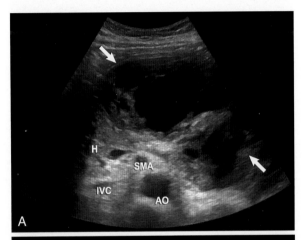

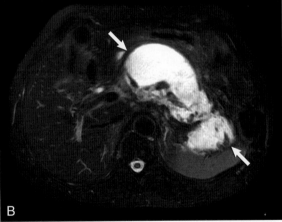

Fig. 18.6 Walled-off pancreatic necrosis. (A) Patient had ERCP-induced pancreatitis 2 months earlier. Now there is a large heterogeneous mass (*arrows*) originating from the body and tail of the pancreas. *AO*, Aorta; *H*, head of the pancreas; *IVC*, inferior vena cava; *SMA*, superior mesenteric artery. (B) Corresponding MRI demonstrates a walled-off heterogeneous mass in the body and tail of the pancreas (*arrows*) corresponding to fluid collections and debris.

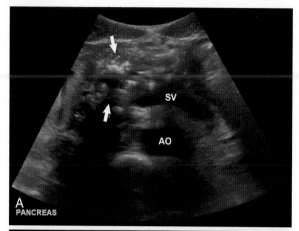

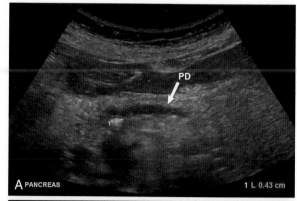

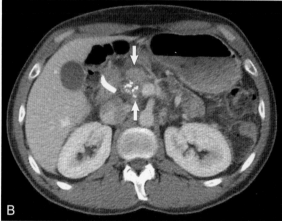

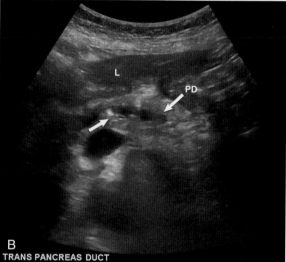

Fig. 18.7 Chronic pancreatitis. (A) Transverse ultrasound of the upper abdomen demonstrating multiple calcifications with shadowing (*arrows*) noted in the head of the pancreas. *AO*, Aorta; *SV*, Splenic vein. (B) Corresponding CT scan demonstrating a calcification in the head of the pancreas (*arrows*) corresponding to chronic pancreatitis.

Fig. 18.8 Chronic pancreatitis with pancreatic ductal stones. (A) Transverse image of the upper abdomen demonstrating echogenic pancreas. Additionally, there is dilatation of the pancreatic duct (*arrow*) as well as a stone (*calipers*) noted in the region of the head of the pancreas. (B) Pancreatic duct stone (*arrow*) is seen causing pancreatic duct (*PD*) dilatation. *L*, Liver.

Chronic Pancreatitis

With recurrent bouts of pancreatitis, there may be fibrosis and atrophy of the pancreas. There can be focal fibrosis with calcifications, which develops in the pancreas (Fig. 18.7). This can appear as a focal mass (Videos 18.4 and 18.5). In chronic pancreatitis, the mass that develops more often has focal calcifications compared with pancreatic cancer, which rarely has calcification. In chronic pancreatitis, there may be secondary pancreatic ductal dilatation from stones or secondary to fibrosis (Fig. 18.8, Video 18.6). These patients may present with pain from the chronic disease, or they can have recurrent bouts of acute pancreatitis superimposed on chronic disease.

PANCREATIC DUCT OR BIDUCTAL OBSTRUCTION

Biductal Dilation

Isolated biliary ductal obstruction may be secondary to choledocholithiasis or other biliary tract diseases. This is better discussed in Chapter 17, on the gallbladder and biliary tract. However, pancreatic adenocarcinoma, which accounts for approximately 90% of all pancreatic neoplasms, can cause biliary and pancreatitis duct dilatation. These patients may present with pain, but may also have painless jaundice. This cancer is most frequently located in the head of the pancreas, and thus biliary ductal, pancreatic ductal, and/or more commonly biductal dilation is present. This tumor can be identified by ultrasound. This mass is most often hypoechoic, although it may be heterogeneous, hyperechoic, or isoechoic. This mass causes an abrupt cutoff of the common bile duct. There will also be pancreatic ductal dilatation (Fig. 18.9, Videos 18.7–18.9). Ultrasound is helpful with use of color Doppler to show a vascular encasement of the vessels. There have been a variety of different Doppler scoring systems that in fact identify either partial or complete encasement of a pancreatic vessel with pancreatic adenocarcinoma. However, there also can be other periampullary neoplasms, including ampullary carcinoma, duodenal carcinoma, distal cholangiocarcinoma, or, rarely, metastatic disease (Fig. 18.10) causing biductal dilatation (Videos 18.10 and 18.11). These tumors may not always be identified with ultrasound, but the biductal dilatation may be seen. Certainly, in these cases, other imaging studies such as CT or magnetic resonance imaging (MRI) are necessary for better evaluation and staging.

Pancreatic Ductal Dilatation

Isolated pancreatic ductal dilatation may be secondary to a mass and/or chronic pancreatitis. There can be pancreatic ductal dilatation with atrophy of the more distal portion of the pancreas, especially with pancreatic cancer.

Patients with chronic pancreatitis will demonstrate a very heterogeneous echotexture to the pancreas, with very irregular margins. They will have pancreatic ductal dilatation and often have echogenic foci representing calculi within the pancreatic duct (see Fig. 18.8, Video 18.6). Adenocarcinomas rarely have calcifications and thus calcifications are most often due to chronic pancreatitis. On occasion, chronic pancreatitis may appear masslike. In these situations, it may be difficult to differentiate adenocarcinoma from focal chronic pancreatitis (see Fig. 18.7). In cases of prior inflammation, strictures may develop in the pancreatic duct (Fig. 18.11). These strictures cannot be identified with ultrasound, but there is usually ductal dilatation in the mid-body or tail of the pancreas. Pancreatic ductal dilatation may occur from a number of other etiologies. For instance, other tumors such as intrapapillary mucinous neoplasms (IPMN), especially of the main duct type, can cause isolated pancreatic ductal dilatation (Fig. 18.12). Although these patients may present with pain, these cysts are often incidental findings. In these situations, correlation with CT or MRI is important.

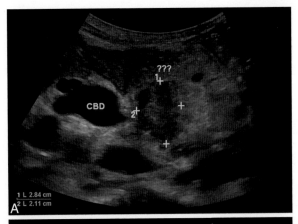

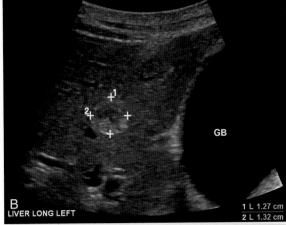

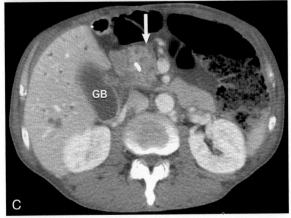

Fig. 18.9 Pancreatic adenocarcinoma. (A) Longitudinal scan of the abdomen demonstrates a dilated common bile duct (*CBD*) with distal obstruction from a mass (*calipers*), corresponding to adenocarcinoma of the pancreas. (B) Ultrasound of the liver in the same patient demonstrates one of many metastases (*calipers*) noted within the liver. *GB*, Gallbladder. (C) Corresponding CT scan demonstrates the patient has had a biliary endoscopy placed stent, noted centrally within the mass (*arrow*) in the head of the pancreas. Also note that in the right lobe of the liver there is still some dilatation of the biliary ductal system. *GB*, Gallbladder.

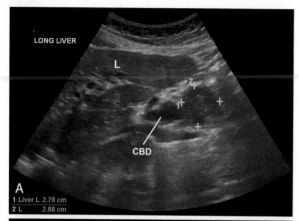

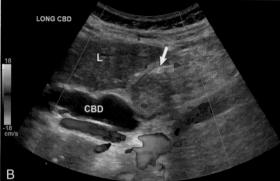

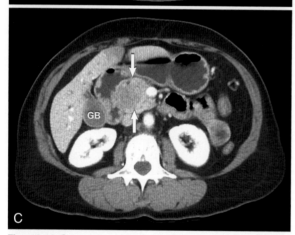

Fig. 18.10 Squamous cell lung carcinoma metastatic to the pancreas. (A) Longitudinal ultrasound of the abdomen demonstrated a mass (*calipers*) obstructing the common bile duct (*CBD*). *L*, Liver. (B) Another image again demonstrating the dilated CBD and the obstructing mass (*arrow*). *L*, Liver. (C) CT scan demonstrating the mass noted within the head of the pancreas (*arrows*). *GB*, Gallbladder.

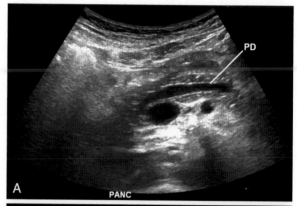

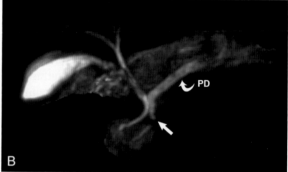

Fig. 18.11 Stricture of the pancreatic duct. (A) Transverse image of the upper abdomen demonstrating the dilated pancreatic duct (*PD*). (B) MRCP demonstrating abrupt cutoff of the pancreatic duct (*straight arrow*), which was shown on ERCP to be a pancreatic stricture from chronic pancreatitis. Also note the normal-appearing common bile duct and the gallbladder. *PD*, Pancreatic duct.

OTHERS

Pancreatic Cysts

As discussed previously, pancreatic pseudocysts are common cystic masses within the pancreas. However, there may be true simple cysts of the pancreas or cystic neoplasms of the pancreas. Some of these can be confused with pancreatic pseudocysts but do have a different prognosis. For instance, in patients with autosomal-dominant polycystic kidney disease or in Von Hippel–Lindau syndrome, multiple cysts can be seen within the pancreas. Some of these cysts can be cystic adenomas. Other cystic pancreatic masses, such as IPMN (see Fig. 18.12), are usually seen as small cysts within the pancreas and can be mistaken for pseudocysts. Likewise, mucinous cystic neoplasm (MCN) are usually larger pancreatic cystic masses.

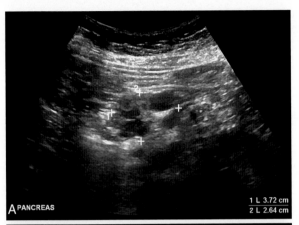

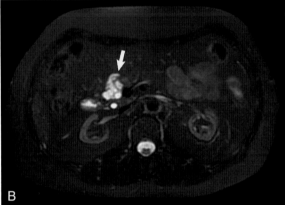

Fig. 18.12 Intraductal papillary mucinous neoplasm (IPMN). (A) There is a multicystic mass (*calipers*) noted in the region of the head of the pancreas. (B) On T2-weighted MRI, this mass (*arrow*) was a cyst that communicated with the pancreatic duct and was an IPMN.

Solid Pancreatic Masses

Most solid pancreatic masses are typically adenocarcinoma. However, enumerable other solid pancreatic masses can be seen. These are not usually encountered on an emergency basis, but could include other solid periampulary tumors, pancreatic endocrine (islet cell) tumors, lymphoma, or metastasis (see Videos 18.7–18.11).

Trauma

The pancreas may also be affected by trauma, which is partially discussed in Chapter 15, on the FAST scan. There may be a resultant hematoma, free fluid, or pancreatitis. There may be iatrogenic causes of pancreatitis, including endoscopic retrograde cholangiopancreatography (ERCP) and surgery, to name a few.

BIBLIOGRAPHY

Alpern MB, Sandler MA, Kellman GM, Madrazo BL. Chronic pancreatitis: ultrasonic features. *Radiology*. 1985;155:215–219.

Banks PA, Bollen TL, Dervenis C, et al. Classification of acute pancreatitis–2012: revision of the Atlanta classification and definitions by international consensus. *Gut*. 2013;62:102–111.

Bollen TL, van Santvoort HC, Besselink MG, van Es WH, Gooszen HG, van Leeuwen MS. Update on acute pancreatitis: ultrasound, computed tomography, and magnetic resonance imaging features. *Semin Ultrasound CT MR*. 2007;28:371–383.

Jeffrey RB Jr, Laing FC, Wing VW. Extrapancreatic spread of acute pancreatitis: new observations with real-time US. *Radiology*. 1986;159:707–711.

Koito K, Namieno T, Nagakawa T, Morita K. Inflammatory pancreatic masses: differentiation from ductal carcinomas with contrast-enhanced sonography using carbon dioxide microbubbles. *AJR Am J Roentgenol*. 1997;169:1263–1267.

Paivansalo M, Suramo I. Ultrasonography of the pancreatic tail through spleen and through fluid-filled stomach. *Eur J Radio*. 1986;6:113–115.

Siddiqi AJ, Miller F. Chronic pancreatitis: ultrasound, computed tomography, and magnetic resonance imaging features. *Semin Ultrasound CT MR*. 2007;28:384–394.

Taylor B. Carcinoma of the head of the pancreas versus chronic pancreatitis: diagnostic dilemma with significant consequences. *World J Surg*. 2003;27:1249–1257.

Yassa NA, Yang J, Stein S, Johnson M, Ralls P. Gray-scale and color flow sonography of pancreatic ductal adenocarcinoma. *J Clin Ultrasound*. 1997;25:473–480.

Zamboni GA, Ambrosetti MC, D'Onofrio M, Pozzi Mucelli R. Ultrasonography of the pancreas. *Radiol Clin North Am*. 2012;50:395–406.

19

Kidney and Renal Transplant

John P. McGahan

NORMAL ANATOMY

Kidneys

The kidneys are retroperitoneal structures and are surrounded by fascial layers, including Gerota's fascia. There is direct supply of the renal arteries and veins to the kidney from the abdominal aorta. The right and left renal arteries lie posterior to the renal veins. Their relationship to each other and the surrounding vascularity is shown in Fig. 19.1. The kidneys consist of the renal parenchyma, which is divided into the outer cortex and the inner medulla. Most of the cortex is peripheral to the medulla, except for the columns of Bertin, which are portions of the cortex that extend between the medullary pyramids. More centrally, the calyces, infundibulum, and renal pyramids are conduits delivering urine to the ureters (Fig. 19.2). The kidneys are approximately 11 cm long in adults, but vary in length from 9 to 12 cm. The renal veins and arteries can be identified with color flow (Video 19.1).

Ureters/Bladder

The ureters are small tubules connecting the retroperitoneally located kidneys to the urinary bladder. In most situations, only the proximal ureter, at the ureteropelvic junction, and the distal ureter, at the ureterovesicular junction, are visualized by ultrasound. The bladder lies deep in the pelvis. The bladder is oval in shape with the ureters entering the posterior lateral bladder wall. More distally, the bladder exits through the urethra. The normal bladder wall is approximately 4 to 6 mm in thickness and is smooth, but bladder wall thickness can increase with inadequate bladder filling. In males, the prostate is seen at the bladder base. In females, the uterus is seen deep to the posterior bladder wall. The urethra in the male is divided into the prostatic, membranous, and penile segments. The female urethra is shorter. Neither is well identified with transabdominal imaging.

NORMAL ULTRASOUND FINDINGS/ TECHNIQUES

Kidney

The kidneys can be imaged with the patient supine, using the liver and spleen as acoustic windows. The left kidney is more problematic to image due to the spleen providing a smaller acoustic window compared with the liver. The upper pole of the left kidney is often a "blind spot," as there is no ideal window for visualization. At times the kidneys, especially the left kidney, may be best visualized with the patient prone. As the superior pole of each kidney is located more medially than the lower pole, the transducer must be angled obliquely to capture the true long axis of the kidney. The kidneys should be scanned in both longitudinal and transverse planes. After longitudinal scanning, the transducer is rotated 90 degrees to the transverse plane, so that both the lower and upper poles of the kidney may be scanned in their entirety. Kidney length typically ranges from 9 to 12 cm, with the right kidney often slightly larger than the left.

The kidneys are usually less echogenic than the liver or spleen. The renal medulla is often hypoechoic compared with the renal cortex, whereas the renal sinus fat is more echogenic than the pyramids. The renal hilum is central and more echogenic than both the cortex and the medulla. The echogenicity is due to the renal sinus fat. The ureter, arteries, and veins are located in the renal hilum. When appropriate settings are used, the entire kidney will fill with color (Fig. 19.3).

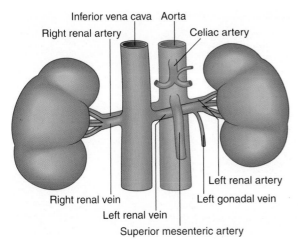

Fig. 19.1 Surface anatomy of the kidney. Diagram showing the relationship of the renal arteries and veins to the kidney. The proximal right renal artery lies posterior to the inferior vena cava (IVC), whereas the distal right renal artery lies posterior to the right renal vein. The left renal artery lies posterior to the left renal vein. The left renal vein lies between the aorta and superior mesenteric artery. (Redrawn with permission from Hertzberg B. *Ultrasound, The Requisites.* 3rd ed. Philadelphia, PA: Elsevier; 2015:133, Fig. 5-75.)

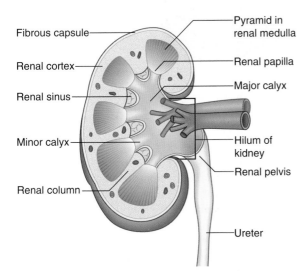

Fig. 19.2 Artist's rendering of a normal kidney. The outer portion of the kidney is the renal cortex, which extends between the renal medulla. The renal medulla filters into the pyramids and the renal papilla, which enter into a minor calyx. The calyceal system drains into the renal pelvis and then connects to the ureter (Redrawn with permission from Soni NJ. *Point of Care Ultrasound.* Philadelphia, PA: Elsevier; 2015:155, Fig. 20.2.)

Certain anatomic variants of the kidney may mimic a renal mass. The kidneys are usually smooth in contour but may have lobulations. These lobulations, when they occur, are numerous and affect both kidneys. There may be a region of prominent cortex or bulge seen in the midportion of the left kidney. This has been termed a *dromedary hump.* This "hump" usually appears as a focal bulge in the left side of the kidney, probably secondary to compression by adjacent structures such as the spleen. This "hump" may be mistaken as for mass (Fig. 19.4). Portions of the cortex extending deep between the medullary pyramids as a column of Bertin may be mistaken for a mass as well. Careful scanning and knowledge of the sonographic appearance of the kidneys will help avoid these pitfalls.

Ureter

The proximal ureter is best visualized in a coronal oblique view using the kidney as an acoustic window. The ureter is very difficult to follow to the bladder because of overlying bowel gas. However, the proximal ureter often can be identified at the ureteropelvic junction. More distally, the ureter can be visualized with a full bladder technique, which may be helpful to identify distal ureteric stones or to see anomalies at the ureterovesicular junction, such as an ureterocele. Additionally, the distal ureter may be identified in women with a transvaginal approach. Color flow ultrasound is useful to identify the distal ureters entering the bladder as color "jets," where the urine enters into the bladder (Fig. 19.5). If these are present, this identifies the ureteric orifice and demonstrates there is no complete ureteric obstruction.

Bladder

The bladder is best evaluated when moderately filled. With underdistention of the bladder, there is suboptimal visualizing of the bladder, bladder masses, or surrounding pelvic structures. Alternatively, an overdistended bladder may cause patient discomfort, which can make scanning difficult. The bladder should be scanned in both the transverse and parasagittal planes. There is constant peristalsis of the ureters as they enter the bladder. Flow of urine from the ureter into the bladder is observed as ureteral "jets" in the bladder with color Doppler ultrasound (see Fig. 19.5). Often, a Foley catheter has been placed in acutely ill patients, introducing a small amount of air into the bladder and making visualization of the bladder or its contents difficult or

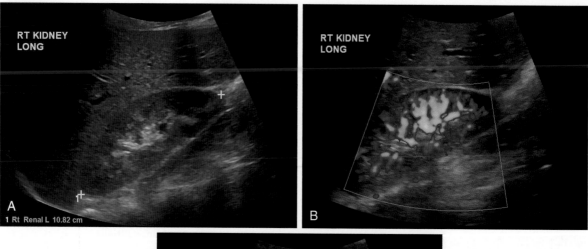

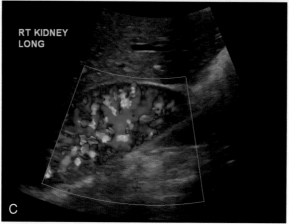

Fig. 19.3 Normal kidney with power and color Doppler. (A) Right renal ultrasound demonstrating normal appearance of the kidney. Liver is anterior. (B) With power Doppler, there is perfusion of the kidney to the renal cortex using the appropriate Doppler settings. (C) With color Doppler ultrasound, there is perfusion of the kidney to the renal cortex.

nearly impossible. As noted previously, the bladder even partially filled may be visualized utilizing a transvaginal approach in women.

ACUTE FLANK PAIN

There are enumerable etiologies of flank pain. Some of these are listed in Table 19.1. The renal etiologies can be basically divided into extraparenchymal renal etiologies and renal parenchymal disease. The major causes that may be detected by ultrasound are often extraparenchymal disease, such as hydronephrosis or stone disease. Parenchymal causes of pain include pyelonephritis, abscess, or renal cysts/masses.

Other etiologies, such as musculoskeletal pain or local trauma, may require nonsonographic methods for detection. Structures that surround the kidney may be the etiology of flank pain.

Hydronephrosis

Although dilatation of the renal collective system usually implies obstruction, dilatation may be secondary to ureteral reflux. A rare abnormality that results in renal dilatation is diabetes insipidus. Different etiologies of renal collecting system dilatation are listed in Table 19.2.

The level of obstruction and the etiology of the hydronephrosis can often be diagnosed by

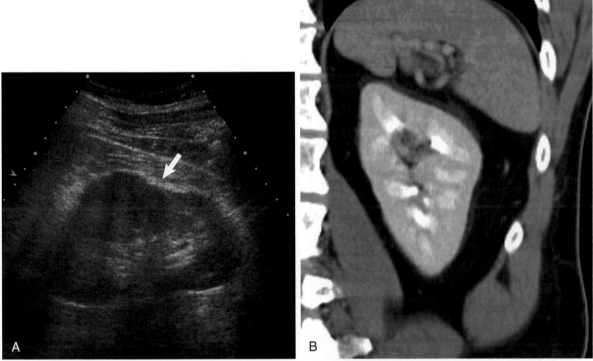

Fig. 19.4 Dromedary hump. (A) Ultrasound of the left kidney demonstrates masslike prominence of the mid-pole of the left kidney (*arrow*), thought to be caused by compression of the spleen on the upper pole of the left kidney. This was thought to be a mass, and a CT scan was obtained. (B) Corresponding CT scan showing prominence of the midpole of the left kidney, but without a mass.

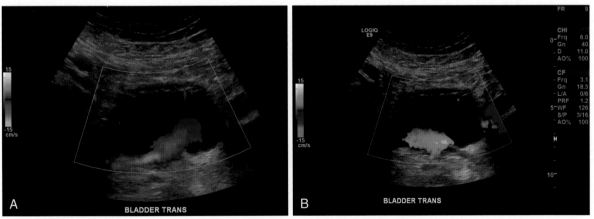

Fig. 19.5 Normal bladder jets. (A) Transverse ultrasound through the bladder demonstrating the right ureteral jet. (B) Transverse ultrasound through the bladder demonstrating the left ureteral jet.

TABLE 19.1 **Potential Etiologies of Right Flank Pain**
I. Extra-Parenchymal renal disease
a. Nephrolithiasis
b. Ureteral stricture/clots
c. Compression (retroperitoneal fibrosis)
d. Bladder outlet obstruction
II. Renal parenchymal disease
a. Pyelonephritis
b. Renal abscess/xanthogranulomatous pyelonephritis
c. Renal infarct
d. Venous obstruction
e. Renal cysts/tumors
III. Others
a. Musculoskeletal
b. Trauma (rib)
c. Radiculopathy
d. Herpes zoster
e. Pleuritis
f. Surrounding organs

TABLE 19.2 **Causes of Renal Collecting System Dilatation**
I. Common
a. Obstruction
b. Previous obstruction
c. Extra renal pelvis
d. Distended bladder
e. Pregnancy
II. Uncommon
a. Diabetes insipidus
b. Reflux nephropathy

sonography. Proximal renal obstruction is most commonly due to stones, but rarely tumors such as a transitional cell carcinoma. If there is ureteric dilatation, then the bladder should always be scanned to potentially diagnose the bladder as the site of obstruction. This is discussed in more detail in the "Bladder" section of the chapter.

There are a variety of different methods of classifying hydronephrosis. In the adult, most hydronephrosis is classified as mild, moderate, or severe (Figs. 19.6 and 19.7). However, in the newborn and pediatric patient, there are other classifications, including that of the Society of Fetal Surgery that grades hydronephrosis from grade 1 to grade 4.

In mild hydronephrosis, there may be more central dilatation of the renal pelvis, with minimal calyceal dilatation. Moderate hydronephrosis in the adult is characterized by more pronounced dilatation of the renal pelvis and progressive dilatation of the calyceal system. The outer cortex is preserved (Fig. 19.7, Video 19.2). Severe hydronephrosis in adults is characterized by more pronounced dilatation of the renal collecting system, as well as marked dilatation of the calyceal system. In these situations, there is distortion of the medullary pyramids and thinning of the renal cortex (Video 19.3).

There are a few pitfalls in the diagnosis of hydronephrosis. These include parapelvic cysts that may mimic hydronephrosis. The cysts are located within the renal pelvis and are fairly smooth walled and rounded or oval. These cysts are fairly localized, except in cases where there are multiple parapelvic cysts, which may mimic hydronephrosis (Fig. 19.8).

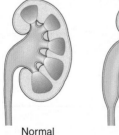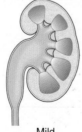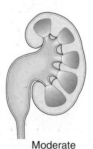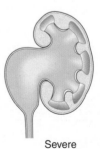

Normal   Mild   Moderate   Severe

Fig. 19.6 Hydronephrosis. Hydronephrosis can be mild, moderate, or severe. In mild hydronephrosis, there are enlarged calyces. In moderate hydronephrosis, there are dilated calyces with obliteration of the papillae and blunted pyramids. In more severe hydronephrosis, there is marked calyceal dilatation, complete obliteration of the papillae and pyramids, and thinning of the renal cortex. (Redrawn with permission from Soni NJ. *Point of Care Ultrasound*. Philadelphia, PA: Elsevier; 2015:157, Fig. 20.6.)

The parapelvic vessels, especially the parapelvic veins, may be mistaken for a dilated renal pelvis. These vessels are easily distinguished from a dilated renal pelvis by use of color flow ultrasound, which clearly demonstrates these are vascular structures (Fig. 19.8).

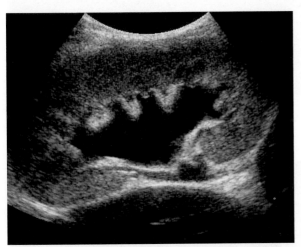

Fig. 19.7 Moderate hydronephrosis. Renal ultrasound dilation demonstrating moderate hydronephrosis with blunting of the calyceal system and more pronounced renal pelvis dilation. (From Middleton W. *General and Vascular Ultrasound*. 2nd ed. Philadelphia, PA: Elsevier; 2007:11.)

Finally, there are different degrees of prominence of the renal pelvis, with some patients having an extra renal pelvis. This may be the normal baseline in these patients, and this should not be confused with hydronephrosis. Comparison with prior studies is often helpful for this distinction.

Renal Stones

Renal stones may be obstructive or nonobstructive. Nonobstructive renal stones appear as an echogenic focus in the kidney. Renal stones are usually composed of calcium oxalate or phosphate. If large enough, they cast an acoustic shadow. Shadowing may be better demonstrated by using a higher-frequency transducer and adjusting the focal zone. Stones will also produce a "twinkle" artifact with color Doppler, seen as alternating color posterior to the stone, compared with the more homogenous color flow of veins and arteries (Fig. 19.9, Videos 19.4–19.6).

Stones may cause obstruction and are a common etiology of flank pain. As discussed previously, obstructing stones associated with hydronephrosis are seen as an echogenic focus with acoustic shadowing. Stones also lodge distally at the ureter–pelvic junction (UPJ). These stones may be seen with transabdominal scanning through the bladder (see Fig. 19.10). Color flow is

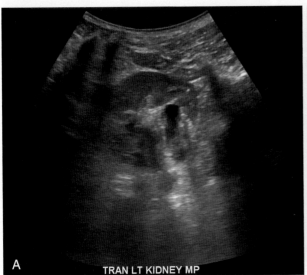

A   TRAN LT KIDNEY MP

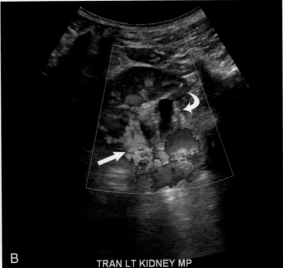

B   TRAN LT KIDNEY MP

Fig. 19.8 Parapelvic cyst and normal renal vein. (A) Real-time ultrasound of the left kidney demonstrates two central hypoechoic structures that were thought to represent renal pelvic dilation. (B) With color flow, one of these structures was noted to be the renal vein (*arrow*), and the other was noted to be an elongated parapelvic cyst (*curved arrow*). No hydronephrosis was identified.

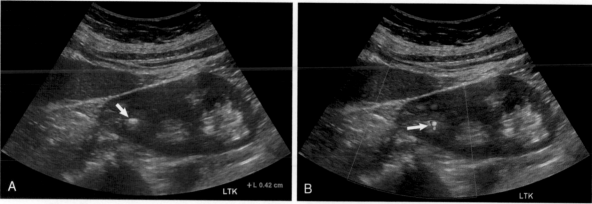

Fig. 19.9 Renal stone plus "twinkle" artifact. (A) This 4-mm stone is well demonstrated by ultrasound calipers (*arrow*), with little shadowing. (B) With color Doppler ultrasound, there is evidence of a "twinkle" artifact at and distal to the stone.

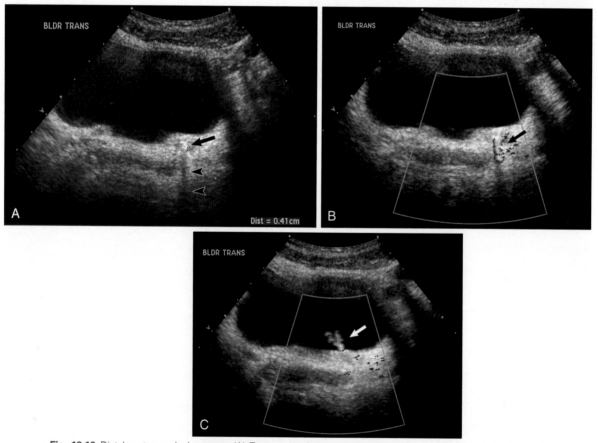

Fig. 19.10 Distal ureterovesicular stone. (A) Transverse ultrasound through the bladder demonstrates a small echogenic focus of a stone lodged in the distal ureter at the ureterovesicular junction (*arrow*). Note the distal acoustic shadowing (*arrowheads*). The stone did not move with patient positioning. (B) With color Doppler, the stone is more evident, showing a "twinkle" artifact distal to the stone (*arrow*). (C) Color Doppler of the ureteric orifice demonstrates flow through the ureter, indicating the stone causes partial and not complete ureteral obstruction.

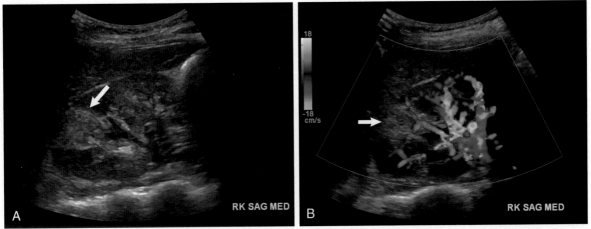

Fig. 19.11 Focal pyelonephritis. (A) Real-time ultrasound examination demonstrates a well-demarcated, echogenic region noted within the upper pole of the right kidney (*arrow*). (B) Color Doppler ultrasound demonstrated this region to be avascular (*arrow*). This region corresponded to an area of focal pyelonephritis. (From McGahan JP, Teefey SA, Needleman L. *General and Vascular Ultrasound*. 3rd ed. Philadelphia, PA: Elsevier; 2016;39, Figs. 19-1, 19-2.)

useful to show the "twinkle" artifact of the stone. If there is complete ureteral obstruction, no color "jet" will be seen. With partial obstruction a "jet" is still present (Fig. 19.10). Rarely, on transvaginal ultrasound, distal ureteric stones may be identified.

Pitfalls of Renal Stones. There are mimics of renal stones. These include vascular calcifications that appear as linear, closely spaced reflections. Although less likely to produce acoustic shadowing, if severe enough, shadowing may be observed with vascular calcifications. Renal sinus fat is more diffuse and should not be confused with renal stones. Usually, the renal medulla is hypoechoic to the renal cortex. However, with renal nephrocalcinosis, the medulla appears to be diffusely echogenic and should not be confused with renal stones, which are a more focal process.

Pyelonephritis

Patients with acute flank pain may be suffering from renal obstruction, but if there is pyuria, or evidence of infection, pyelonephritis may be considered. Acute pyelonephritis is an infection of the renal parenchyma and collecting system most commonly secondary to lower urinary tract infection. The etiology is usually a bacterial infection from *Escherichia coli*. With mild pyelonephritis, the kidney may appear sonographically normal. There may be some perinephric fluid,

renal enlargement, and decreased visualization of the renal sinus fat. Focal pyelonephritis may result in areas of decreased or increased echogenicity (Fig. 19.11, Video 19.7). There also may be decreased distinction of the renal medulla and cortex. In these situations there may be swelling of a portion of the renal parenchyma, resulting in a differentiation from the rest of the renal parenchyma. This region is usually avascular (Video 19.8). With treatment of pyelonephritis, the kidney will eventually appear normal. Contrast-enhanced computed tomography (CT) is more sensitive than ultrasound in demonstrating focal pyelonephritis. Contrast-enhanced ultrasound shows promise in the detection of pyelonephritis. Eventually, these focal areas of pyelonephritis can resolve or develop into renal abscesses. These are usually hypoechoic and avascular areas within the kidney (Fig. 19.12). Color flow may demonstrate surrounding hyperemia. Contrast-enhanced CT or contrast-enhanced ultrasound may be helpful to better identify focal pyelonephritis or a focal renal abscess (see Fig. 19.12).

Emphysematous pyelonephritis is uncommon but is a severe infection where there is formation of an abscess with gas. This gas may appear echogenic with dirty shadowing. It is better depicted with CT.

Xanthogranulomatous pyelonephritis (XGP) is a chronic infection secondary to renal stone disease and will be discussed in the "Chronic Renal Obstruction" section.

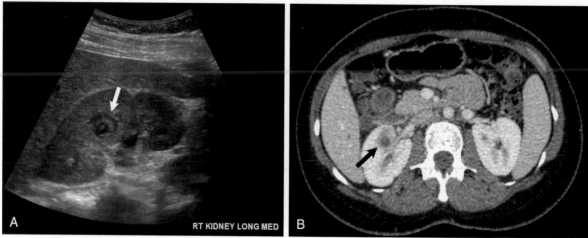

Fig. 19.12 Renal abscess. (A) A real-time ultrasound examination of the right kidney demonstrates a complex, well-demarcated mass in the midpole of the right kidney (*arrow*). (B) Corresponding CT scan demonstrates an area of decreased density within the kidney (*arrow*), which corresponds to a small renal abscess. (From McGahan JP, Teefey SA, Needleman L. *General and Vascular Ultrasound.* 3rd ed. Philadelphia, PA: Elsevier; 2016:276, Figs. S19-3, S19-4.)

CHRONIC FLANK PAIN/HEMATURIA

Chronic Renal Obstruction/Xanthogranulomatous Pyelonephritis

Renal stones are common etiologies of chronic renal obstruction. Chronic renal obstruction may be focal or diffuse, if secondary to a stone. This will lead to hydronephrosis, as previously described. Eventually, this can lead to Xanthogranulomatous pyelonephritis (XGP). This is a chronic infection of the kidney caused by a renal stone. There is a resultant hydronephrosis with chronic infection caused by *E. coli* or *Proteus mirabilis*. This results in either a focal or diffuse renal abscess. There is an enlarged hypoechoic-appearing kidney with a central echogenic focus with acoustic shadowing (Fig. 19.13). The renal parenchyma may appear hypoechoic secondary to a single or multiple areas of pyonephrosis/abscess.

Renal Masses/Cysts

Renal masses may be divided into renal cysts, complex cysts, and solid masses. These may have an etiology of chronic flank pain or hematuria. Simple renal cysts are commonly identified within the kidneys. These are thin-walled, smooth, anechoic masses with posterior acoustic enhancement (Fig. 19.14, Video 19.9). There is a Bosniak classification based upon the CT appearance of the

cysts, which classifies renal cysts as simple (Bosniak 1), mildly complex (Bosniak 2), more complex (Bosniak 3), and mixed solid and cystic (Bosniak 4). A Bosniak 2 cyst has a slightly thick septation with only a slight risk of malignancy. Ultrasound is more sensitive than CT in identifying septations within renal cysts. Cysts that are Bosniak 3 and/or 4 are more complex and have a high rate of malignancy and must be further evaluated with other imaging, such as contrast-enhanced magnetic resonance imaging (MRI) or CT. As discussed previously, parapelvic cysts are similar to cortical cysts but often are elongated and occur in the parapelvic region and may be confused with hydronephrosis. Multiple bilateral renal cysts occur with autosomal-dominant polycystic renal disease. In this entity, cysts are of various sizes and the kidneys are usually large (Fig. 19.15). This entity may be a cause of renal failure. Any renal cyst may be a cause for more acute flank pain, as there can be hemorrhage into the cyst.

Ultrasound alone cannot differentiate benign from malignant solid renal masses. The differential for renal masses is broad, but usually includes primary renal cell carcinoma (RCC), angiomyolipoma, oncocytoma, or metastatic disease. RCC can appear hyperechoic, isoechoic, or hypoechoic. Alternatively, angiomyolipomas (AML) are usually hyperechoic, but on occasion, the RCC may be hyperechoic and may be difficult to

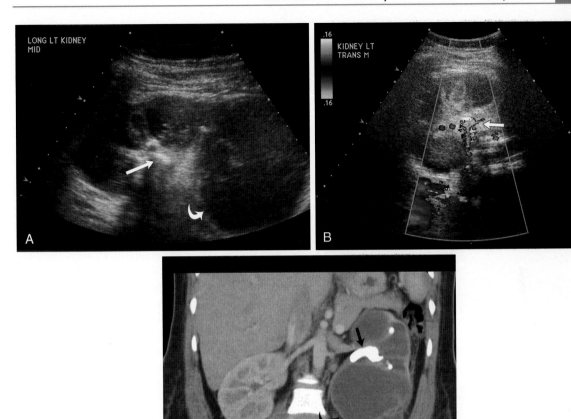

Fig. 19.13 Xanthogranomalatous pyelonephritis (XGP). (A) Longitudinal ultrasound demonstrating enlarged kidney with central echogenic focus (*arrow*), with some acoustic shadowing. Note masslike appearance to the lower pole of the left kidney (*curved arrow*). (B) Using color Doppler ultrasound, the renal stone is identified with a typical "twinkle" artifact (*arrow*). (C) Corresponding CT scan demonstrating a large central stone (*arrow*), which caused chronic obstruction of the left kidney with multiple abscesses (*curved arrow*). (From McGahan JP, Teefey SA, Needleman L. *General and Vascular Ultrasound*. 3rd ed. Philadelphia, PA: Elsevier; 2016: p. 345, Figs. S119-1, S119-2.)

differentiate from a fat-containing AML. A patient with a solid renal mass is often asymptomatic, but they may have hematuria or flank pain. If a renal mass is identified, examination of the renal vein and surrounding structures is important, as RCCs may invade the renal vein and cause local or more distant metastasis (Fig. 19.16, Videos 19.10 and 19.11).

ACUTE RENAL INSUFFICIENCY

Probably the most common etiology for acute renal insufficiency is decompensation of renal function in a patient with intrinsic renal disease, such as chronic glomerulonephritis or nephrosclerosis. In these entities the kidneys are small and echogenic. Etiologies such as hypertensive nephropathy or nephrosclerosis or hereditary nephritis usually have a bilateral decrease in renal size. Other etiologies of renal failure, such as acute nephrogenic toxicity, may have no changes in the appearance of the kidneys. In some cases of renal failure, there may be distinguishing features, such as multiple cysts with autosomal-dominant polycystic kidney disease (see Fig. 19.15).

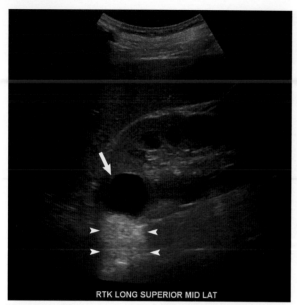

Fig. 19.14 Simple cyst. Longitudinal ultrasound demonstrated a well-demarcated, hypoechoic structure with smooth walls (*arrow*) and distal acoustic enhancement (*arrowheads*) consistent with a simple renal cyst.

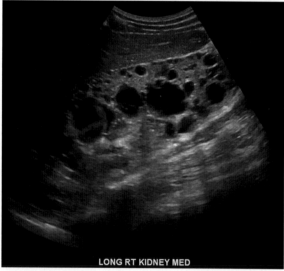

Fig. 19.15 Polycystic renal disease. Longitudinal ultrasound examination demonstrates an enlarged echogenic kidney with multiple cysts of differing sizes in autosomal-dominant polycystic renal disease.

The focus of ultrasound in cases of acute renal insufficiency is to exclude potential treatable etiologies, such as acute bilateral hydronephrosis or renal vein thrombosis. Hydronephrosis has been discussed in detail. Use of color flow may be helpful to identify the normal renal vein and excluded renal vein thrombosis (see Fig. 19.8).

BLADDER

Acute Infectious Cystitis

Females are more prone to bladder infection, although in males simultaneous prostatitis and cystitis are common. The most common organism found in cases of cystitis is *E. coli*. Patients may present with bladder irritability, frequency, and hematuria, and may be febrile with a left shift in the white blood cell count. There may be echogenic debris within the bladder in patients with acute cystitis (Fig. 19.17). This debris moves with positioning and has no increased vascularity (Videos 19.12 and 19.13). However, echogenic debris in the bladder may be a nonspecific finding or may be secondary to a number of etiologies, including hematuria (Video 19.14).

There may be diffuse bladder wall thickening in patients with chronic cystitis. However, there are a number of different etiologies for bladder wall thickening or bladder masses (Table 19.3).

Emphysematous Cystitis

Emphysematous cystitis is a more serious infection, often occurring in patients who are diabetic. Again, the most common offending organism is *E. coli*. Intramural gas is present within the wall of the bladder, associated with dirty shadowing. Also, there may be intraluminal gas present in these cases. Remember, intraluminal gas may be secondary to placement of a Foley catheter. Often, the bladder wall, if identified, is thickened and echogenic (see Table 19.3).

Chronic Cystitis

Chronic cystitis occurs after multiple bouts of acute cystitis. Chronic cystitis may produce more bladder thickening. The bladder may be smaller than normal because of repeated infections. In chronic cystitis, there may be invagination of portions of the uroepithelium into the lamina propria of the bladder wall. These are called *Brunn's epithelial nests,* which can result in multiple small cysts within the bladder, called either *cystitis cystica* or *cystitis glandularis*. These may be manifested as bladder wall cysts or solid papillary masses. Solid papillary masses within the bladder wall may be secondary to chronic cystitis, but they also may be due to other etiologies and may be difficult to differentiate from a

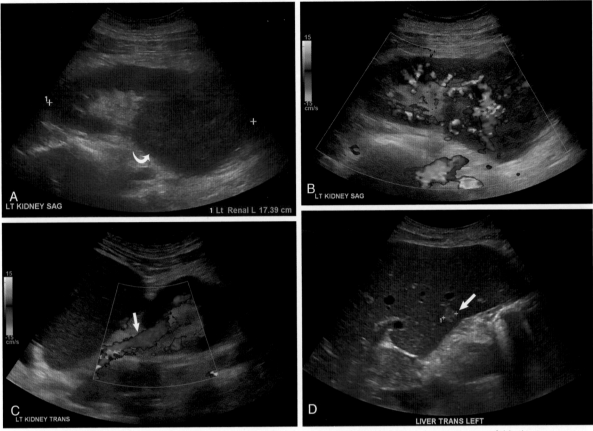

Fig. 19.16 Renal cell carcinoma. (A) Longitudinal images of the left kidney demonstrate a fairly large, hypoechoic mass (*curved arrow*) noted in the lower pole of the left kidney. (B) Longitudinal ultrasound with color demonstrates marked hypervascularity of the mass. (C) Transverse ultrasound image demonstrating a patent renal vein (*arrow*). (D) Incidental note is made of multiple echogenic masses (*arrow*) within the liver, which corresponded to metastasis from the left renal cell carcinoma.

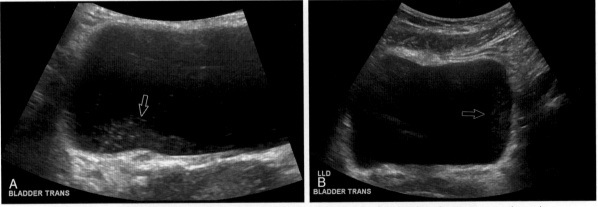

Fig. 19.17 Bladder debris in a patient with cystitis. (A) Transverse scan of the bladder demonstrates echogenic material noted in the posterior aspect of the bladder (*arrow*). There was no color flow. (B) The patient was placed in the left lateral decubitus position, and the bladder debris were noted to become dependent (*arrow*).

bladder neoplasm. Cystoscopy may be needed for precise diagnosis. Filling defects in the bladder are listed in Table 19.3.

Calculi

Bladder calculi may be secondary to migration of stones from the kidney into the bladder. Ureteric stones may pass into the bladder, but on occasion they become lodged at the ureterovesicular junction. Such stones may be visualized by scanning through the bladder or may be seen with transvaginal scanning in the female. These stones may demonstrate a "twinkle" artifact, and if they are totally

TABLE 19.3 **Potential Causes of Bladder Wall Thickening and Masses**	
Nonmalignant	**Malignant**
Chronic cystitis	Primary bladder tumors
Bladder outlet obstruction	Prostatic cancer
Postradiation	Lymphoma
Postoperative	Metastasis
Adherent blood clot	Cancer from contagious organs
Endometriosis	
Neurofibromatosis	
Benign prostatic hypertrophy	
Bladder calculi	

obstructive, they produce hydronephrosis and ureteric dilation. A ureteric jet may be identified with incomplete obstruction, but not seen with complete obstruction (see Fig. 19.10). These stones, unlike bladder stones, do not move with patient positioning. It is helpful to distinguish a distal ureterovesicular junction stone from a bladder stone by having the patients change position. A bladder stone will be mobile, whereas a distal ureterovesical stone will not move (see Figs. 19.10 and 19.18). Additionally, bladder calculi can occur because of urinary stasis within the bladder. Patients who have indwelling catheters may develop stones surrounding those catheters. These are similar to stones identified elsewhere, which are echogenic with acoustic shadowing (Fig. 19.18).

Tumor

Transitional cell carcinoma of the bladder is the most common malignant tumor of the bladder. Many patients present with hematuria, but can have generalized bladder complaints, including frequency and dysuria. Ultrasound may be helpful to identify a solid polypoid bladder tumor. These masses are noted to be nonmobile with increased color flow (Fig. 19.19). Some of these tumors are flat and appear as focal thickening. The differential for a bladder mass or focal thickening of the bladder is fairly broad (see Table 19.3). Squamous cell carcinoma is a rare tumor arising within the bladder, usually secondary to prior infection. Rarely, adenocarcinoma of

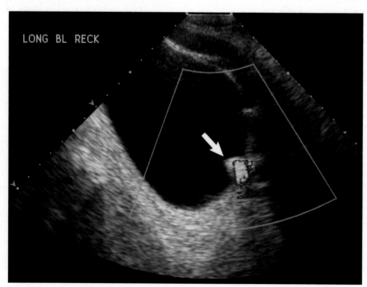

Fig. 19.18 Bladder stone. Echogenic focus (*arrow*) within the bladder, with a "twinkle" artifact. Note: This stone moved with positioning of the patient.

the bladder may be seen, usually in urachal remnants. Occasionally, debris in the bladder may appear as a mass. Debris is void of color and moves with patient positioning (see Fig. 19.17).

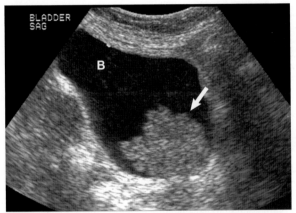

Fig. 19.19 Bladder cancer. Longitudinal ultrasound examination of the bladder (B) demonstrates a nonmobile polypoid mass (*arrow*). Color flow was noted in the mass. (From McGahan JP, Teefey SA, Needleman L. *General and Vascular Ultrasound*. 3rd ed. Philadelphia, PA: Elsevier; 2016:35, Fig. 17-1.)

RENAL TRANSPLANT: TYPES OF TRANSPLANTS

Anatomy and Scanning Technique

Most renal transplants are from adult donors and are placed into the right and/or left iliac fossa. The transplant renal artery is typically anastomosed to the external iliac artery. The transplant renal vein is typically anastomosed to the external iliac vein. The transplant ureter is tunneled into either the right or the left side of the dome of the bladder (Fig. 19.20).

More recently, pediatric en bloc renal transplants have been performed. In this situation, both kidneys from the donor are harvested with the donor aorta. Thus the donor renal vein is anastomosed to the left and/or right external iliac vein, and the donor aorta is anastomosed to the external iliac artery. There are two separate ureters, which are attached to separate tunnels in either the right or left side of the dome of the bladder (Fig. 19.21).

When imaging the transplant kidneys, higher-frequency transducers may be utilized. Linear array transducers using higher frequencies may be appropriate for the transplant kidney, as the kidney is superficially located. In adult donors, the superior portion of the

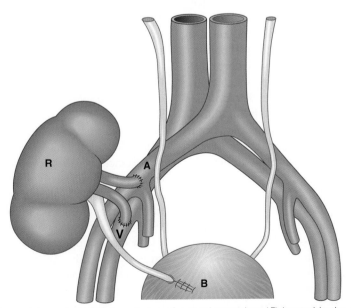

Fig. 19.20 Adult renal transplant. Artist rendering of a renal transplant (*R*) located in the right iliac fossa. The transplant renal artery is typically anastomosed to the external iliac artery (*A*). The transplant vein (*V*) is typically anastomosed to the external iliac vein. The transplant ureter is connected to the native bladder (*B*).

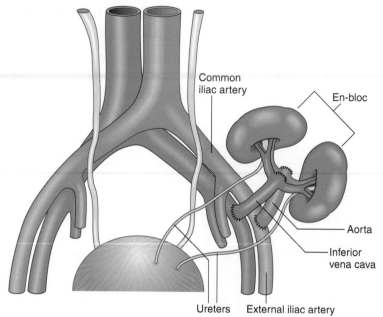

Fig. 19.21 Illustration of anatomy of pediatric en bloc kidney transplant. In this figure, kidney transplant is in the left lower quadrant with donor aorta anastomosed to the external iliac artery; the inferior vena cava was anastomosed to the left external iliac vein. (Redrawn with permission from Fananapazir G, Tse G, Corwin MT, et al. Pediatric en bloc kidney transplants: clinical and immediate postoperative US factors associated with vascular thrombosis. *Radiology.* 2016;279(3):935–942.)

transplant kidney is located laterally and the inferior pole of the kidney is medial. Therefore the transducer must be angled appropriately to obtain the long-axis measurement of the kidney. Both longitudinal and transverse images of the transplant kidney should be obtained. Imaging of the pediatric en bloc is more problematic, as these kidneys are often in a superior and inferior relationship to each other. Thus careful scanning is needed to locate both the superior and inferior kidney. Also, with en bloc kidneys, complications may occur to one and/or both of these kidneys, making scanning more difficult than with an adult transplant kidney.

Common Complications

Hydronephrosis. Hydronephrosis is one of the complications that may occur with a renal transplant. There may be mild prominence of the pelvicalyceal system from edema at the ureteral anastomosis site in the early postoperative period. Also, there may be some redundancy of the collecting system in the later postoperative period, which can cause mild renal pelvicalyceal dilatation. Moderate or severe hydronephrosis can be a complication

that occurs with implantation of the ureter into the bladder and can be easily recognized by ultrasound (Fig. 19.22, Video 19.3). When it is unclear if the etiology of hydronephrosis is from a functional obstruction, renal scintigraphy can be utilized.

Fluid Collections. Renal transplant fluid collections are very common. Small hematomas are identified in the postoperative period. However, sonography has been noted to miss small hematomas or postoperative fluid collections. These hematomas are probably not of importance until they compress the kidney, ureter, and/or the collecting system (Fig. 19.23). Acute hematomas may be difficult to detect, as they may be isoechoic to the surrounding peritoneal fat or muscle (see Fig. 19.23). Thus if a hematoma is suspected, rescanning at a later date is important, as these hematomas become more cystic with anechoic regions (see Fig. 19.23). Subscapular hematomas may be so large that they compress the kidney and decrease arterial flow to the kidney during diastole (Fig. 19.24). This has been termed a *page* kidney.

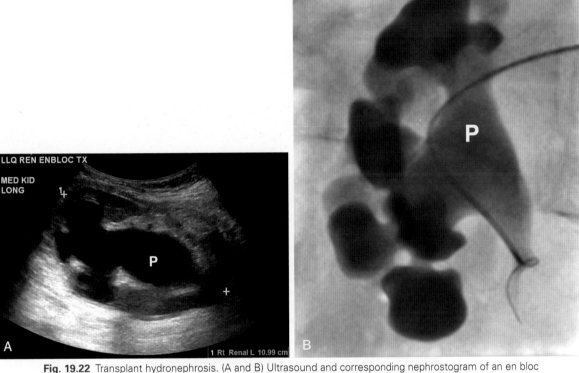

Fig. 19.22 Transplant hydronephrosis. (A and B) Ultrasound and corresponding nephrostogram of an en bloc transplant with severe dilatation of the renal pelvis (*P*) and calyceal blunting in one of the two kidneys from pediatric en bloc.

Urinomas may be of more clinical significance. These are due to urine extravasation, and under most circumstances require surgical intervention. Urinomas typically occur as a result of the breakdown of the anastomosis of the ureteric implantation into the bladder. Urinomas occur most commonly in the first 2 postoperative weeks. Aspiration of fluid with laboratory analysis is diagnostic. Renal scintigraphy may be helpful to identify the urine leak.

Lymphoceles are the most common fluid collections seen later in transplant patients. They may occur as early as 1 to 3 weeks postoperatively and can vary in size from a small fluid collection to fairly large collections (Fig. 19.25, Video 19.15). These are usually of minimal significance unless they compress the renal collection system or cause pain.

Finally, abscesses may result from infected transplant fluid collections. These fluid collections are different in appearance than urinomas or lymphoceles, as they often have subtle internal debris (Fig. 19.26). They may be very difficult to differentiate from postoperative hematomas. However, hematomas resolve with time, whereas abscesses may become more well demarcated with time. Aspiration may be necessary for diagnosis or treatment of a paranephric fluid collection.

Vascular Complications. The most common vascular complication of renal transplant is renal artery stenosis. These can be seen within weeks of surgery or may take years to develop. Renal artery stenosis is identified by angle-correcting Doppler of the transplant renal artery to observe elevation of the peak systolic velocities within

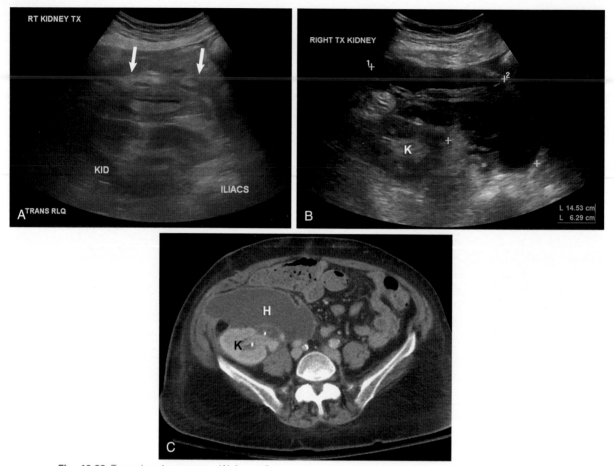

Fig. 19.23 Transplant hematoma. (A) Immediate posttransplant ultrasound showing isoechoic hematoma (*arrows*), which was difficult to appreciate. *KID,* Kidney. ILIACS, Iliac vessels. (B) Two weeks later the hematoma is hypoechoic (*calipers*), noted anterior to the kidney (*K*). (C) Corresponding CT showing hematoma (*H*) and the transplant kidney (*K*).

the renal artery and identifying spectral broadening. Spectral broadening indicates a wide range of Doppler velocities at or just past the site of narrowing. Criteria for diagnosis of renal artery stenosis include (1) elevated systolic velocities in the main renal artery of over 300 cm/sec, (2) spectral broadening, and (3) a tardus parvus appearance to the parenchymal renal arteries. *Tardus* refers to a delay in the upstroke of the waveform, and *parvus* refers to a decreased peak velocity of the waveform (Figs. 19.27 and 19.28). A time from end diastole to peak systole over 0.1 seconds has been found to be a useful value in defining the tardus in parenchymal arteries. No identification of (1) elevated renal artery velocity, (2) spectral broadening, or (3) parenchymal

tardus parvus deformity places the patient at low risk for significant renal artery stenosis. However, identification of all three of these markers places the patient into a high-risk group for renal artery stenosis. Complete discussion of renal artery stenosis is beyond the scope of this chapter.

A more precipitous finding in the renal transplant patient that may require immediate recognition is renal vein thrombosis. This occurs in up to 5% of transplant patients and usually within the first few days of surgery. These patients may present with either oliguria or anuria. This diagnosis is suggested if there is reversal of flow within the main renal artery and lack of flow within the renal vein.

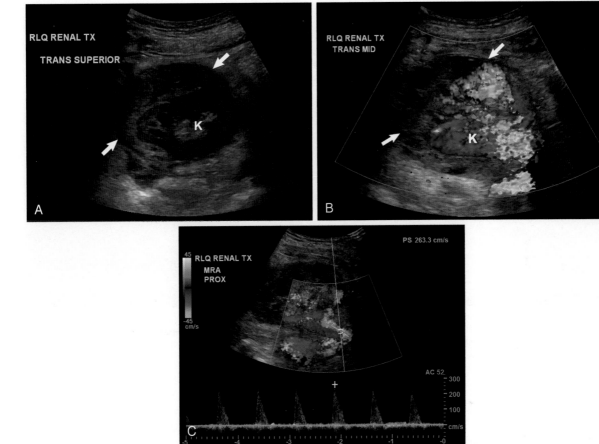

Fig. 19.24 Perinephric hematoma affecting blood flow. (A) Real-time imaging showing hematoma (*arrows*) surrounding the kidney (*K*). (B) Color Doppler showing the hematoma (*arrows*), which is void of color flow surrounding the vascular kidney (*K*). (C) Doppler of the main renal artery shows reversal of flow in the artery, due to compression of the kidney by the hematoma.

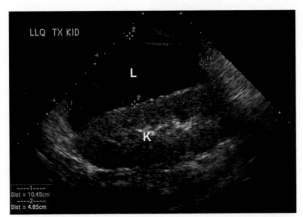

Fig. 19.25 Lymphocele. Real-time ultrasound showing large fluid collection surrounding the kidney (*K*), which corresponds to a lymphocele (*L*).

Arteriovenous Malformation and Pseudoaneurysms. Both arteriovenous malformations (AVMs) and/or pseudoaneurysms are common in renal transplant patients because these patients have routine biopsy of the transplant kidney. AVMs are diagnosed by an unusual color Doppler pattern within the kidney, including color Doppler aliasing, and noting increased velocity and decreased resistance to flow in the renal artery. There is also increased velocity with turbulence and arterialization noted within the draining vein (Fig. 19.29).

Rejection/Acute Tubular Necrosis. Parenchymal processes in renal transplant are usually diagnosed by renal biopsy. However, analysis of the waveform of the parenchymal arteries may be useful to obtain an arterial

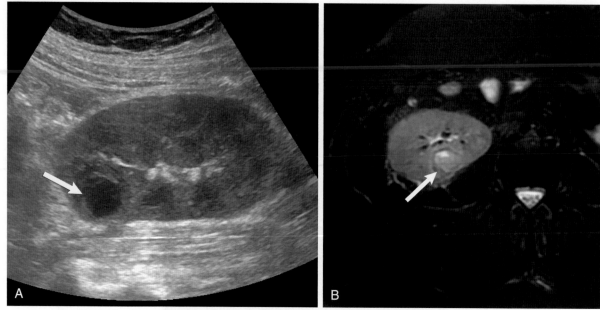

Fig. 19.26 Renal transplant abscess. (A) Longitudinal ultrasound demonstrated a new hypoechoic structure with some internal echoes (*arrow*). (B) Transverse T2-weighted MRI of the kidney shows the mass to be nearly isointense to the surrounding kidney, but with a fluid–debris level and a hypointense rim. This corresponded to a renal abscess, which was percutaneously aspirated.

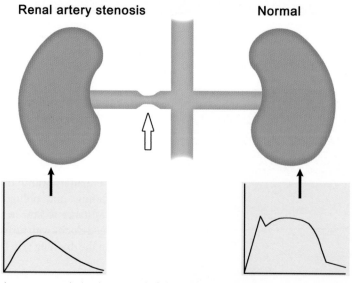

Fig. 19.27 Renal artery stenosis (tardus parvus). Schematic diagram of renal artery Doppler tracings. Right side of the image: Tracing from a normal renal artery. Note the early systolic upstroke. Left side of the image: Tracing shows the dampened systolic upstroke (tardus) and a smaller systolic velocity (parvus) waveform downstream from the stenosis.

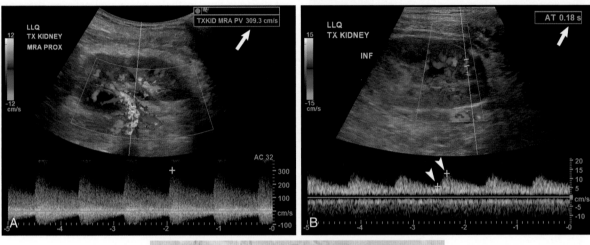

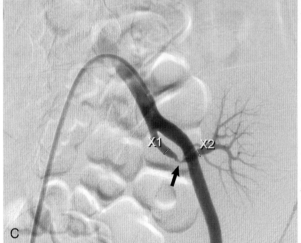

Fig. 19.28 Renal artery stenosis. (A) Elevated peak systolic velocity over 300 cm/sec (*arrow*) with spectral broadening. (B) Tardus parvus waveform in the parenchymal artery with an acceleration time of 0.18 seconds (*arrow*). (C) Corresponding angiogram demonstrating the renal artery stenosis.

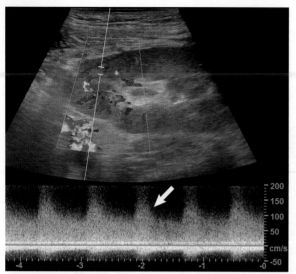

Fig. 19.29 Arterial venous fistula in transplant kidney postbiopsy. Note the unusual color Doppler pattern within the kidney at the site of the pulsed Doppler gate on the real-time image. Also note the increased velocity of over 200 cm/sec, with turbulence and arterialization noted within the draining vein (*arrow*).

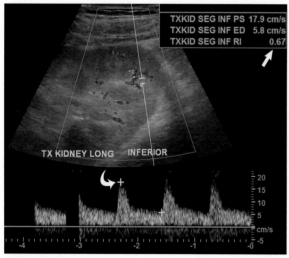

Fig. 19.30 Normal resistive index in parenchymal artery. On the Doppler tracing, a cursor is automatically placed on the peak systolic velocity of 17.9 cm/sec (*curved arrow*), and another arrow is placed on the smallest diastolic velocity at 5.8 cm/sec. The resistive index is automatically calculated at 0.67, which is a normal value (*arrow*).

waveform. A Doppler sample of the parenchymal artery is sampled and an arterial waveform is obtained. This waveform may be measured by obtaining its resistive index. The resistive index is defined as the peak systolic velocity minus the lowest diastolic velocity divided by the peak systolic velocity (Fig. 19.30). When there is an increased resistive index greater than 0.8 or loss of diastolic flow in the parenchymal arteries, these are nonspecific findings but may include acute tubular necrosis (ATN) or rejection. In these instances, if there is clinical suspicion of rejection or ATN, a biopsy of the transplant is needed to confirm the diagnosis.

BIBLIOGRAPHY

Ascenti G, Zimbaro G, Mazziotti S, Gaeta M, Lamberto S, Scribano E. Contrast-enhanced power doppler US in the diagnosis of renal pseudotumors. *Eur Radiol.* 2001;11:2496–2499.

Bosniak MA. The Bosniak renal cyst classification: 25 years later. *Radiology.* 2012;262:781–785.

Bredemeyer M. ACR Appropriateness Criteria for acute onset of flank pain with suspicion of stone disease. *Am Fam Physician.* 2016;94:575–576.

Choong KK. Sonographic detection of emphysematous cystitis. *J Ultrasound Med.* 2003;22:847–849.

Coursey CA, Casalino DD, Remer EM, et al. ACR Appropriateness Criteria(R) acute onset flank pain--suspicion of stone disease. *Ultrasound Q.* 2012;28:227–233.

Dubinsky TJ, Sadro CT. Acute onset flank pain—suspicion of stone disease. *Ultrasound Q.* 2012;28:239–240.

Fananapazir G, Rao R, Corwin MT, Naderi S, Santhanakrishnan C, Troppmann C. Sonographic evaluation of clinically significant perigraft hematomas in kidney transplant recipients. *AJR Am J Roentgenol.* 2015;205:802–806.

Fananapazir G, Tse G, Corwin MT, et al. Pediatric en bloc kidney transplants: clinical and immediate postoperative US factors associated with vascular thrombosis. *Radiology.* 2016;279:935–942.

Fontanilla T, Minaya J, Cortes C, et al. Acute complicated pyelonephritis: contrast-enhanced ultrasound. *Abdom Imaging.* 2012;37:639–646.

Fritzsche P, Amis Jr ES, Bigongiari LR, et al. Acute onset flank pain, suspicion of stone disease. American College of Radiology. ACR Appropriateness Criteria. *Radiology.* 2000;215 (suppl:683–686).

Granata A, Andrulli S, Fiorini F, et al. Diagnosis of acute pyelonephritis by contrast-enhanced ultrasonography in kidney transplant patients. *Nephrol Dial Transplant.* 2011;26:715–720.

Hazewinkel MH, Gietelink L, van der Velden J, Burger MP, Stoker J, Roovers JP. Renal ultrasound to detect hydronephrosis: a need for routine imaging after radical hysterectomy? *Gynecol Oncol.* 2012;124:83–86.

Herbst MK, Rosenberg G, Daniels B, et al. Effect of provider experience on clinician-performed ultrasonography for hydronephrosis in patients with suspected renal colic. *Ann Emerg Med.* 2014;64:269–276.

Herndon CD. The role of ultrasound in predicting surgical intervention for prenatal hydronephrosis. *J Urol.* 2012;187:1535–1536.

Kim J. Ultrasonographic features of focal xanthogranulomatous pyelonephritis. *J Ultrasound Med.* 2004;23:409–416.

Lee JY, Kim SH, Cho JY, Han D. Color and power Doppler twinkling artifacts from urinary stones: clinical observations and phantom studies. *AJR Am J Roentgenol.* 2001;176:1441–1445.

Maizels M, Reisman ME, Flom LS, et al. Grading nephroureteral dilatation detected in the first year of life: correlation with obstruction. *J Urol.* 1992;148:609–614; discussion 15–6.

McArthur C, Baxter GM. Current and potential renal applications of contrast-enhanced ultrasound. *Clin Radiol.* 2012;67:909–922.

Moore CL, Scoutt L. Sonography first for acute flank pain? *J Ultrasound Med.* 2012;31:1703–1711.

Nicolau C, Bunesch L, Peri L, et al. Accuracy of contrast-enhanced ultrasound in the detection of bladder cancer. *Br J Radiol.* 2011;84:1091–1099.

Riddell J, Case A, Wopat R, et al. Sensitivity of emergency bedside ultrasound to detect hydronephrosis in patients with computed tomography-proven stones. *West J Emerg Med.* 2014;15:96–100.

Rodgers SK, Sereni CP, Horrow MM. Ultrasonographic evaluation of the renal transplant. *Radiol Clin North Am.* 2014;52:1307–1324.

Stunell H, Buckley O, Feeney J, Geoghegan T, Browne RF, Torreggiani WC. Imaging of acute pyelonephritis in the adult. *Eur Radiol.* 2007;17:1820–1828.

Tiu CM, Chou YH, Chiou HJ, et al. Sonographic features of xanthogranulomatous pyelonephritis. *J Clin Ultrasound.* 2001;29:279–285.

Wong-You-Cheong JJ, Woodward PJ, Manning MA, Davis CJ. From the archives of the AFIP: inflammatory and nonneoplastic bladder masses: radiologic-pathologic correlation. *Radiographics.* 2006;26:1847–1868.

20

Abdominal Aorta

Mindy Lipsitz, Zachary Soucy

INTRODUCTION

Patients with aortic pathology often present with non-specific complaints or presentations such as back pain, abdominal pain, myocardial infarction (MI), or even stroke, making the diagnosis difficult. The adage of "abdominal pain plus one other organ system" should prompt the physician to consider aortic pathology as the unifying diagnosis. The level and acuity of pain often is secondary to the etiology of the pain. For example, chronic pain may be secondary to an expanding aortic aneurysm, whereas more acute pain may be secondary to aortic dissection or traumatic aortic rupture. Abnormalities of the liver, spleen, and colon should also be considered in the differential listed in Box 20.1.

NORMAL ANATOMY

The aorta originates from the left ventricle of the heart and ascends, giving off branches to supply blood to the upper body and brain. The ascending aorta courses left and caudally, forming the aortic arch and the descending aorta. The aorta tapers as it descends from the thoracic into the abdominal cavity, ultimately bifurcating into the common iliac arteries (Fig. 20.1).

The first and most proximal branch of the abdominal aorta is the celiac axis. It divides into three main branches: the splenic, common hepatic, and left gastric arteries. The left branch becomes the splenic artery, and the right branch the common hepatic artery. There is a smaller division of the celiac axis, the left gastric artery, which is often not well visualized on ultrasound.

The second large branch of the abdominal aorta, approximately 1 to 2 cm caudal but sometimes abutting the celiac axis, is the superior mesenteric artery (SMA), which lies anterior to the aorta. The splenic vein passes over the SMA, emptying into the portal vein just right of midline. The left renal vein passes between the SMA and the aorta before emptying into the inferior vena cava (IVC).

SONOGRAPHIC FINDINGS

Imaging of the aorta is normally performed using a curved array transducer, typically 3 MHz frequencies, depending on body habitus. The probe indicator should face the patient's head for coronal and sagittal views or the anatomic right side for axial views. It is important to image the entirety of the abdominal aorta in both long and short axis, starting superiorly in the epigastric region and scanning through the proximal common iliac vessels. As the aorta descends, it follows the lordosis of the spine, allowing for more superficial ultrasound imaging.

It is best to start the examination by identifying posterior landmarks such as the vertebral body, a rounded, hyperechoic structure with posterior shadowing. Depth is typically set in the 20- to 30-cm range to identify these structures and set the far field, depending on abdominal girth. Once the vertebral body is identified, the depth can be adjusted to visualize the structures of interest, keeping the vertebral body visible (Fig. 20.2, Video 20.1).

The aorta will rest anterior and to the anatomic left of the vertebral body. On the right, the IVC runs alongside the aorta; thus the two structures must be sonographically distinguished from one another. The IVC is usually respirophasic, thin walled, and collapsible, depending on patient's hydration status and phase of respiration. The aorta is thicker walled, non-collapsing, and pulsatile. When pulse wave Doppler is placed on an aorta with normal flow, it has a triphasic appearance (Fig. 20.3A) compared with the IVC, which has a monophasic waveform of differing morphology, depending on the phase of respiration (see Fig. 20.3B).

The major branches of the aorta often have characteristic sonographic appearances. The axial view of the celiac axis originating from the aorta is commonly known as a *seagull sign* (Fig. 20.4, Video 20.2). The axial view of the SMA takeoff surrounded with hyperechoic fatty tissue is known as the *Mantel clock sign*. The pancreas and the liver are tissues anterior to the splenic vein that can be seen at the level of the SMA (Fig. 20.5, Video 20.3).

Several centimeters inferior to the takeoff of the SMA, the origin of the right and left renal arteries are seen (Fig. 20.6, Video 20.4). The abdominal aorta ultimately bifurcates into the right and left common iliac arteries (Fig. 20.7, Video 20.5).

ULTRASOUND TECHNIQUE AND TIPS

Visualization of the abdominal aorta can be challenging, depending on the patient's body habitus, bowel contents, and specific anatomy. The patient should be supine, and it may be advantageous to have the patient bend their knees with the feet on the bed. This rocks the pelvis posteriorly, allowing the rectus abdominal muscles to relax, giving the operator improved ability for bowel compression.

To visualize the proximal aorta, the liver can be utilized as an acoustic window. Asking the patient to take a deep breath lowers the diaphragm and liver, creating a larger acoustic window. If the proximal aorta is not readily visualized in the upper abdomen, the patient can be rolled to the left lateral decubitus position to displace bowel gas. If still having difficulty with visualization, the probe can be placed in the right midaxillary line to utilize the right lobe of the liver as an acoustic window. In this view, the aorta will appear in the far field, with the IVC in the near field. Alternatively, the abdominal aorta may be imaged left parasagittally, where the rectus

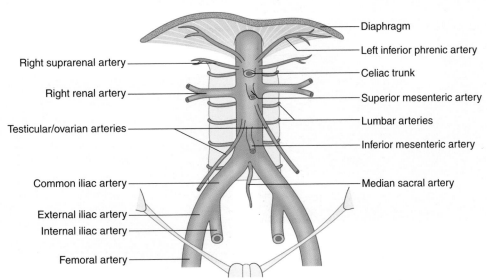

Fig. 20.1 Normal anatomy of the aorta, including major branch vessels.

Right suprarenal artery

Right renal artery

Testicular/ovarian arteries

Common iliac artery

External iliac artery

Internal iliac artery

Femoral artery

Diaphragm

Left inferior phrenic artery

Celiac trunk

Superior mesenteric artery

Lumbar arteries

Inferior mesenteric artery

Median sacral artery

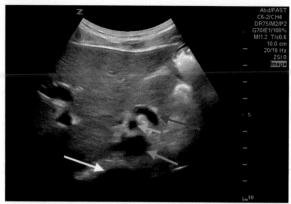

Fig. 20.2 Transverse view of the aorta with the spine in the far field (*white arrow*), aorta (*red arrow*), superior mesenteric artery (*orange arrow*) and splenic artery (*blue arrow*).

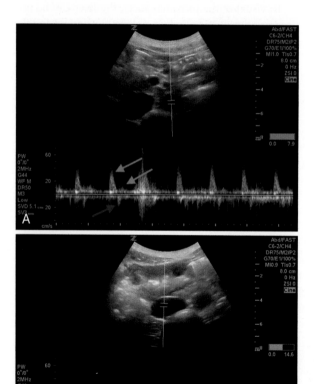

Fig. 20.3 (A) Pulse wave Doppler with gate over the aorta demonstrating normal physiologic triphasic arterial flow. *Red arrows* represent forward flow, with the *blue arrow* representing retrograde flow. (B) Pulse wave Doppler with gate over the IVC demonstrating monophasic waveforms.

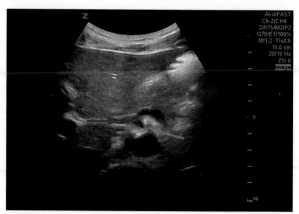

Fig. 20.4 Celiac axis originating from the proximal aorta (*red arrow*) branching into the splenic (*blue arrow*) and common hepatic arteries (*purple arrow*), often referred to as "seagull sign."

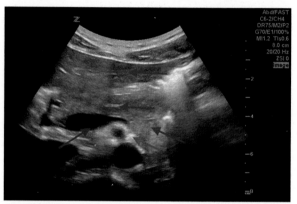

Fig. 20.5 SMA demonstrating the "mantel clock sign" (*red arrow*) with overlying splenic vein (*blue arrow*), liver (*purple arrows*), and pancreatic body and tail (*green arrows*).

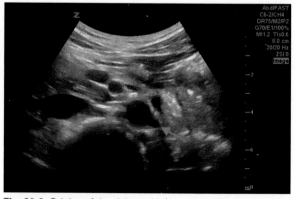

Fig. 20.6 Origins of the right and left renal arteries (*red arrows*) arising from the aorta.

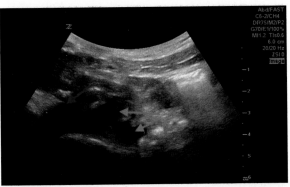

Fig. 20.7 Distal aortic bifurcation into the right and left common iliac arteries (*red arrows*) with the IVC (*blue arrow*).

TABLE 20.1	Risk Factors for AAAs

Age
Male gender
Smoking
Hypertension
Hyperlipidemia
Inherited genetic defects (Marfan's syndrome,
    Ehlers-Danlos syndrome, Turner's syndrome)
Intramural hematoma
Penetrating atherosclerotic ulcer
Atherosclerotic disease
Inflammatory and infectious aortitis along with an
    underlying aortic dissection

abdominis meets the oblique abdominal musculature. Angling the probe toward the spine in this position helps undercut anterior gaseous distention of the bowel.

If the patient's abdominal girth prohibits acceptable image acquisition, using the lowest-frequency probe on the lowest-frequency setting can help penetrance and improve visualization. If bowel gas proves a challenge, use graded compression with the ultrasound probe. Applying gentle, steady compression can dissipate bowel gas by physically displacing the intestine in the mid-to-lower abdomen. Bowel gas in the upper abdomen is more difficult to avoid, as the proximal duodenum is tethered by its retroperitoneal segments and is not easily moved.

PATHOLOGY

Abdominal Aortic Aneurysm

An abdominal aortic aneurysm (AAA) occurs when there is a focal enlargement of the abdominal aorta >3 cm or >50% enlargement of the normal diameter. AAAs are usually asymptomatic until they are large or rupture. Risk factors for AAA are shown in Table 20.1. A transverse view of the aorta will identify both saccular—a focal outpouching of the aortic wall (Fig. 20.8A, Video 20.6)—and fusiform—concentrically dilated—aneurysms, as shown in Fig. 20.8B, and Video 20.7. Measurement of the AAA should occur in the short-axis view to avoid the cylinder tangent error of a long-axis view, with the calipers placed on the anterior outer wall to the posterior outer wall (Fig. 20.9). Ninety percent of AAAs occur below the level of the renal arteries.

As AAAs enlarge, a palpable mass on physical examination may be appreciated, although evaluation may be limited by body habitus. Sensitivity for detection of AAA on physical examination increases by 50% as AAA diameter increases from 3 cm to >5 cm, facilitating easier sonographic identification (see Fig. 20.9, Video 20.8). However, one study found that of patients with ruptured AAA, only 18% had palpable abdominal masses on physical examination, making physical examination alone extremely unreliable. Any patient with suspected AAA should have point-of-care ultrasound (POCUS), as early ultrasound in patients with ruptured AAA has been shown to decrease mortality by approximately 30%. In addition, it is important to appreciate the proximity of the aorta to the kidney (Fig. 20.10, Video 20.9). A large AAA may compress the ureters, leading to hydronephrosis visualized on POCUS. Thus, if left-side hydronephrosis is identified, AAA should be considered.

Aneurysmal Leak or Rupture

An aneurysmal leak occurs when a AAA develops a tear, and aneurysmal rupture occurs when the AAA bursts. Both usually occur when mechanical stress exceeds aortic wall strength. Aneurysmal tears usually occur at a weak point in the vessel wall or within an intraluminal thrombus. Tears and ruptures can be demonstrated on POCUS, as seen in grayscale ultrasound (Fig. 20.11, Video 20.10), and can be confirmed by placing color Doppler over the AAA and assessing for flow outside of the aortic lumen. When using color Doppler, adjustment to low-velocity scales may be necessary to register leaks or extravasation with low flow rates.

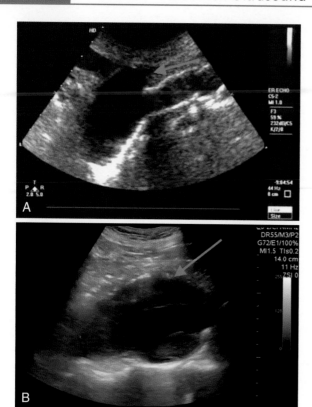

Fig. 20.8 (A) Long-axis view of saccular aortic aneurysm demonstrating the utility of this view. (B) Long-axis view of fusiform aortic aneurysm (*red arrow*).

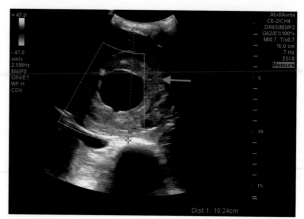

Fig. 20.9 Appropriate outside anterior–to–outside posterior measurement of AAA with intramural thrombus (*red arrow*) in transverse view. The AAA is large, displacing intraabdominal contents, and can be easily visualized on POCUS.

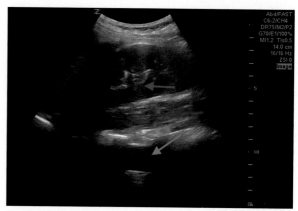

Fig. 20.10 Demonstration of proximity of abdominal aorta (*red arrow*) to hilum of the kidney (*purple arrow*), which projects medially onto the psoas muscle (*blue arrow*).

Patients with aneurysmal rupture develop hypovolemic shock and require prompt surgical intervention, as in-hospital mortality approaches 90%. There are two types of ruptures, retroperitoneal (RP) and intraperitoneal, described in Table 20.2. Most ruptured AAAs leak into the left retroperitoneum and therefore infrequently cause intraperitoneal free fluid visualized on focused assessment with sonography for trauma (FAST) examination. RP free fluid is visualized in less than 5% of ruptured cases on POCUS. Indirect evidence of RP hemorrhage includes elevation or anterolateral displacement of the left kidney. Though inferior to computed tomography (CT), ultrasound performed by radiologists was found to be 76% sensitive for aortic rupture with contained or RP hemorrhage and useful in the acute setting.

Intramural and Intraluminal Thrombus

Intramural (IM) thrombi are blood clots that form within the aortic wall (see Fig. 20.9, Video 20.8), and intraluminal (IL) thrombi are clots that occur within the lumen of the aorta (see Fig. 20.11, Video 20.10). Most IM thrombi are seen with atherosclerotic vascular disease but can occur secondary to aneurysms, trauma, malignancy, dissections, systemic fungal infections, or in hypercoagulable states. Smoking and hyperlipidemia are the greatest risk factors for IM thrombi.

The sonographic findings of IM thrombi are echogenic material within the walls of the aorta. The use of color Doppler can aid in the diagnosis and, if completely occlusive, reveal lack of flow within the lumen of the aorta. Early recognition of IM thrombi in severe stenosis or occlusion can be assessed with two-dimensional

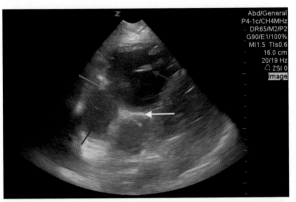

Fig. 20.11 AAA with large defect in the posterior right aortic wall (*red arrow*) with retroperitoneal hemorrhage (*blue arrow*), intraluminal clot (*purple arrow*), and anterior aspect of vertebral body (*white arrow*).

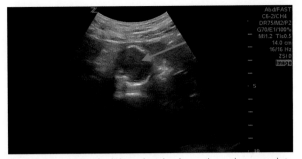

Fig. 20.12 Intraluminal thrombus (*red arrow*) causing complete aortic occlusion, which was evident on examination and confirmed on CT.

TABLE 20.2 Intraperitoneal vs. Retroperitoneal Ruptures

Intraperitoneal	Retroperitoneal
Blood free in intraperitoneal cavity	Blood "contained" by surrounding structures
Lower chance of survival	Higher chance of survival
Presents with abdominal pain	Presents with back pain
Acutely unstable on examination	Pulsatile abdominal mass on examination

(2D) and color Doppler POCUS, with a sensitivity and specificity of 91% and 93%, respectively. In this instance, the ultrasonographer should pay particular attention to measure from outer wall to outer wall of the AAA, to avoid errantly measuring the IL diameter. Gain should be optimized to elucidate the contrast between the IM thrombus, IL blood, or lack thereof and structures external to the aorta.

IL thrombi are clots within the lumen of the aorta. IL thrombus growth rates are important to measure, as they can be associated with an increased risk of rupture. If left undetected, IL thrombi can also lead to complete occlusion of the aorta (Fig. 20.12, Video 20.11), which carries a mortality rate of 31% to 52% in patients with inadequate collateral flow. Complete occlusion is rare, but occurs most often in middle-aged women with a smoking history and in a low-flow state. The imaging modality of choice remains computed tomographic angiography (CTA) or magnetic resonance angiography (MRA) for IM and IL thrombi; however, POCUS can be used to expedite care and involvement of vascular surgery if indicated. A majority of thrombi are managed expectantly because a IL thrombus does not typically preclude forward blood flow.

Aortic Dissection

The aorta is made up of three layers (Fig. 20.13). An aortic dissection can either occur in the posttraumatic or nontraumatic setting when blood enters between the tunica media and intimal layers, forcing these layers apart. The most common risk factors for dissection are arterial hypertension or any cause of medial disruption, such as genetic disorders, drug use, or inflammatory vascular disease. Blood in the false lumen of the aorta decreases blood flow to the rest of the body. Patients classically describe a tearing pain radiating to the back and may present with hypotension, stroke, mesenteric ischemia, renal failure, or MI if the dissection flap involves the coronary arteries. Aortic dissections have a high mortality rate of up to 1% per hour over the first several hours. Depending on institutional protocols, cardiothoracic or vascular surgery should be promptly consulted in any case where a patient is hemodynamically unstable with sonographic findings of AAA or aortic dissection.

Sonographic evidence includes direct visualization of the dissection flap in either the longitudinal or transverse views, though it is ideal for each view to corroborate the finding (Fig. 20.14A, Video 20.12 and Fig. 20.14B, Video 20.13). Indirect sonographic

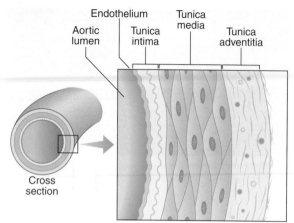

Fig. 20.13 Depiction of the three layers of the aortic wall.

evidence of dissection includes ascending aorta dilatation, aortic valve insufficiency, pericardial effusion, or tamponade. Color Doppler may highlight a dissection flap and nonlaminar flow (Fig. 20.15, Video 20.14).

Endovascular Aortic Grafts

Endovascular aortic grafts (endografts) are commonly deployed during endovascular aortic repair (EVAR) techniques commonly used to treat AAAs and can also be used to treat some types of aortic dissections and aortic rupture (Fig. 20.16, Video 20.15). Endovascular leaks (endoleaks) occur when there is persistent blood flow and pressure within the aneurysmal sac after endograft placement. Patients can present with insidious onset of symptoms, and diagnosis of endoleak can be difficult. There are several types of endoleaks described in Table 20.3. Postsurgical surveillance after EVAR is important, as endoleak rates post-procedure occur in up to 39% of patients.

Currently, CTA is the preferred modality to assess for endoleaks. If a patient is unstable, 2D color Doppler can be used to visualize the endoleak. It may demonstrate blood flow around or through the stent but will not determine the type of endoleak present (Fig. 20.17). When present, endoleaks can increase the size of an aneurysm, putting the patient at risk for aortic rupture.

Ultrasound imaging is neither sensitive nor specific in determining the type of endoleak; thus this pathology cannot be definitively ruled out. Management of potential endograft complication or endoleak involves prompt discussion with a vascular surgeon.

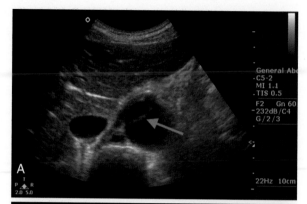

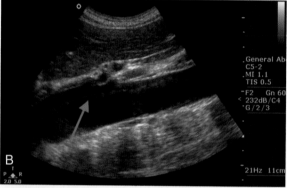

Fig. 20.14 (A) Transverse view of an abdominal aortic dissection flap (*red arrow*). (B) Longitudinal view of an abdominal aortic dissection flap (*red arrow*).

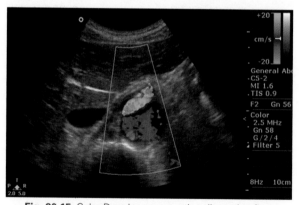

Fig. 20.15 Color Doppler accentuating dissection flap.

OTHER ETIOLOGIES

With careful scanning, other etiologies of chest, back, or abdominal pain may be identified. Among these etiologies are cardiac, intraperitoneal hemorrhage, and hepatobiliary pathologies presented in Chapters 9, 15, and 17.

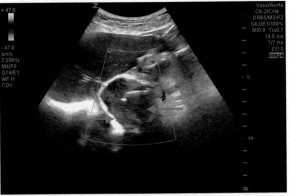

Fig. 20.16 Aortic endograft lying within an AAA. Stent highlighted (*red arrows*).

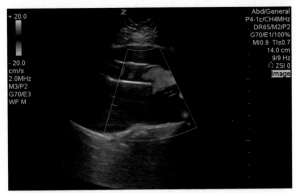

Fig. 20.17 Endograft leak with color Doppler demonstrating flow outside the endograft.

TABLE 20.3 **Types of Endoleaks**

Type	Incidence	Etiology
Type I	10% of cases	Inadequate seal at the site of graft attachment; stent migration
Type II	80% of cases	Retrograde flow through branch vessels fills the aneurysmal sac
Type III	Unknown	Mechanical failure of stent graft; improper overlap during insertion
Type IV	Unknown	Blood leaks across the graft due to porosity of graft
Type V	Unknown	Expansion of the sac without evidence of leak site

(Data from Nicholls SC, Gardner JB, Meissner MH, H Johansen K. Rupture in small abdominal aortic aneurysms. *J Vasc Surg.* 1998;28[5]:884–888; Galland RB, Whiteley MS, Magee TR. The fate of patients undergoing surveillance of small abdominal aortic aneurysms. *Eur J Vasc Endovasc Surg.* 1998;16[2]:104–109; Jones A, Cahill D, Gardham R. Outcome in patients with a large abdominal aortic aneurysm considered unfit for surgery. *Br J Surg.* 1998;85[10]:1382–1384.)

Renal abnormalities, such as pyelonephritis and hydronephrosis, may present with flank or abdominal pain. Ultrasound can be used in distinguishing renal pathology from other etiologies of back and flank pain. These are presented in more detail in Chapter 19.

Gastrointestinal abnormalities should be considered in the differential, but less commonly or inconsistently have sonographic features. Two prominent exceptions include small bowel obstruction and appendicitis, for which ultrasound is useful. These pathologies are covered in Chapter 21.

Upper abdominal pain may be secondary to pancreatic abnormalities. These can include pancreatitis, pancreatic masses, or pseudocysts, which may cause biliary obstruction. Acute pancreatic disease is presented in more detail in Chapter 18.

BIBLIOGRAPHY

Battaglia S, Danesino GM, Danesino V, Castellani S. Color Doppler ultrasonography of the abdominal aorta. *J Ultrasound.* 2010;13(3):107–117. https://doi.org/10.1016/j.jus.2010.10.001.

Bertino R, Saucier N, Barth D. The retroperitoneum. In: Rumack C, Wilson S, Charboneau JW, Levine D, eds. *Diagnostic Ultrasound.* 4th ed. Philadelphia (PA): Elsevier Mosby; 2011:447–485.

Bhatt S, Ghazale H, Dogra VS. Sonographic evaluation of the abdominal aorta. *Ultrasound Clin.* 2007;2:437–453.

Braverman Alan. Acute aortic dissection. *Circulation.* 2010;122:184–188.

Burger T, Meyer F, Tautenhahn J, et al. Ruptured infrarenal aortic aneurysm—a critical evaluation. *Vasa.* 1999;28:30–33.

Catalano O, Siani A. Ruptured abdominal aortic aneurysm: categorization of sonographic findings and report of 3 new signs. *J Ultrasound Med.* 2005;24:1077–1083.

Efstratiadis G, Kiirmiziz D, Papazoglou K, Economidou D, Memmos D. The walking man with a completely occluded aorta. *Nephrol Dial Transplant.* 2004;19(1):227–229.

Ernst CB. Abdominal aortic aneurysm. *N Engl J Med.* 1993;328(16):1167–1172.

Golledge J, Abrokwah J, Shenoy KN, et al. Morphology of ruptured abdominal aorti aneurysms. *Eur J Vasc Endovasc Surg*. 1999;18:96–104.

Hirsch AT, Miedema MD. Infrarenal aortic occlusion. *N Engl J Med*. 2008;359:735.

Labruto F, Blomqvist L, Swedenborg J. Imaging the intraluminal thrombus of abdominal aortic aneurysms: techniques, findings, and clinical implications. *J Vasc Interv Radiol*. 2011;22(8):1069–1075.

Langsfeld M, Nepute J, Hershey FB, et al. The use of deep duplex scanning to predict hemodynamically significant aortoiliac stenoses. *J Vasc Surg*. 1988;7:395–399.

Lederle FA, Parenti CM, Chute EP. Ruptured abdominal aortic aneurysm: the internist as diagnostician. *Am J Med*. 1994;96(2):163–167.

LeFevre ML. Screening for abdominal aortic aneurysm: U.S. Preventive services task force recommendation statement. *Ann Intern Med*. 2014;161(4):281–290.

Ma OJ, Mateer JR, Reardon RF, Joing S. Aorta. In: *Ma and Mateers Emergency Ultrasound*. New York: McGraw-Hill; 2014.

Marston WA, Ahlquist R, Johnson G, Meyer AA. Misdiagnosis of ruptured abdominal aortic aneurysms. *J. Vasc. Surg*. 1992;16(1):17–22.

Nair, Vaishnavi, Jan 8 2015 slide presentation entitled: "Ruptured Aneurysms of the Aorta". https://www.slideshare.net/marina761/ruptured-abdominal-aortic-aneurysmppt-ruptured-abdominal-aortic.

O'Leary SA, Kavanagh EG, Grace PA, McGloughlin TM, Doyle BJ. The biaxial mechanical behaviour of abdominal aortic aneurysm intraluminal thrombus: classification of morphology and the determination of layer and region specific properties. *J Biomech*. 2014;47(6):1430–1437. https://doi.org/10.1016/j.jbiomech.2014.01.041. Epub 2014 Feb 7.

Plummer D, et al. Emergency department ultrasound improves time to diagnosis and survival of abdominal aortic aneurysm. *Acad Emerg Med*. 1998;4(41).

Raman KG, Missig-Carroll N, Richardson T, Muluk SC, Makaroun MS. Color-flow duplex ultrasound scan versus computed tomographic scan in the surveillance of endovascular aneurysm repair. *J Vasc Surg*. 2003;38(4):645–651.

Reardon R, Clinton M, Madore F, Cook T. Abdominal aortic aneurysm. In: Ma OJ, Mateer J, Reardon R, Joing S, eds. *Emergency Ultrasound*. 3rd ed. New York (NY): McGraw-Hill Education; 2014:225–245.

Rose J, Civil I, Koelmeyer T, Haydock D, Adams D. Ruptured abdominal aortic aneurysms: clinical presentation in Auckland 1993-1997. *ANZ J Surg*. 2001;71(6):341–344.

Sato M, Imai A, Sakamoto H, Sasaki A, Watanabe Y, Jikuya T. Abdominal aortic disease caused by penetrating atherosclerotic ulcers. *Ann Vasc Dis*. 2012;5(1):8–14.

Satta J, Laara E, Juvonen T. Intraluminal thrombus predicts rupture of an abdominal aortic aneurysm. *J Vasc Surg*. 1996;23:737–739.

Sawhney NS, DeMaria AN, Blanchard DG. Aortic intramural hematoma: an increasingly recognized and potentially fatal entity. *Chest*. 2001;120:1340–1346.

Stenbaek J, Kalin B, Swedenborg J. Growth of thrombus may be a better predictor of rupture than diameter in patients with abdominal aortic aneurysms. *Eur J Vasc Endovasc Surg*. 2000;20:466–469.

Sukharev II , Guch AA, Novosad EM, Vlaikov GG. Ultrasonic duplex scanning in occlusion of abdominal aorta, arteries of iliac segment and of lower extremities. *Klin Khir*. 2000;12:17–18.

Valente T, Giovanni R, Lassandro F, et al. MDCT evaluation of acute aortic syndrome. *Br J Radiol*. 2016;89(1061).

Vorp DA, Mandarino WA, Webster MW, Gorcsan 3rd J. Potential influence of intraluminal thrombus on abdominal aortic aneurysm as assessed by a new non-invasive method. *Cardiovasc Surg*. 1996;4(6):732–739.

21

Lower Abdomen and Bowel

Kenn Ghaffarian, Thomas Ray Sanchez

BOWEL ULTRASOUND

Normal Anatomy

The small bowel consists of the bowel distal to the stomach and proximal to the colon. It is approximately 5 meters long and includes the duodenum, jejunum, and ileum. The small bowel contains prominent mucosal folds known as *plicae circulares* or *valvular connvinetes*. The jejunum has the most developed and highest concentration of these folds, which remain present even in distended bowel (Fig. 21.1). The plicae circulares decrease in density as you move distally to a nearly smooth distal ileum. The mucosal layer of small bowel contains finger-like projections into the lumen called *villi*.

The large bowel begins with the cecum and includes the entire colon and rectum (Fig. 21.2). At the point where the ileum joins the cecum, a sphincter is present (ileocecal valve) that prevents the backflow of contents into the small bowel. The cecum is a pouchlike structure that usually contains gas. The large bowel does not contain villi, and there are no major mucosal folds (excluding the rectum). The wall of the colon is creased by its muscular layer, including its serosa, into small sacs called *haustra*. This gives the colon a segmented appearance.

Ultrasound Techniques and Normal Findings

Imaging of the bowels is performed using a low-frequency transducer, such as a curvilinear probe (typically 3- to 6-MHz frequency), which allows for good penetration and a large field of view. The higher-frequency linear array can be used to evaluate thin or pediatric patients and to examine bowel adjacent to the abdominal wall in greater detail.

The bowel should be evaluated in a systematic fashion with the patient supine. One technique is described as the "lawn mower" pattern (Fig. 21.3). In this method, begin in the right lower quadrant with the probe held in a transverse orientation (indicator directed to the patient's right) and scan superiorly toward the right upper quadrant. The probe is then moved slightly medially and now scanned inferiorly, parallel to the original path. This pattern is repeated until the whole abdominal surface has been covered.

As the sonographer moves the probe across the abdomen, he or she will hold steady, consistent, posteriorly directed pressure into the abdomen at 1- to 2-cm intervals. This technique, known as *graded compression*, is performed in an attempt to disperse bowel gas and to bring the probe closer to the abdominal contents by compressing abdominal wall soft tissue toward muscular structures of the back.

The bowel is often filled with gas. This gas creates a shadow artifact that prevents visualization of any structures posterior to this artifact. This shadow is typically of mixed echogenicities ("dirty shadow"), as opposed to the typically anechoic shadows ("clean shadow") of bone or calcium stones. However, bowel can be visualized when it is filled with liquid, semisolid, or solid material.

The duodenum is difficult to see on ultrasound, but a transverse segment can be seen on the caudal edge of the liver (Fig. 21.4). The jejunum contains plicae circulares seen 3 to 5 mm apart. This can create a "feather-like" or "herring-bone" appearance (Fig. 21.5). The ileum has fewer of these mucosal folds and may have a smooth appearance. At the terminal ileum, a

Jejunum

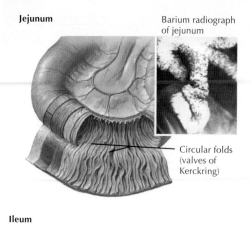

Ileum

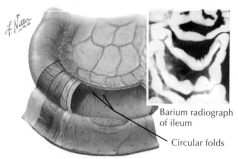

Barium radiograph of jejunum

Circular folds (valves of Kerckring)

Barium radiograph of ileum

Circular folds

Fig. 21.1 Normal small bowel containing plicae circulares (circular folds), also called *valves of Kerckring*. The jejunum has the highest concentration of these mucosal folds, which decrease in density in the ileum. (Reprinted from Netter Anatomy Illustration Collection. ©Elsevier Inc. All Rights Reserved.)

hypoechoic "halo" may be seen representing the muscular lips of the ileocecal valve. These sonographic findings should be combined with the anatomic location of the bowel to determine the bowel loop under examination. The appendix will be discussed in the next section.

The large bowel has a similar appearance to the small bowel but is distinguished by periodic indentations every 3 to 5 cm apart corresponding to haustral sacculations (Fig. 21.6). The large bowel does not contain plicae circulares. The colon can usually be evaluated from the cecal pole to the rectum. The transverse and descending colon may be difficult to examine, given the variable location and abundant echogenic fat surrounding the lumen, respectively. Valves of the rectosigmoid colon and rectum may be visible when the lumen is filled with fluid. Again, correlate the sonographic findings with the anatomic location (paracolic regions) to determine the loop under examination.

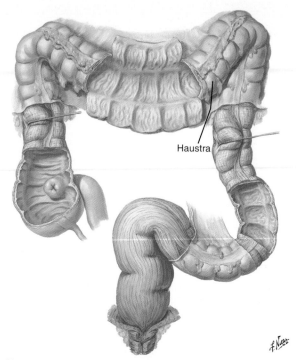

Fig. 21.2 The large bowel contains haustra, which are folds in the wall that create its segmented appearance. (Reprinted from Netter Anatomy Illustration Collection. ©Elsevier Inc. All Rights Reserved.)

Haustra

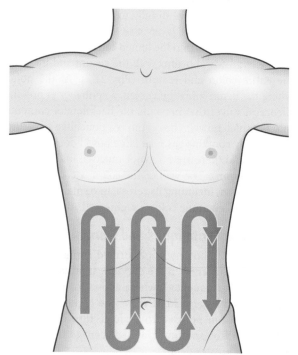

Fig. 21.3 Projected path of the probe when evaluating bowel. The bowel is examined in a systemic fashion, which is sometimes described as a "lawn mower pattern."

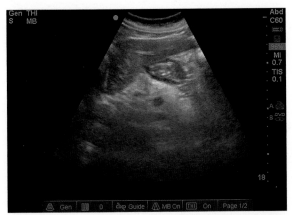

Fig. 21.4 Sonographic image of the duodenum. The duodenum is seen posterior to the gallbladder on the caudal edge of the liver.

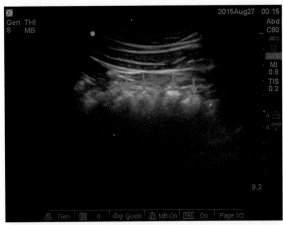

Fig. 21.6 Sonographic image of large bowel. The large bowel has periodic indentations in the wall, creating segments known as *haustra* (*arrows*). The air-filled transverse colon is demonstrated here.

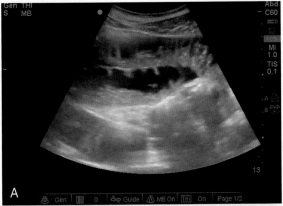

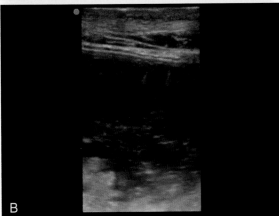

Fig. 21.5 Sonographic image of the jejunum. The jejunum contains a high density of mucosal folds known as *plicae circulares* (A). These are demonstrated in higher resolution with a high-frequency linear probe (B).

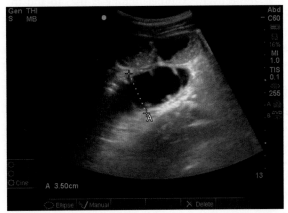

Fig. 21.7 Dilated small bowel. Long-axis sonographic image of dilated small bowel measuring 3.5 cm (35 mm) concerning for small bowel obstruction. Above this is bowel containing fluid and semisolid contents.

Small Bowel Obstruction

The hallmark finding of small bowel obstruction (SBO) is fluid-filled, dilated loops of bowel. The small bowel is considered dilated when greater than 25 mm in diameter (Fig. 21.7). Some studies use a lower threshold for the ileum (15 mm). Some studies include a required length of dilated bowel. Other findings include collapsed bowel distal to the areas of dilation or absent/decreased peristalsis distal to the obstruction and the presence of peristalsis in the dilated loops. In a recent meta-analysis by Gottlieb et al., the pooled sensitivities and specificities of ultrasound for the diagnosis of SBO were 92% and

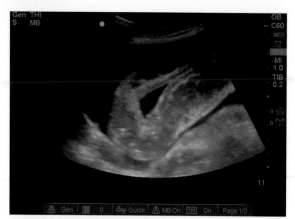

Fig. 21.8 Large bowel obstruction. The large bowel is dilated and contains dense echoes in the lumen concerning for large bowel obstruction. There is surrounding free fluid.

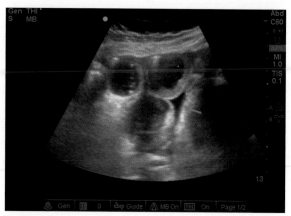

Fig. 21.9 Strangulated bowel. Multiple, dilated bowel loops with thickened walls (>3 mm) with surrounding intraperitoneal fluid suggestive of bowel strangulation. Note the triangular wedge of intraperitoneal fluid also known as a *tanga sign* (*arrow*).

97%, respectively. Another finding is the "to-and-fro" sign, where intraluminal contents are seen in real time first moving distally, and seconds later the same echoes are visualized moving proximally in the direction from which they originated.

Ileus

Criteria differentiating ileus from SBO have not been well established. One group suggests that the presence of dilated small bowel loops with abundant gas and the absence of peristalsis with a colon filled with gas, fluid, or stool is suggestive of ileus. There have been case reports of ultrasound demonstrating gallstone ileus.

Large Bowel Obstruction

Large bowel obstruction is also defined by dilated bowel with a cutoff of greater than or equal to 50 mm located proximal to normal or collapsed large bowel. The bowel is filled with dense spot echoes and located on the periphery of the abdomen (Fig. 21.8).

Strangulation of Bowel

Strangulated bowel loops will be dilated and lack peristalsis. According to Schmutz and colleagues, as opposed to ileus, the distal bowel loops will be collapsed, and the colon will lack intraluminal contents. The bowel wall may become thickened (>3 mm) and lose its mucosal folds (Fig. 21.9). There may be intraperitoneal fluid around the dilated loops of bowel. This free fluid may form a triangular wedge, termed *the tanga sign* after a similarly shaped bikini (see Fig. 21.9).

Etiologies of Bowel Obstruction

Although adhesions are one of the most common etiologies of bowel obstruction, this cannot be visualized using ultrasound. However, other etiologies may be seen, including intussusception, external incarcerated hernias, tumors of the bowel, and gallstone ileus.

APPENDIX

Clinical Correlation

Patients may present with acute or chronic right lower quadrant abdominal pain. Etiologies of this pain can be from several different organ systems, including intestinal, urologic, and genitourinary conditions (Box 21.1). One entity that should be considered is appendicitis. Ultrasound may be used as the initial or even definitive modality of imaging to confirm this diagnosis. However, ultrasound findings can sometimes be indeterminate, or visualization of the appendix may not be possible. In these cases, computed tomography (CT) or magnetic resonance imaging (MRI) may be required and can lead to alternative diagnoses.

Normal Anatomy

The normal appendix is 6 to 9 cm in length. It is an oval-shaped structure with defined layers (serosa, muscularis, submucosa, mucosa) and is typically less than 6 mm in diameter. The appendix is a blind-looped, vestigial organ that arises off the cecum. It is classically described as being located at McBurney's point, which

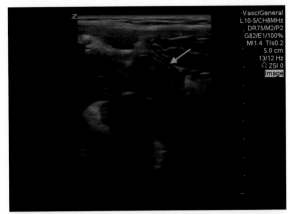

Fig. 21.11 Ultrasound image of the normal appendix demonstrating its blind end. This image shows a long-axis view of the appendix (*arrow*) located anteriorly to the iliac artery.

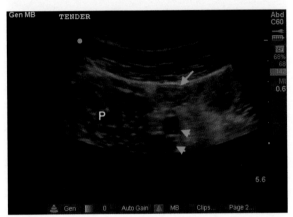

Fig. 21.10 Transverse image of the right lower quadrant of the abdomen. This transverse image using a low-frequency curvilinear probe demonstrates landmarks for identifying the appendix, including the psoas (*P*) and iliac vessels (*arrowheads*). Also seen is a portion of ileum (*arrow*).

is one-third the distance from the anterior-superior iliac spine (ASIS) and the umbilicus on surface anatomy. Autopsy and imaging studies have demonstrated that the appendix is found at this location in only 30% to 40% of patients and is more likely to be oriented in a retrocecal location (up to 65%). The appendix will often lie superficial to the psoas muscle or iliac vessels (Fig. 21.10). The normal appendix lacks peristalsis and will collapse with compression.

Ultrasound Techniques and Normal Findings

Imaging of the appendix is typically performed using a high-frequency linear array transducer (typically 9–12 MHz). However, in patients with more abdominal wall soft tissue, the curvilinear probe (typically 3–6 MHz) may be required for further penetration but comes at the expense of lower resolution.

The patient is most commonly in the supine position during examination. However, a recent study shows promise that dynamic patient positioning can increase visualization of the appendix. One approach to finding the appendix is to begin the examination by placing the probe where the patient reports maximal pain. This region is then evaluated using graded compression, which involves slow, steady pressure into the abdomen using the transducer. This technique will decrease the distance between the appendix and the probe, as well as dissipate bowel gas and its problematic shadow artifact. The examination is continued in a systematic fashion in the right lower quadrant of the abdomen until the appendix is visualized. Once a loop of bowel is identified as probable appendix, it is critical to trace this segment to confirm that it is blind-ending (Fig. 21.11). Otherwise, a loop of small bowel can be mistaken for the appendix. The appendix is often found overlying the right psoas muscle or the iliac vessels. Once the appendix is identified, it should be visualized in both its long and short axes (Fig. 21.12). The diameter of the appendix should be measured from outer wall to outer wall at its maximal thickness. An attempt should be made to compress the appendix. Color Doppler may be used as an adjunct as is described later.

If the appendix cannot be found in the prior manner, an alternative technique can be used. Begin in the right upper quadrant with the probe indicator in a cranial orientation and identify bowel gas and haustra from the ascending colon. Again, bowel gas has a hyperechoic stripe superficially with a "dirty shadow" (mixed

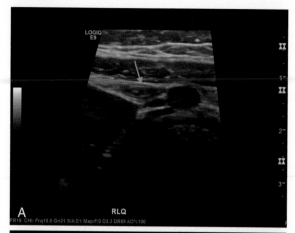

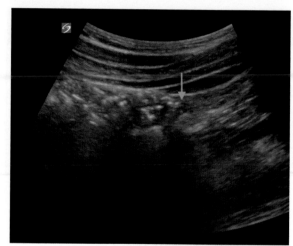

Fig. 21.13 Ultrasound image of the edge of the cecal pouch. The probe is moved from the right upper quadrant down to right lower quadrant tracing the path of the ascending colon. At the edge of the cecum there is a transition between bowel gas and abdominal contents (*arrow*).

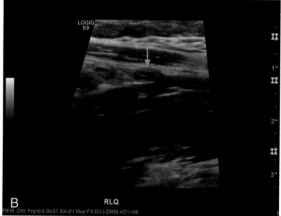

Fig. 21.12 Ultrasound images of the normal appendix in (A) long-axis and (B) in short-axis views (*arrow*).

echogenicity shadow) posteriorly. The probe is then slid caudally toward the right lower quadrant, following the previously identified bowel gas. At the inferior end of the ascending colon, a transition point is encountered where bowel gas ends and abdominal contents are now able to be visualized (Fig. 21.13). This represents the border of the cecum. Now that the cecum is identified, the probe is then moved in a medial and superior fashion to identify the appendix as it arises from the cecal pouch.

Visualization of the appendix is not only a technically challenging study for the operator but is also very dependent on patient factors such as body habitus and ability to comply with the examination. Obesity will add layers of soft tissue between the abdominal wall and the appendix, decreasing resolution and the ability to perform adequate graded

compression. Appropriate analgesics before scanning is important so that the patient can tolerate the additional abdominal wall pressure during the graded compressions. If the appendix is not visualized using ultrasound, CT or MRI (pediatric, pregnant) may be necessary.

Pathology

Appendicitis. The hallmark imaging features of an inflamed appendix are (1) a dilated appendix that is greater than 6 mm in diameter and (2) is noncompressible (Fig. 21.14). Again, it is of critical importance that the appendix is confirmed as having a closed end, as small bowel can easily be mistaken for the appendix on ultrasound imaging. The appendix should be visualized to its distal end, as appendicitis localized to the distal tip has been described. Other potential findings include periappendical fluid (Fig. 21.15), which is an anechoic stripe or wedge adjacent to the appendix, or periappendical fat stranding (Fig. 21.16). Fat stranding has a similar appearance to early edematous soft tissue (see Chapter 27). Fat stranding will be homogenous, hyperechoic haziness with loss of its naturally distinctive layers. Color Doppler may be used as an adjunct. When visualized in its short axis, the inflamed appendix will demonstrate increased flow circumferentially

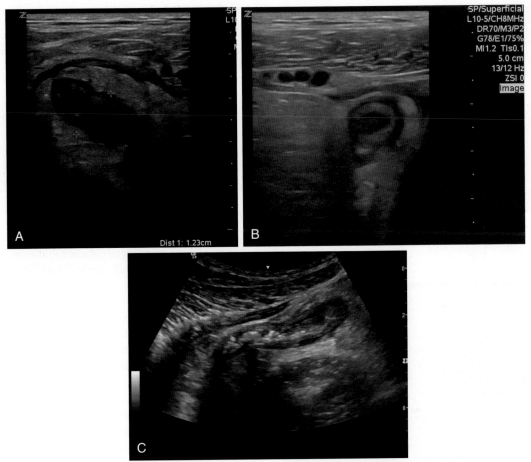

Fig. 21.14 Ultrasound image of the inflamed appendix. (A) Note the long-axis view of the dilated appendix, which measures greater than the 6-mm cut-off. (B) An example of a transverse view of the inflamed appendix. (C) The curvilinear probe demonstrating a long-axis view of a dilated appendix. The inflamed appendix should also not be compressible with external force from the probe.

along its wall and give it a "ring of fire" appearance (Fig. 21.17).

Appendicolith. In up to 33% of patients, a fecalith may be visualized. This has a similar sonographic appearance as a gallstone—hyperechoic focus with a shadow artifact—located within the lumen of the appendix (Fig. 21.18).

Appendiceal Abscess. Appendiceal abscesses are the most common complication of acute appendicitis. Appendiceal abscesses occur secondary to rupture of the inflamed appendix and have variable sonographic appearances. Some are hypoechoic, well-circumscribed fluid collections adjacent to the appendix. Others may be ill-defined and irregular in shape. The appendix itself may be difficult to visualize if an appendiceal abscess is present.

Other Etiologies

Ureterolithiasis may present as acute right lower quadrant abdominal pain. Although the stone itself is often not visualized on ultrasound, the sequela of ureteral obstruction (hydronephrosis) can be identified on renal ultrasound. Details are presented in Chapter 19.

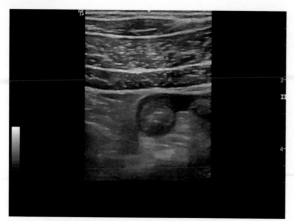

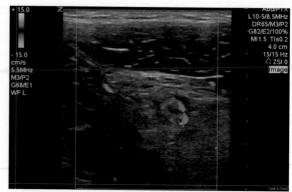

Fig. 21.17 "Ring of fire" appearance of the inflamed appendix in short-axis view using color Doppler mode.

Fig. 21.15 Ultrasound image of periappendical fluid. To the right of this appendix in the short-axis view is an anechoic wedge representing free fluid.

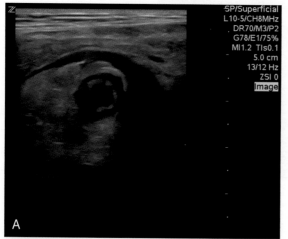

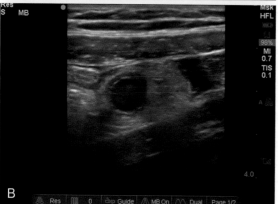

Fig. 21.16 Ultrasound image of fat stranding adjacent to the appendix. The tissues surrounding this inflamed appendix are homogenous, hyperechoic, and hazy. This is best demonstrated to the left of the appendix on (A) and on the right of (B).

Hernias cause a variety of patient complaints, including right lower quadrant abdominal pain. Hernias may be acute or chronic; they may become incarcerated or even strangulated.

In females, ovarian and adnexal pathology may also mimic appendicitis. Pathology can include ovarian torsion, ectopic pregnancy, and ovarian cysts. Some of these abnormalities may be seen on ultrasound (see Chapter 23 and 24).

In males, scrotal and testicular pathology may cause referred pain to the abdomen. Sonographic findings can range from testicular torsion to epididymitis-orchitis. Male genitourinary ultrasound is discussed in Chapter 22.

PEDIATRIC ABDOMEN

Acute Appendicitis in Pediatrics

In contrast to adults, appendicitis in children is often associated with appendicoliths (Fig. 21.19A). Periappendiceal edema is the most reliable sign of acute appendicitis (Fig. 21.19B), and the walls of the appendix can sometimes show hypervascularity on color Doppler, which is another sign of inflammation (Fig. 21.19C). Diagnosis of appendicitis in children is often delayed and mostly due to the inability of young children to clearly communicate their symptoms in addition to a challenging physical examination. This is one reason why appendiceal rupture is more common in children. Early rupture is suggested when the walls of the appendix are ill-defined or discontinuous (Fig. 21.20). Focal fluid collection adjacent to a distended or collapsed appendix is also suggestive of appendiceal

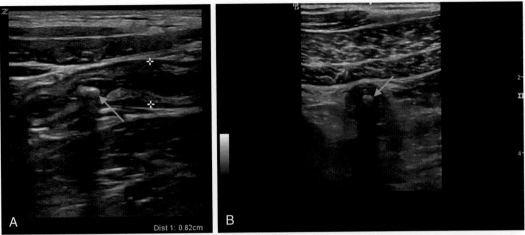

Fig. 21.18 Ultrasound image of an appendix with fecalith. Note the hyperechoic focus of the fecalith with its posterior shadow artifact seen within the appendix visualized in (A) long-axis and (B) short-axis views.

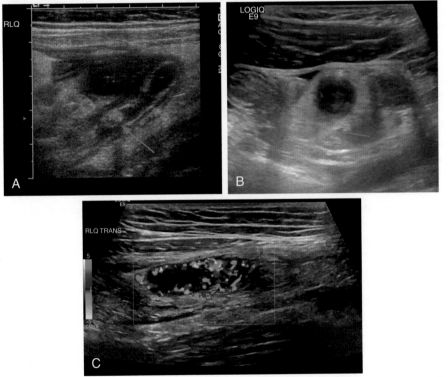

Fig. 21.19 Acute appendicitis. (A) Distended appendix with appendicolith (*arrow*). (B) Dilated appendix with surrounding mesenteric edema (*arrow*). (C) Appendicitis with hypervascular walls on Doppler.

rupture. It is important to scan not only the right lower quadrant but also the entire abdomen and pelvis if ruptured appendicitis is suspected to look for other fluid collections or abscesses elsewhere. The presence of multiple or large collections of abscesses will alter the acute management and will now require percutaneous abscess drainage and postponement of appendectomy. Additional findings of distended and hypoactive bowels

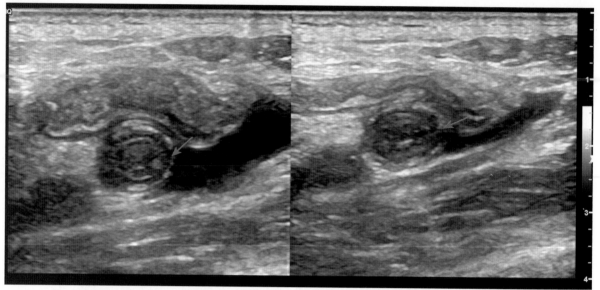

Fig. 21.20 Discontinuity in the mucosa at the tip of the distended appendix (*short arrows*) with adjacent fluid consistent with perforation.

indicate an adynamic ileus secondary to peritonitis and support the diagnosis of ruptured appendicitis.

Hypertrophic Pyloric Stenosis

Clinical Correlation. Presenting patients are typically very young, around 2 to 8 weeks old, and often male. Parents will describe projectile nonbilious vomiting and weight loss. On examination, infants are usually not lethargic and will vigorously suck when fed. Sometimes, an "olive-shaped" mass can be felt in the epigastric region representing the thickened pylorus.

Normal Anatomy. The pylorus is a channel that connects the stomach to the duodenum. Circular smooth muscle forms the pylorus, which allows food to enter the duodenum when it relaxes. The normal pyloric channel is short, measuring less than 10 mm, and a single layer of pyloric muscle is thin, measuring less than 2 mm from serosa to mucosa. Unimpeded flow of fluid should be seen across the pylorus when the gastric antrum contracts. The normal pylorus therefore is difficult to measure.

Imaging. Examination is performed using a high-resolution linear transducer (9–12 MHz). The pylorus is located medial and posterior to the gallbladder and

can be imaged in the transverse oblique plane just lateral to the epigastrium. A very distended stomach will displace the pylorus posteriorly, making it difficult to image. Positioning the patient on the left lateral oblique can be helpful in trying to find the pylorus. Infants who just vomited before the ultrasound examination often will have a collapsed stomach. Administration of oral fluid (e.g., Pedialyte) is helpful not only in outlining the gastric antrum that leads to the pylorus but also in assessing flow across the pyloric channel.

Pathology. Hypertrophic pyloric stenosis (HPS) is an acquired disorder secondary to progressive thickening of the pyloric muscle leading to circumferential narrowing of the pyloric channel and resulting in gastric outlet obstruction. The exact cause of HPS is unknown but is thought to be related to infantile hyperacidity leading to pyloric spasm and eventually hypertrophy of the pyloric muscle. The diagnosis of HPS relies on two key findings: pyloric muscle thickness >3 mm and pyloric canal length >17 mm. A single layer of the pyloric muscle is measured from mucosa to serosa on both transverse and longitudinal views (Fig. 21.21). A value of >3 mm is considered diagnostic and has been reported to be

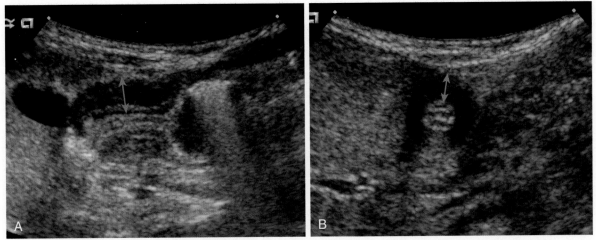

Fig. 21.21 Hypertrophic pyloric stenosis (HPS). (A) Longitudinal scan of the pylorus with a single layer of pyloric muscle measuring 4 mm (*double-headed arrow*). (B) Transverse scan showing the "donut appearance" of the thick pyloric muscle and central redundant mucosa (*double-headed arrow*).

almost 100% sensitive and specific for pyloric stenosis. Measurement of the pyloric canal length is less reliable and frequently underestimates its true length, often due to a distended stomach that displaces the pylorus posteriorly. Other secondary findings that support HPS include (1) prominent and redundant mucosa protruding into the gastric antrum, (2) thick pyloric muscle indenting the gastric antral contour—the so-called *cervix sign*, and (3) failure of the pylorus to open with absence or paucity of fluid passing through into the duodenum (Fig. 21.22). Treatment of HPS is pyloromyotomy, a surgical incision of the pyloric muscle that relieves the obstruction.

Pylorospasm is a related entity representing a transient form of gastric outlet obstruction in infants. It often resolves but can sometimes progress to HPS. Clinical presentation is similar to HPS, but the ultrasound findings are less severe. The pyloric muscle thickening is mild and <3 mm, usually in the range of 2 to 2.5 mm. Stomach contents can also be seen passing through the pylorus into the duodenum.

Pitfalls. One common pitfall in the imaging of HPS is to mistake the collapsed gastric antrum for the thickened pyloric muscle (Fig. 21.23). It is therefore important to orally administer a small amount fluid (e.g., Pedialyte) if the stomach is empty to fully evaluate the pylorus and differentiate it from the

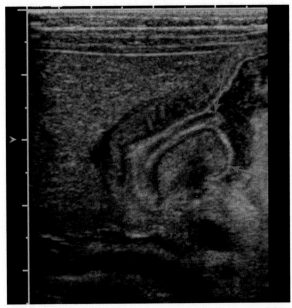

Fig. 21.22 HPS with prominent and redundant mucosa (*short arrow*) with thick pyloric muscle representing the "cervix sign" (*long arrow*).

fluid-filled gastric antrum. Care must be made not to overdistend the stomach, as this will displace the pylorus posteriorly, making it difficult to image and measure appropriately.

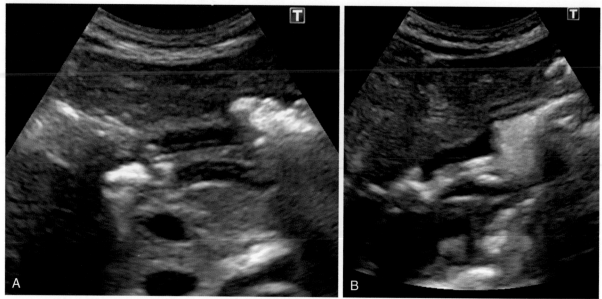

Fig. 21.23 Pitfall in pyloric imaging. (A) Gastric antrum mimicking the pylorus when collapsed. (B) After oral fluid, the pylorus opens and shows fluid across the normal pylorus into the duodenum.

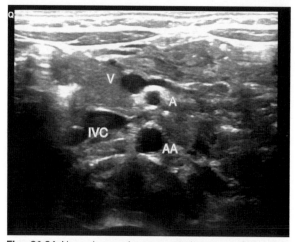

Fig. 21.24 Normal superior mesenteric artery (SMA) and superior mesenteric vein (SMV) orientation. The SMV is anterior and to the right of the SMA. A left-sided SMV is highly associated with malrotation. *A,* Superior mesenteric artery; *AA,* abdominal aorta; *IVC,* inferior vena cava; *V,* superior mesenteric vein.

Other Etiologies. Gastroesophageal reflux is the most common cause of nonbilious vomiting in infants. It is frequent during the first few months of life due to the immaturity of the lower esophageal sphincter. Imaging is not necessary, but in severe cases pyloric stenosis needs to be ruled out by ultrasound. An upper

gastrointestinal (GI) study using barium or water-soluble contrast under fluoroscopy can confirm the clinical suspicion.

Malrotation is a congenital disorder resulting from the abnormal rotation of the bowels during fetal development. The mesentery ends up having a short root and becomes prone to volvulus. Infants present with acute-onset bilious vomiting. An upper GI study under fluoroscopy is required to evaluate this emergent condition. Ultrasound can be useful in the assessment of the superior mesenteric vein (SMV) and superior mesenteric artery (SMA) relationship (Fig. 21.24).

Intussusception

Clinical Correlation. Intussusception is a common cause of bowel obstruction in children younger than 5 years. Abdominal pain, vomiting, and "currant jelly stools" are the classic triad of symptoms. A "sausage-shaped abdominal mass" can be seen or palpated in some patients. Gross blood is sometimes present on rectal examination.

Imaging. The sensitivity and specificity of ultrasound in diagnosing intussusception is close to 100%, making it the preferred imaging modality in the initial evaluation of patients suspected to have intussusception. The high-resolution linear transducer

(9–12 MHz) is primarily used in evaluating the right lower quadrant. The terminal ileum is identified in the right lower quadrant as the peristalsing segment of bowel that connects to the pouchlike cecum. It is important to scan the right lower quadrant first to identify the terminal ileum and cecum and then the entire abdomen, following the course of the colon to look for the leading edge of the intussusception. The rest of the abdomen should be scanned for evidence of lead points such as duplication cysts or masses.

Pathology. Intussusception happens when a loop of bowel telescopes into an adjacent bowel segment and can result in bowel obstruction. Several types of intussusception include ileoileal, ileocolic, ileoileocolic, and colocolic, and are named based on which segments of bowels are involved. Ileocolic intussusception is the most common type in children and occurs when the terminal ileum telescopes into the cecum. Both segments of bowels can migrate distally and in severe cases can even prolapse into the rectum. The feared complication of intussusception is bowel ischemia and perforation. The most common cause is "idiopathic" but likely secondary to enlarged mesenteric lymph nodes acting as lead points. The classic "target sign" is produced by the alternating mucosal, muscular, and serosal layers of the telescoped bowels (Fig. 21.25A), and the "sandwich sign" is observed on the longitudinal scan showing the outer receiving intussuscipiens and the telescoped bowel inside representing the intussusceptum (Fig. 21.25B). Measuring the transverse diameter of the intussusception from serosa to serosa is helpful in differentiating small bowel intussusception. An ileocolic intussusception will often measure more than 2.5 cm, whereas small bowel–to–small bowel intussusception typically measures less than 2.0 cm (Fig. 21.26). An ileocolic intussusception also frequently contains lymph nodes and significant mesenteric fat, whereas small bowel intussusceptions often do not. This differentiation is important in deciding management because ileocolic intussusception needs to be reduced emergently to prevent bowel ischemia and perforation, whereas small bowel intussusceptions are frequently transient and will reduce spontaneously. Color Doppler can also be helpful in determining the reducibility of the intussusception and integrity of bowel. Absence of

blood flow in the bowel walls is concerning for bowel ischemia and is correlated with a lower success rate and increased chance of perforation during attempted nonoperative reduction. The presence of lead points such as duplication cysts, vascular malformations, Meckel's diverticulum, and polyps can also be seen on ultrasound and would indicate the need for surgical management (Fig. 21.27).

Management. Nonsurgical reduction of intussusception is the preferred method of treatment. Although fluoroscopy is the most popular imaging used to monitor nonoperative management, ultrasound offers a radiation-free alternative with the same success rate. Saline from an enema bag is introduced through a rectal catheter, and ultrasound is used to monitor the reduction process. A successfully reduced intussusception will show (1) fluid-filled cecum, (2) thickened but patent ileocecal valve, and (3) free flow of fluid into the distal small bowels (Fig. 21.28). Sonography can also easily distinguish an edematous ileocecal valve from a residual intussusception, which can be at times difficult to reliably differentiate on fluoroscopy. The presence of significant or increasing amount of free fluid in the abdomen and pelvis is concerning for perforation and can be easily monitored during ultrasound-guided reduction.

Other Etiologies. Meckel's diverticulum is a congenital distal small bowel outpouching that results when the omphalomesenteric duct (vitelline duct) fails to involute. The diverticulum can contain heterotopic gastric or pancreatic mucosa that can cause bleeding. Bacterial overgrowth can lead to Meckel's diverticulitis, presenting clinically as abdominal pain. The diverticulum itself can act as a lead point and cause intussusception.

Mesenteric Adenitis
Clinical Correlation. Mesenteric adenitis results from inflammation of mesenteric lymph nodes, usually as a reaction to underlying bowel disease. Symptoms include abdominal pain and fever, making it difficult to differentiate from early appendicitis, especially if the pain is predominantly in the right lower quadrant.

Normal Anatomy. Mesenteric lymph nodes represent groups of lymphatic tissue found between layers of bowel

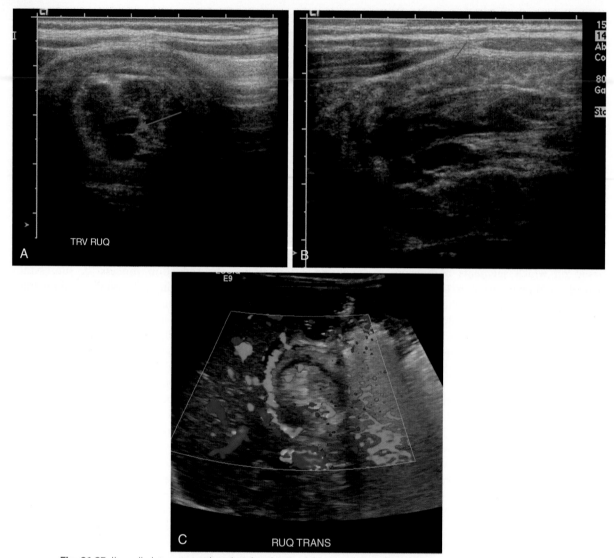

Fig. 21.25 Ileocolic intussusception showing the receiving intussuscipiens (*inner arrow*) and the telescoped intussusceptum inside (*outer arrow*), shown in both (A) a transverse axis and (B) long axis. (B) Long views of intussusception demonstrate a classic "sandwich sign" compared to (A & C) transverse views, which demonstrate a "target sign." Color Doppler can aid in evaluation, demonstrating color flow in perfused bowel (C) and reduced or no color flow in ischemic bowel.

mesentery and act in defense against microbial infection. These are usually small in size and measure between 3 and 5 mm in the short-axis dimension. Distinction between a normal and pathologic mesenteric lymph node is often based on size. Reactive lymph nodes often measure >10 mm in the long-axis and 5 to 10 mm in the short-axis dimensions.

Imaging. A high-resolution (9–12 MHz) linear probe is used in the examination. In a supine position, apply light compression, beginning at the area where pain is reported. The most common concentration of these lymph nodes is in the right lower quadrant. Careful evaluation of the proximal colon, terminal ileum, and appendix in that region is important

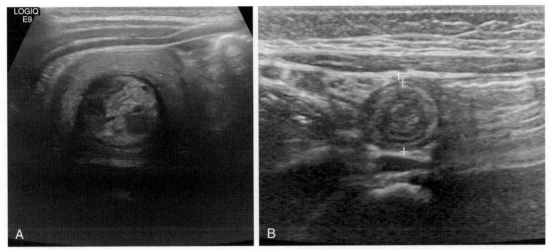

Fig. 21.26 Ileocolic vs. ileoileal intussusception. (A) Ileocolic intussusception measuring 3.5 cm and containing lymph nodes and mesenteric fat. (B) Small bowel intussusception measuring 1.2 cm and having no significant mesenteric fat or lymph nodes inside.

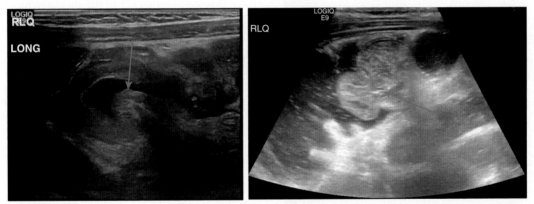

Fig. 21.27 Lead points of intussusception. (A) Meckel's diverticulum (*arrow*) within an intussusception. (B) Colonic polyps (*arrow*) causing recurrent colocolic intussusception in a child.

because any inflammatory conditions involving these segments of bowel can result in mesenteric lymph node enlargement. Doppler examination often will show hypervascularity but can be challenging in the uncooperative child.

Pathology. Although it has been documented that even small nodes less than 5 mm can be symptomatic, mesenteric adenitis typically presents as clusters of three or more lymph nodes individually measuring 5 to 10 mm in the short axis and 10 to 20 mm in the long axis (Fig. 21.29). Demonstration of tenderness during

the examination by light compression can also be helpful. The adjacent mesentery can appear echogenic, reflecting the surrounding inflammatory reaction. Hypervascularity of these lymph nodes on Doppler imaging indicates an underlying inflammatory process (Fig. 21.30). Although the lymph nodes are enlarged, more rounded, and hypoechoic, mesenteric adenitis typically will not become massively enlarged, calcify, or show central necrosis. The presence of these unusual nodal characteristics should lead one to suspect a more aggressive process such as malignancy (e.g., lymphoma) or unusual/aggressive infection.

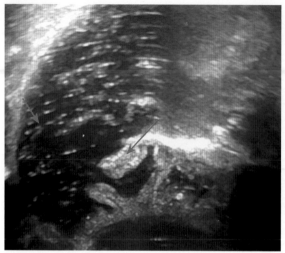

Fig. 21.28 Successful ultrasound-guided reduction of intussusception. (A) Fluid-filled cecum (*short arrow*) and thick but patent ileocecal valve (*long arrow*).

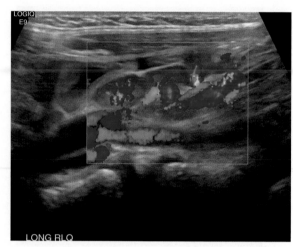

Fig. 21.30 Hypervascularity of the nodes are evident on Doppler evaluation.

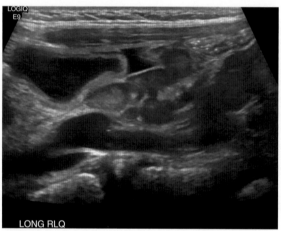

Fig. 21.29 Mesenteric adenitis. Clusters of enlarged lymph nodes in the right lower quadrant.

Other Etiologies. Appendicitis can be difficult to differentiate from mesenteric adenitis because both can present as right lower quadrant abdominal pain. It is therefore important to confirm that the appendix is normal or, if not visualized, that there are no secondary signs of appendicitis before making a diagnosis of mesenteric adenitis in a technically adequate examination.

Inflammatory bowel disease (IBD), such as Crohn's disease, can present with enlarged mesenteric lymph nodes. Bowel wall thickening of the terminal ileum and/or ascending colon can lead one to suspect IBD and can

be confirmed by either CT of the abdomen or magnetic resonance enterography (MRE).

BIBLIOGRAPHY

Chang ST, Jeffrey RB, Olcott EW. Three-step sequential positioning algorithm during sonographic evaluation for appendicitis increases appendiceal visualization rate and reduces CT use. *AJR Am J Roentgenol.* 2014;203(5):1006–1012. https://doi.org/10.2214/AJR.13.12334.

Dias SC, Swinson S, Torrao H, et al. Hypertrophic pyloric stenosis: tips and tricks for ultrasound diagnosis. *Insights Imaging.* 2012;3:247–250.

Fleischer AC, Dowling AD, Weinstein ML, James AE. Sonographic patterns of distended, fluid-filled bowel. *Radiology.* 1979;133(3 Pt 1):681–685. https://doi.org/10.1148/133.3.681.

Fox C, Solley M, Anderson C, Zlidenny A, Lahham S, Maasumi K. Prospective evaluation of emergency physician performed bedside ultrasound to detect acute appendicitis. *Eur J Emerg Med.* 2008. https://doi.org/10.1097/MEJ.0b013e328270361a.

Gottlieb M, Peksa GD, Pandurangadu AV, Nakitende D, Takhar S, Seethala RR. Utilization of ultrasound for the evaluation of small bowel obstruction: a systematic review and meta-analysis. *Am J Emerg Med.* 2017. https://doi.org/10.1016/j.ajem.2017.07.085.

Hernanz-Schulman M. Hypertrophic pyloric stenosis. *Radiology.* 2003;227:319–331.

Hryhorczuk AL, Strouse PJ. Validation of US as the fist-line diagnostic test for assessment of pediatric ileocolic intussusception. *Pediar Radiol.* 2009;39:1075–1079.

Ko YT, Lim JH, Lee DH, Lee HW, Lim JW. Small bowel obstruction: sonographic evaluation. *Radiology*. 1993;188:649–653.

Lahham S, et al. *Introduction to Abdominal Ultrasound* Version 1.0. iBooks; 2015.

Lioubashevsky N, Hiller N, Rozovsky K, Segev L, Simanovsky N. Ileocolic versus small-bowel intussusception in children: can US enable reliable differentiation? *Radiology*. 2013;269:266–271.

Mallin M, Craven P, Ockerse P, et al. Diagnosis of acute appendicitis by bedside ultrasound in the emergency department. *Acad Emerg Med*. 2014. https://doi.org/10.1111/acem.12365.

Mallin, M., Dawson, M. *Introduction to Bedside Ultrasound: Volume 2. Chapter 13: Appendicitis*. Version 1.34. Emergency Ultrasound Solutions (2013). iBooks.

Mallin, M., Dawson, M. *Introduction to Bedside Ultrasound: Volume 2. Chapter 14: Small Bowel Obstruction*. Version 1.34. Emergency Ultrasound Solutions (2013). iBooks.

Ogata M, Mateer JR, Condon RE. Prospective evaluation of abdominal sonography for the diagnosis of bowel obstruction. *Ann Surg*. 1996;223(3):237–241. https://doi.org/10.1097/00000658-199603000-00002.

Puylaert JB. Acute appendicitis: US evaluation using graded compression. *Radiology*. 1986;158(2):355–360. https://doi.org/10.1016/0736-4679(86)90023-5.

Puylaert JB. Mesenteric adenitis and acute terminal ileitis: US evaluation using graded compression. *Radiology*. 1986;161(3):691–695. https://doi.org/10.1148/radiology.161.3.3538138.

Roccarina D, Garcovich M, Ainora ME, et al. Diagnosis of bowel diseases: the role of imaging and ultrasonography. *World J Gastroenterol*. 2013;19(14):2144–2153. https://doi.org/10.3748/wjg.v19.i14.2144.

Sanchez TR, Corwin MT, Davoodian A, Stein-wexler R. Sonography of abdominal pain in children. Appendicitis and its common mimics. *J Ultrasound Med*. 2016;35:627–635.

Sanchez TR, Potnick A, Graf JL, Abramson LP, Patel CV. Sonographically guided enema for intussusception reduction: a safer alternative to fluoroscopy. *J Ultrasound Med*. 2012;31:1505–1508.

Scheible W, Goldberger L. Diagnosis of small bowel obstruction: the contribution of diagnostic ultrasound. *AJR Am J Roentgenol*. 1979;133:685.

Schmutz GR, Benko A, Fournier L, Peron JM, Morel E, Chiche L. Small bowel obstruction: role and contribution of sonography. *Eur Radiol*. 1997;7(7):1054–1058. https://doi.org/10.1007/s003300050251.

Simanovsky N, Hiller N. Importance of sonographic detection of enlarged abdominal lymph nodes in children. *J Ultrasound Med*. 2001;7(26):581–584.

Sivit CJ, Newman KD, Chandra KS. Visualization of enlarged mesenteric lymph nodes at US examination: clinical significance. *Pediatr Radiol*. 2009;39:1075–1079.

Taylor GA. Suspected appendicitis in children: in search of the single best diagnostic test. *Radiology*. 2004;231:293–295.

Trout AT, Towbin AJ, Zhang B. Journal club: the pediatric appendix – defining normal. *AJR Am J Roengenol*. 2014;202:936–945.

Wale A, Pilcher J. Current role of ultrasound in small bowel imaging. *Semin Ultrasound CT MR*. 2016;37(4):301–312. https://doi.org/10.1053/j.sult.2016.03.001.

Pelvis Ultrasound

22

Male Pelvis

Eugenio O. Gerscovich, John P. McGahan

SCROTUM

Normal Anatomy

The surface of the testis is surrounded by the tunica vaginalis, which extends to the inner surface of the scrotal wall in continuity. A trace amount of fluid in between both layers allows a high mobility of the testis. This arrangement is similar to the pleura with the visceral and parietal layers that allow the lung excursion. Adult measurements of the testis are variable, in the range of 3 to 5 cm in length, 2.5 cm in anteroposterior diameter, and 3 cm in transverse diameter. The testis is surrounded by a fibrous capsule, the tunica albuginea. It cannot be recognized as such on scanning, but it is important because its smooth contour is disrupted with testicular trauma. The seminiferous tubules of the testes are separated by septa. They drain into the rete testes and then into the epididymis (Fig. 22.1). The epididymis sits along the surface of the testis. It is classically divided in a head, body, and tail, from superior to inferior. Normally, only the head is visualized, measuring approximately 1 to 2 cm in diameter. The vascularity of the epididymis is less than that of the adjacent testis. The tail of the epididymis drains into the vas deferens, located in the spermatic cord. The testis is suspended by the spermatic cord that descends from the abdomen into the scrotum through the inguinal canal. The cord contains the vas deferens carrying the sperm to the ejaculatory ducts, the spermatic artery to the testis, other arteries, pampiniform plexus (venous), lymphatics, and nerves (see Fig. 22.1).

Ultrasound Technique/Findings

The patient should be in the recumbent position with the scrotum exposed over a towel. Starting with an axial view of both testes in grayscale and color Doppler, the procedure should be done with a high-resolution convex or linear transducer with convex settings. The grayscale comparison views of each testis are helpful to show symmetry between the two testes. The comparison color flow views of the testes are extremely helpful to detect potential abnormalities associated with either increased or decreased flow. With those views, the imager should get an immediate understanding of asymmetries in echogenicity, size, and perfusion between both sides (Figs. 22.2 and 22.3).

Then, with a high-resolution linear transducer, each testis, epididymis, tunica vaginalis, scrotal wall, and spermatic cord should be examined in grayscale and color Doppler. On ultrasound, the multiple histologic layers of the scrotal sac are seen as a single layer. Only with scrotal edema is the multilayered appearance of the scrotal sac seen, resembling an "onion skin." The examination should include longitudinal views of each testis, including the epididymis, using both grayscale and color flow. Begin with the nonaffected side to set the technical parameters before examining the side of concern. Both testes are oval structures of homogeneous, midlevel echogenicity with their long axis in the superoinferior body direction (Fig. 22.4). This is important in cases of torsion, where the long axis

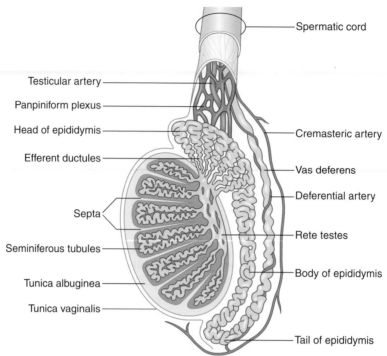

Spermatic cord

Testicular artery

Panpiniform plexus

Head of epididymis

Efferent ductules

Cremasteric artery

Vas deferens

Deferential artery

Septa

Rete testes

Seminiferous tubules

Tunica albuginea

Body of epididymis

Tunica vaginalis

Tail of epididymis

Fig. 22.1 Normal scrotal anatomy. The seminiferous tubules in the testicle converge centrally into the rete testis. These tubules connect to the epididymis and eventually to the vas deferens. (Redrawn from Sudokoff GS, Quiroz F, Karcaaltincaba M, Foley WD. Scrotal ultrasonography with emphasis on the extratesticular space: anatomy, embryology and pathology. *Ultrasound Q.* 2002;18:255–273; Rumack CM, Levine D. *Diagnostic Ultrasound.* 5th ed. Philadelphia, PA: Elsevier; 2018:841.)

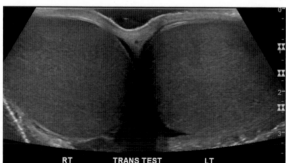

RT   TRANS TEST   LT

Fig. 22.2 Grayscale axial view of both testes. Observe a symmetrical appearance of both testes. This is an important view to note any differences in the appearance to the testes.

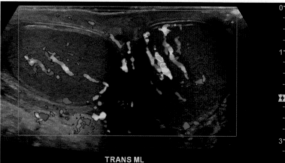

TRANS ML

Fig. 22.3 Color Doppler view of both testes. Observe a fairly symmetrical perfusion of both testes. This is important to document in cases where there may be increased or decreased flow to one of the testes.

of the testis may rotate 90 degrees. A linear area of echogenicity in the periphery of the testis represents the mediastinum, where the seminiferous tubules and vascular structures exit and enter the testis (not to be confused with a testicular laceration) (Fig. 22.5). Flow to the testes should be evaluated with color and pulsed wave Doppler, as the normal testis normally shows forward flow in systole and diastole, as do all other

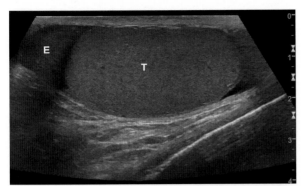

Fig. 22.4 Normal scrotal anatomy in an adult. Longitudinal ultrasound of the scrotum showing the homogeneous appearance to the testis (*T*) and the head of the epididymis (*E*).

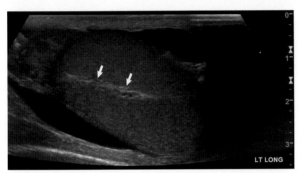

Fig. 22.5 Normal anatomy of the testis. The mediastinum of the testis (*arrows*) is where the rete testis converges and is seen as an echogenic band extending in a cranial-caudal direction.

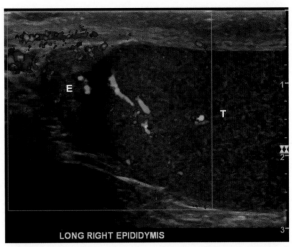

LONG RIGHT EPIDIDYMIS

Fig. 22.6 Normal anatomy. Color Doppler. Color flow is identified in both normal testis (*T*) and epididymis (*E*).

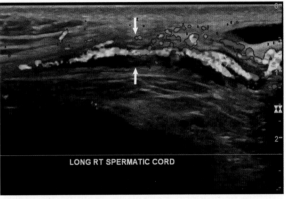

LONG RT SPERMATIC CORD

Fig. 22.7 Normal anatomy of the spermatic cord with color Doppler. The spermatic cord has smooth boundaries that are parallel (*arrows*). The cord includes the vas deferens, testicular artery, other arteries, the pampiniform plexus, lymphatics, and the ilioinguinal nerve.

organ parenchyma. There is color flow in both the normal testis and the epididymis (Fig. 22.6). Any reduction, absence, or reversal of diastolic flow is indicative of high resistance to flow such as seen with edema, ischemia, or venous compromise. The epididymis is isoechoic or slightly less echogenic than the testis. On ultrasound, the spermatic cord is observed as a laminar structure, not exceeding a caliber of 1 cm, without twists (important in cases of torsion). It is easier to identify with deep breaths, as the cord is observed moving up and down (Fig. 22.7, Video 22.1).

Acute Scrotum: General Considerations

Acute scrotum is defined as an acute painful swelling of the scrotum or its contents accompanied by local signs and possible general symptoms. Possible etiologies

include epididymo-orchitis, testicular ischemia, trauma, torsion of testicular appendages, and complicated inguinal/femoral hernias. The incidence is variable, but their early correct diagnosis is extremely important because of a possible testis loss in cases of mismanagement.

Since the advent of medical diagnostic ultrasound several decades ago, this tool has remained the best modality in the diagnosis of scrotal/inguinal pathology, despite the development of newer and more complex tools, such as computed tomography (CT), magnetic resonance imaging, and positron emission tomography.

These modalities are of value when scrotal pathology extends beyond this region, such as with metastatic tumors.

As is well known, ultrasound has an exquisite image resolution in the range of millimeters, has the capability of real-time imaging (useful to observe changes with the Valsalva maneuver), and demonstrates blood flow (useful in cases of ischemia or inflammation). It is readily available at most medical institutions; it is less expensive than the other mentioned modalities and does not expose the patient to ionizing radiation.

Inflammation: Epididymitis and Epididymo-orchitis.

Inflammatory changes of the scrotum are mostly bacterial in origin. It is one of the most common diagnoses in men from the teenage years to middle age. The most common presentation is in the form of acute epididymitis, which may extend to the testis, resulting in epididymo-orchitis. In sexually active patients, it results from bacteria ascending in the urethra through the vas deferens and reaching the epididymis. The main causal etiology in men younger than 35 years is *Chlamydia*, followed by *Neisseria gonorrhoeae*, *Treponema pallidum*, *Trichomonas*, and *Gardnerella vaginalis*. Urinary coliforms such as *Escherichia coli*, *Pseudomonas* species, *Proteus* species, and *Klebsiella* are seen in children and older men. In homosexual males, coliforms are prevalent.

In young children, infection may be due to congenital malformations. In older men, it may be due to bladder outlet obstruction or be secondary to urethral stricture or prostatic hyperplasia, resulting in urinary reflux into the ejaculatory ducts and vas deferens. Other causes of infection in the older group are urethral/prostatic instrumentation and bladder catheterization.

Infrequent isolated orchitis, without epididymitis, may be seen with mumps, with a preceding general malaise and parotiditis.

Clinical presentations favoring inflammatory disease rather than torsion are the following: gradual progression of unilateral scrotal pain and swelling, urinary symptoms, urethral discharge, possible fever/chills (more so in children), and absence of nausea/vomiting.

The ultrasound appearance of epididymitis includes edema and hypervascularity of the epididymis with enlargement, decreased/heterogeneous echogenicity, and increased Doppler flow (Fig. 22.8, Video 22.2). When the inflammation extends to the testis, similar findings to those in the epididymis are observed in

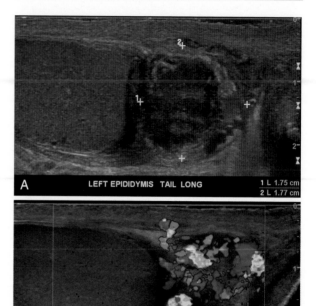

Fig. 22.8 Epididymitis. (A) Grayscale, longitudinal view showing the epididymal tail to be enlarged and heterogeneous (*calipers*). (B) This long-axis view shows the epididymal tail to be markedly hypervascular.

the testis (Fig. 22.9, Video 22.3). Frequent associated findings are reactive hydrocele, pyocele, and scrotal wall edema/hyperhemia (Fig. 22.10). With reactive hydrocele, the fluid is clear. With pyocele, the fluid is echogenic with pseudomembranes (fibrin). Possible complications of inflammation are abscess (Fig. 22.11) and testis ischemia, resulting in segmental or complete testis infarction.

In immunosuppressed patients, inflammation may lead to gangrene with gas-forming organisms (Fournier gangrene). In addition to the classic inflammatory findings, ultrasound shows gas in the form of bright echogenic foci with an artifact posterior to the echogenic-appearing gas (Fig. 22.12).

Testicular Ischemia and Torsion.

Ischemia is defined as an insufficient blood supply to an organ, in this case, to the testis. Possible causes of testis ischemia are torsion, inflammation, trauma, surgical complication of inguinal hernia repair, and vasculitis. The former is the most common.

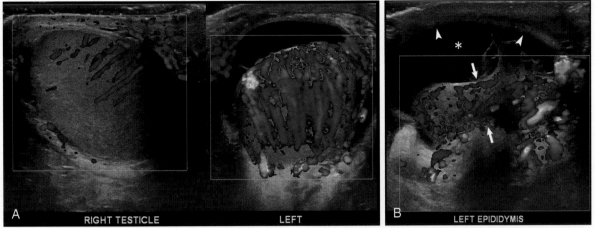

Fig. 22.9 Epididymo-orchitis with color Doppler. (A) Axial view of both testes showing increased vascularity of the left testis compared with the right testis. Also note the associated hydrocele. (B) Long-axis view of the left epididymis. Observe the thickened (edematous) body of the epididymis with increased vascularity (*arrows*), a reactive hydrocele/pyocele (*asterisk*), and scrotal wall thickening (*arrowheads*).

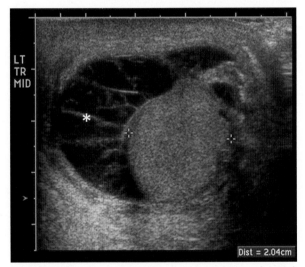

Fig. 22.10 Epididymo-orchitis. Grayscale. Axial view of the left scrotum. Observe the multiseptated fluid collection (*asterisk*) corresponding to a pyocele surrounding the testis (*calipers*).

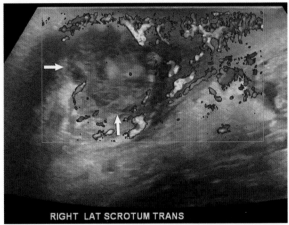

Fig. 22.11 Scrotal wall abscess. Color Doppler. Axial view. Hypoechoic, heterogeneous, and hypoperfused area (*arrows*), corresponding to an abscess that was within the scrotal wall, which is surrounded by reactive hypervascularity.

Testicular torsion results from torsion of the spermatic cord from which the testis is suspended and carries its blood supply. The cord may make a partial/complete single turn (360 degrees) or two or more turns. Infrequently, it may detorse spontaneously. The reported annual incidence of testicular torsion is 3.8/100,000 in patients younger than 18 years.

Torsion can occur at any age, but there are two peaks: one in the newborn period and the other one in adolescence. In general, in the former, torsion occurs above the tunica vaginalis. In the latter, torsion is within the tunica vaginalis. In adolescents, torsion may be spontaneous or related to physical activity. Clinically, it presents as sudden unilateral scrotal pain with progressive scrotal swelling. Additional possible features at presentation are an elevated testis (the torsion shortens the spermatic cord), nausea/vomiting (resulting from a visceral reflex), and absent cremasteric reflex in older children.

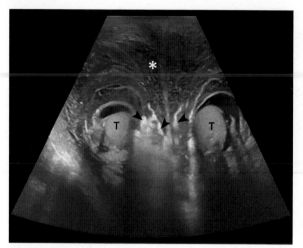

Fig. 22.12 Fournier gangrene in an immunosuppressed patient. Grayscale. Observe the marked scrotal wall edema with "onion skin" appearance (*asterisk*) and bright echogenic foci with posterior artifact, representing interstitial gas (*arrowheads*). Testes (*T*). There are bilateral hydroceles or pyoceles.

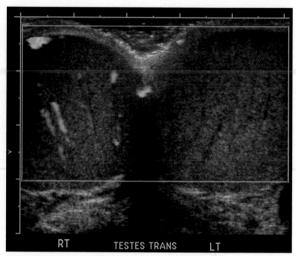

Fig. 22.13 Early testis torsion. Color Doppler. Axial view of both testes. Observe the hypoperfusion of the left testis compared with the right one. There is a symmetrical grayscale appearance of both testes and no associated findings.

The prognosis of testis torsion and the related damage are related to the number of twists of the cord and the time since the beginning of the scrotal pain. Early diagnosis and treatment are essential, because the chance of testis salvage is estimated to be close to 100% in the first 6 hours, but it decreases rapidly afterwards.

Testicular torsion, even when the testis is saved, results in subsequent abnormal spermatogenesis in about half of the patients and borderline impairment in another 20%. Of interest is the fact that contralateral testicular biopsies at the time of torsion are abnormal in 57% to 88% of patients, indicating an underlying pathology in both testes. Some studies suggest that leaving a damaged testis in place increases the damage to the contralateral testis. Testicular hormonal function is preserved in cases of early treatment of torsion, but it is abnormal in cases of late intervention or testis atrophy. The mechanism of injury is attributed to ischemia and reperfusion. Functionally, a blood–testis barrier (Sertoli cell barrier), protecting the testis, is described. It breaks during torsion and ischemia, exposing antigenic material from the damaged testis to the immune system, with the newly formed antibodies attacking the contralateral testis.

As expected, testis torsion is a dynamic process, and the ultrasound appearance depends on the time of imaging. It is very important to obtain comparison images of both testes, in grayscale and color Doppler.

At the beginning, the torsion of the spermatic cord first compromises the venous return and progressively increases the resistance to flow in the artery, manifested as decreased or reversed diastolic flow and then to its absence. This is observed on pulsed Doppler waveforms. Color Doppler shows decreased or absent perfusion of the affected testis, compared with the normal one. At this early stage, grayscale images are normal or may show a slightly increased size of the torsed testis (Fig. 22.13). As time progresses, additional grayscale findings develop: hydrocele, epididymal edema, and scrotal wall edema. Next, the testis necrotizes and becomes heterogeneous (Fig. 22.14).

In practical terms, on imaging, the torsed testis has a chance of being salvaged only when the only abnormal finding is decreased or absent perfusion on Doppler and the grayscale images are normal. The chances of salvage rapidly decrease when the described additional grayscale findings are observed.

A very useful tool in the diagnosis of testicular torsion is the examination of the spermatic cord. It should be examined superiorly up to the entrance into the inguinal canal. Normally, it shows a linear course with vessels and vas deferens in parallel. When torsed, it loses this appearance and shows what has been described as the "whirlpool" sign, with the appearance of a knot. This finding has been observed in classic cases of complete torsion, in incomplete torsion (less than 360 degrees),

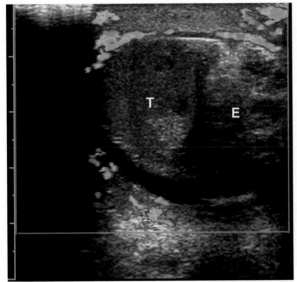

Fig. 22.14 Late testis torsion. Color Doppler. Axial view of the left testis (*T*) and an epididymis (*E*). Observe hypoperfusion of the testis and epididymis. There is edema of the epididymis and slight heterogeneity of the testis.

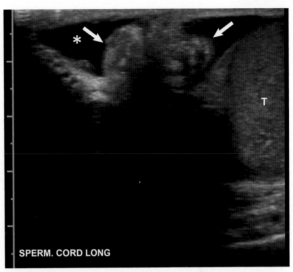

SPERM. CORD LONG

Fig. 22.15 Testis torsion with a spermatic cord twist, or "knot." Long axis. The normal linear appearance of the cord is lost, and a convoluted appearance is observed immediately above the upper pole of the testis (*arrows*). Testis (*T*). Hydrocele (*asterisk*).

and in the torsion-detorsion sequence (testis spontaneously detorsing) (Fig. 22.15, Video 22.4).

Trauma

The scrotum is an infrequent site of injury, reported to be less than 1% of all injuries. The low rate of injury is attributed to the testes being protected by surrounding muscles and due to their high mobility. Clinical presentation indicates the type of injury: blunt, penetrating, degloving (avulsion), and, rarely, electrical burn. Blunt trauma is the most common one and most commonly related to sports or a direct kick. The key role of ultrasound is to diagnose or exclude injury to the testis itself. In blunt trauma, surgical indications are suspicion of testis rupture, enlarging hematoma, and nonreducible testis dislocation (observed in motorcycle crashes). Penetrating injuries are usually related to gunshots, stab wounds, and self-mutilation. Since 2001, a new source of penetrating scrotal injuries has been combat wounds by improvised explosive devices (IEDs). This requires surgical exploration. Degloving is seen with scrotal trapping in machinery and also requires surgical intervention.

Similarly to the situation with testis ischemia, when indicated, prompt intervention is necessary to save the involved and contralateral testes from possible infection,

atrophy, necrosis, and loss of spermatogenesis. Possible ultrasound findings with scrotal trauma include the following:

Scrotal wall and extratesticular hematomas: They appear as focal or diffuse tissue thickening with early high/iso-echogenicity and then evolving to low echogenicity or fluid. They are hypovascular.

Hematoceles: They appear as complex fluid within the tunica vaginalis. Like other blood collections, at presentation, they are echogenic and progress to low echogenicity, septation, and possible fluid/fluid levels (hematocrit effect). They are hypovascular.

Epididymal injuries are commonly associated with testicular injuries. Epididymides appear enlarged and heterogeneous. Vascularity is variable.

Testicular injuries are the most relevant to the ultrasound examination. A fractured testicle appears as a linear, hypoechoic band in the parenchyma with a normal testis contour and intact tunica albuginea. They are difficult to visualize because of their association with intra- and extratesticular hematomas (Fig. 22.16). Color Doppler helps evaluate the vascular integrity of the testis. Testis rupture results from discontinuity of the testicular capsule (tunica albuginea) and extrusion of parenchyma into the adjacent tissues. It appears as loss of definition of

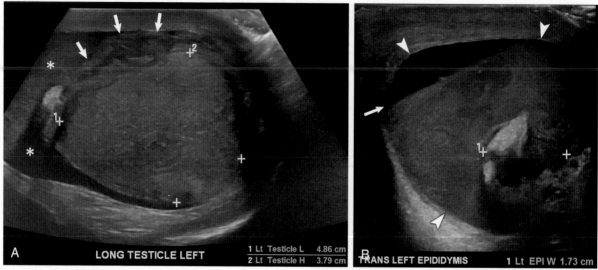

Fig. 22.16 Testicular rupture. (A) Long axis. Grayscale. The continuity of the contour of the testis (*calipers*) is disrupted (*arrows*), and the parenchyma is heterogeneous. Hematocele (*asterisk*). (B) Axial view. Grayscale. Heterogeneous epididymis (*calipers*) and large hematocele (*arrowheads*) with hematocrit effect (fluid/fluid level) (*arrow*) is seen in this image.

its contour and heterogeneous parenchyma representing hemorrhage and infarction (see Fig. 22.16, Video 22.5). It is associated with scrotal wall hematoma and hematoceles. As the blood vessels to the testis run immediately under the tunica albuginea in what it is called the *tunica vasculosa*, a tear of the former results in extensive bleeding and hypoperfusion of the parenchyma.

Doppler examination helps define these areas. Surgical exploration is mandatory to debride the ischemic tissue and preserve the viable portions.

In major trauma to the scrotum, the earlier described findings may coexist.

Scrotal injuries are frequently associated with injuries of adjacent structures such as the urethra, rectum, and femoral vessels.

Torsion of Testicular Appendages

Torsion of the testicular appendages is one of the leading causes of acute scrotum in children. These appendages are embryonic remnants. Four of them are anatomically described, but only two have clinical significance: the appendix testis is in the upper pole of the testis and is present 92% of the time, and the appendix epididymis is usually located in the region of the head and is present 23% of the time. More than 80% of cases of appendageal torsion occur between the ages of 7 and 14. The

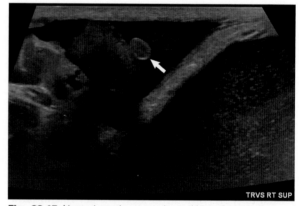

Fig. 22.17 Normal testis appendage. Note the small round structure (*arrow*), corresponding to a normal appendage of the testis, which is attached to the upper portion of the testis. It is visualized due to the accompanying hydrocele.

appendages measure a few millimeters and are usually pedunculated. Normally, they are collapsed against the testis and are not visualized. Only when a hydrocele is present does the fluid in the tunica vaginalis allow these small appendages to be observed (Fig. 22.17). Torsion of the pedicle of the appendage results in ischemia and necrosis with secondary reactive inflammation. Findings on ultrasound are observed as hyperemia of epididymis and scrotal wall that surround the enlarged hypovascular appendage (larger than 5.6 mm).

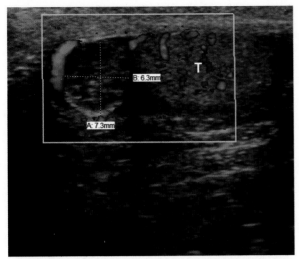

Fig. 22.18 Twisted testis appendage. Color Doppler. Long-axis view showing a rather enlarged and hypovascular structure corresponding to torsion of the appendage of the testicle (*calipers*). Testis (*T*). (Courtesy Dr. Chirag V. Patel, University of California, Davis.)

There is an associated thickening of the epididymis and hydrocele with torsion of the appendages (Fig. 22.18, Video 22.6). Blood flow to the testis itself remains normal (unlike in testis torsion). Clinically, torsion of testicular appendages manifests as gradually increasing pain localized to the upper pole of the testis, unlike the pain in testis torsion, which is sudden and involves the whole testis. Many times, the external appearance of the scrotum is normal, but inflammatory signs may be observed, as described earlier. In about 20% of cases a "blue dot" can be clinically observed in the upper pole of the testis, corresponding to the infarcted testicular appendage, as seen through the translucent skin of the scrotum. Besides testicular torsion, the differential diagnosis includes epididymitis/orchitis (infrequent in children).

Other Possible Findings in the Scrotum

Other entities may be encountered when examining the scrotum. These can include extratesticular abnormalities such as spermatoceles, hydroceles, or varicoceles. Each of these has a different appearance.

Hydroceles are fluid collections that surround the testis and are located within the tunica vaginalis. They are usually small and go unnoticed, but if large enough, the patient may present with a mass. Simple hydroceles are anechoic and surround the testis, but they can contain sediment or crystals, which can be seen.

Spermatoceles probably are the most common scrotal mass and present in the head of the epididymis. These are usually small, mainly anechoic structures, but they may contain spermatozoa and thus have internal echoes in the fluid. When color Doppler is placed on a spermatocele, a color signal may be seen, called *acoustic streaming*. This should not be confused with true vascular flow.

Within the spermatic cord, there are veins that can dilate, representing a "**varicocele**." This is usually caused by incompetent valves in the testicular veins. They are usually more common on the left side compared with the right side. The upper limit of the normal diameter of these veins is 2 mm. They are usually chronic, but if acute, this may be secondary to obstruction of the vein within the abdomen. In these cases, ultrasound of the inferior vena cava or renal veins may be indicated.

Patients with **testicular tumors** may present with a scrotal mass, noticed after minor trauma. These tumors are usually germ cell tumors and can be confused with testicular abscesses or testicular trauma. These masses may have a variety of appearances, including increased color flow, and may show cystic/solid components and calcifications.

INGUINAL AND FEMORAL HERNIAS

Normal Anatomy

A hernia is defined as a protrusion of a structure through a wall that normally surrounds or covers that structure. In the groin area, the most common ones are inguinal hernias, of which there are two types: indirect and direct. Femoral hernias are less frequent. When uncomplicated, hernias manifest as discomfort or moderate pain. When complicated, such as with incarceration (nonreducible), intestinal obstruction, or strangulation (vascular compromise), the pain becomes severe. Clinical history and physical examination are very important to understand the urgency of the situation. Ultrasound is helpful when the anatomy is relatively preserved, but in some cases the anatomic detail becomes distorted, and CT becomes the modality of choice. CT is helpful for evaluation of the local anatomy and pathology of the groin but also assesses the abdomen and pelvis for possible complications, including but not limited to intestinal obstruction and peritonitis.

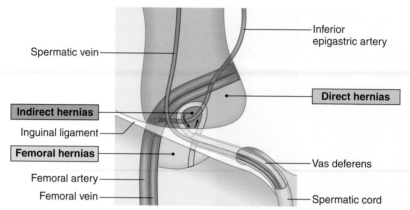

Fig. 22.19 Diagram of the normal anatomy of the right groin. Note the relationship between a direct hernia lying medial to the inferior epigastric artery and an indirect hernia lying lateral to the inferior epigastric artery. Note the location of the femoral hernia in relationship to the femoral vessels.

Ultrasound Findings. For the ultrasound evaluation, the anatomy of the inguinal and femoral canals must be understood (Fig. 22.19). For that, it is important to become familiar with a few anatomic landmarks. The inguinal ligament is the thickened inferior edge of the external oblique muscle aponeurosis of the abdomen. It runs from the anterosuperior iliac spine to the pubic tubercle. A second landmark is the inferior epigastric vessels (one artery and two veins). They measure a few millimeters and originate from the external iliac artery and vein, immediately above the inguinal ligament. They ascend medially toward the posterior aspect of the rectus abdominis. The inguinal canal is a short oblique tunnel running parallel and above the inguinal ligament, through the lower abdominal wall. It has a superficial medial ring (opening) and a deep, more lateral ring. The latter is located lateral to the inferior epigastric vessels. In a male, the inguinal canal contains the spermatic cord, arteries and veins to the scrotum, and the ilioinguinal nerve. In a female, it contains the round ligament and the ilioinguinal nerve.

The femoral canal lies below the inguinal ligament and contains the femoral artery and vein (medial).

Indirect inguinal hernias originate lateral to the inferior epigastric vessels and descend in the inguinal canal. Direct inguinal hernias originate medial to those vessels. Both of them are located above the inguinal ligament. Femoral hernias originate medial to the femoral vein and below the inguinal ligament.

The ultrasound examination is performed in supine and standing positions, with and without the Valsalva

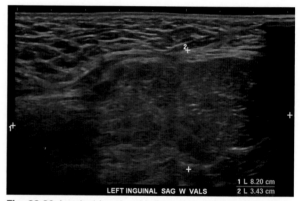

Fig. 22.20 Inguinal hernia with fatty contents (*calipers*). Grayscale view. Note the hernia sac. To the left is the neck of the hernia, and the entire sac is measured with calipers.

maneuver. Several parameters of a hernia should be analyzed:

1. The maximum size of the hernia sac in three dimensions and of the neck (open defect) (Fig. 22.20)
2. The type of sac content: fat (preperitoneal or omentum), small or large bowel (depending on the presence or absence of peristalsis), peritoneal fluid
3. Mobility, regarding the possibility of returning its contents to the abdominal cavity: reducible (it can be completely returned), nonreducible (it cannot be returned at all), partially reducible (part of it can be returned) (Video 22.7)

Complications include herniated fat or bowel with edema, ischemia, and necrosis/perforation.

SUMMARY

In the evaluation of the emergent pathology of the scrotum, ultrasound plays an important role in the differential diagnosis, evaluation of the severity, and evolution of the problem of concern.

BIBLIOGRAPHY

Baldisserotto M, de Souza JC, Pertence AP, Dora MD. Color doppler sonography of normal and torsed testicular appendages in children. *AJR Am J Roentgenol.* 2005;184:1287–1292.

Beni-Israel T, Goldman M, Bar Chaim S, Kozer E. Clinical predictors for testicular torsion as seen in the pediatric ED. *Am J Emerg Med.* 2010;28:786–789.

Hadway P, Reynard JM. The six-hour rule for testis fixation in testicular torsion: is it history? *J Clin Urol.* 2013;6:84–88.

Horstman WG, Middleton WD, Melson GL. Scrotal inflammatory disease: color doppler US findings. *Radiology.* 1991;179:55–59.

Rao MS, Arjun K. Sonography of scrotal trauma. *Indian J Radiol Imaging.* 2012;22:293–297.

Sharp VJ, Kieran K, Arlen AM. Testicular torsion: diagnosis, evaluation, and management. *Am Fam Physician.* 2013;88:835–840.

Vijayaraghavan SB. Sonographic differential diagnosis of acute scrotum: real-time whirlpool sign, a key sign of torsion. *J Ultrasound Med.* 2006;25:563–574.

Visser AJ, Heyns CF. Testicular function after torsion of the spermatic cord. *BJU Int.* 2003;92:200–203.

Yoong P, Duffy S, Marshall TJ. The inguinal and femoral canals: a practical step-by-step approach to accurate sonographic assessment. *Indian J Radiol Imaging.* 2013;23: 391–395.

23

Female Pelvis, Nonpregnant

Simran Sekhon

NORMAL ANATOMY

The uterus is composed of the muscular layer, or myometrium. The body is the main portion of the uterus. The fundus is a more superior portion above the body of the uterus. The areas of the uterus where the fallopian tubes enter are called the *cornua.* The inferior portion of the uterus is the cervix. Peritoneal reflections are noted both anterior to the uterus, called the *vesicouterine pouch,* and posterior to the uterus, called the *retrouterine recess* or, more commonly, the *posterior cul-de-sac.* The central lining of the uterus is the endometrium, which is firmly adherent to the myometrium. The endometrium varies significantly in thickness in the menstruating female but is more stable in size in a postmenopausal female.

Some of the portions of the female pelvis, such as the broad ligaments and round ligaments, are poorly visualized by imaging. The fallopian tubes run laterally from the upper margins of the uterus. Different segments of the fallopian tube are lateral near the ovaries to medial near the uterus: the infundibulum with its associated fimbriae near the ovary; the ampullary region that represents the major portion of the lateral tube; the isthmus, which is the narrower part of the tube that links to the uterus; and the interstitial (also known as *intramural*) part that transverses the uterine musculature.

The ovaries are elliptical in shape, with the long axis oriented vertically. However, the ovaries may be variable in location. In the nulliparous female, the ovary is located along the lateral pelvic wall called the *ovarian fossa.* This is bounded anteriorly by the obliterated umbilical artery, posteriorly by the ureter and the internal iliac artery, and superiorly by the external iliac vein.

The arterial supply to the uterus is primarily from the uterine artery, which is a major branch of the internal iliac artery. The ovaries have a dual arterial supply, with the main ovarian artery arising from the aorta laterally and slightly inferior to the renal arteries (Fig. 23.1).

NORMAL ULTRASOUND FINDINGS/ TECHNIQUE

The two main approaches for visualization of the pelvic organs are use of transabdominal or transvaginal sonography. Both of these techniques are used extensively in the evaluation of the female pelvis. The transabdominal approach visualizes the entire pelvis and gives a global overview. In an emergency situation, the main limitation of this technique is the inability of the patient to have a full bladder. Additionally, visualization of the deep pelvis in certain patients may be limited using the transabdominal approach, as lower-frequency transducers are often utilized. Transvaginal sonography has the benefit of using high-frequency transducers, which produce much better resolution. Small endometrial, adnexal, or ovarian abnormalities are much better delineated with the transvaginal technique. Large masses, such as large fibroids, may be out of the field of view of transvaginal sonography and may be better identified on abdominal sonography.

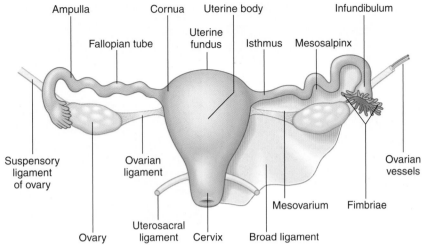

Fig. 23.1 Female reproductive organs. (Redrawn from Rumack CM, Levine D. *Diagnostic Ultrasound.* 5th ed. Philadelphia, PA: Elsevier; 2018: 528–563, Fig.15-1.)

Transvaginal sonography better distinguishes intrauterine fluid collections and adnexal masses from loops of bowel. Both techniques may be utilized depending on the situation.

UTERUS

The uterus may be visualized using either the transabdominal and/or the transvaginal technique. The transabdominal technique is optimally performed with a distended urinary bladder. In situations in which transvaginal sonography cannot be fully performed in a timely fashion, a Foley catheter may be used to distend the bladder with saline. The highest-frequency transducer should be used to examine the uterus and ovaries. Usually, this is a 3.5- to 5-MHz transducer. Imaging of the uterus is performed in both longitudinal and transverse planes.

The uterus lies in the true pelvis between the bladder anteriorly and the rectosigmoid colon posteriorly. The uterus may be in variable positions. When describing the uterus, *flexion* refers to the axis of the uterine body relative to the cervix, whereas *version* refers to the axis of the cervix relative to the vagina. The uterus is usually anteverted and anteflexed but may appear retroflexed on transabdominal sonography due to

displacement by the fluid-filled bladder. The size and shape of the uterus vary with age. In the neonatal stage, the uterus is 2.3 to 4.6 cm in length. It grows in size to approximately 8 cm in length by 5 cm in width and 4 cm in the anteroposterior dimension in the adult. In the multiparous female, the uterus increases both in length and in width with each pregnancy. In the postmenopausal female, the uterus atrophies and ranges in size from 3.5 to 6.5 cm in length in patients over 65 years of age.

On ultrasound (US), the uterus appears fairly homogeneous in appearance. The echogenic line noted centrally within the myometrium is the endometrium. The endometrium varies in size and appearance throughout the menstrual cycle. During the proliferative phase, it begins to thicken in the range of 4 to 8 mm, and by the secretory phase it may range in thickness from 7 to 14 mm (Figs. 23.2 and 23.3).

OVARY

The position of the ovaries is variable. Normally, the ovaries are identified laterally or posterolaterally to the anteflexed midline uterus. However, as the uterus changes position, the ovaries may also change position. At times the ovaries are displaced

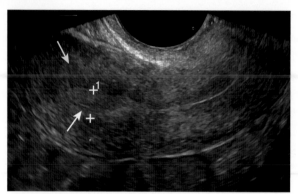

Fig. 23.2 Transvaginal longitudinal image of the uterus shows normal myometrium (*yellow arrow*) and endometrium (*white arrow*). Calipers measure endometrial thickness.

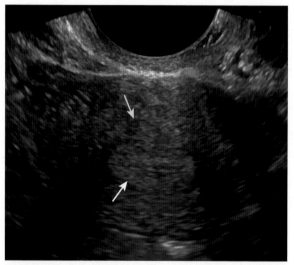

Fig. 23.3 Transvaginal transverse image of the uterus shows normal myometrium (*yellow arrow*) and endometrium (*white arrow*).

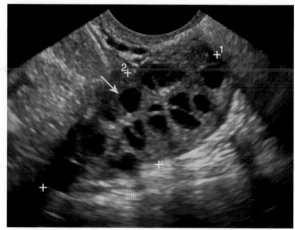

Fig. 23.4 Normal premenopausal ovary with multiple follicles (*yellow arrow*). Calipers and numerals measure ovarian size.

within the ovary. Ovarian size varies with the age of the patient. Ovarian volume in the premenarchal female is up to 8 cc. In a menstruating female, normal ovaries may have a volume up to 22 cc. Visualization of the postmenopausal ovaries is more difficult due to atrophy.

HEMORRHAGIC OVARIAN CYST

Hemorrhage into a follicular cyst or corpus luteum generates pain and may lead to an emergent presentation. The US pattern varies according to the age of the hemorrhage and the degree of clot formation. The typical appearance is that of a complex mass with internal echoes and some degree of posterior through-transmission. Although fresh blood may be anechoic initially, a hemorrhagic cyst is defined by low-level echogenicity in a fine, lacelike, reticular pattern for the first 24 hours, and this pattern is diagnostically specific (Fig. 23.5). As clot retraction occurs, US may depict triangular or curvilinear echogenic regions at the cyst wall (Fig. 23.6). Fluid-debris levels develop as the clot liquefies. Rupture of a hemorrhagic cyst may be associated with sexual intercourse, exercise, trauma, and pregnancy, and it may involve the right ovary more frequently because the left ovary is protected by a cushion of sigmoid colon. Although cyst rupture may cause massive hemoperitoneum, most patients can be followed with conservative treatment unless they are in unstable condition (Fig. 23.7).

from the lower pelvis and are best visualized on the transabdominal approach. In these cases, the ovaries may be out of the field of view using transvaginal sonography. On sonography, the ovary has a variable appearance. During the proliferative phase of the cycle, many follicles are identified within the ovary (Fig. 23.4). Before ovulation, one follicle becomes dominant and reaches the size of 2 to 2.5 cm in diameter. Other follicles become atretic. After ovulation, the corpus luteum develops and may be identified by US as a hypoechoic or sometimes isoechoic lesion located

ENDOMETRIOMAS

Endometriosis affects an estimated 10% of premenopausal women. Ectopic endometrial tissue is estrogen sensitive, and it proliferates and bleeds synchronously with the endometrium. Without the normal drainage pathway of the vagina, bleeding from endometrial implants in the adnexa, uterosacral ligaments, or peritoneum often causes cyclic pelvic pain. As much as 80% of ectopic endometrial tissue is found in the ovaries. When larger focal deposits of endometrial tissue are present in the ovary, these endometriomas are detectable at imaging.

Spontaneous rupture of an endometrioma may lead to acute presentation but is uncommon. It causes severe, acute abdominal pain due to chemical peritonitis from the leakage of old blood. A ruptured endometriotic cyst is associated with pregnancy and the large size of the cyst. In nonpregnant patients, rupture commonly occurs at menstruation due to an increase in internal pressure.

Torsion of an endometriotic cyst rarely occurs because of adhesions; therefore severe abdominal pain

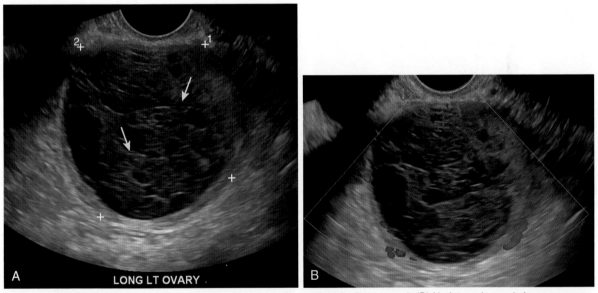

Fig. 23.5 (A) Hemorrhagic cyst with reticular lacelike pattern (*yellow arrows*). (B) No internal vascularity or solid component.

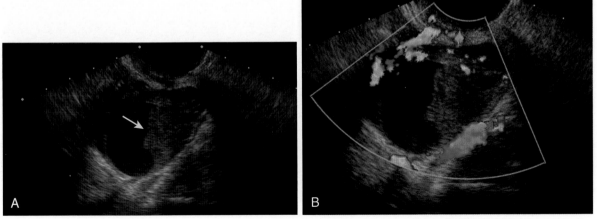

Fig. 23.6 (A) Retracting clot (*yellow arrow*) within a hemorrhagic cyst. (B) No blood flow within the clot.

and the typical findings of ovarian endometriotic cysts are indicative of rupture rather than torsion.

Endometriomas have a variety of appearances on US, ranging from an anechoic cyst to a complex cystic mass with septations and heterogeneous echogenicity. The most typical appearance on an endometrioma is that of a homogeneously hypoechoic, cystic mass with diffuse, low-level internal echoes and posterior acoustic enhancement. This homogeneous appearance has been termed the *ground glass pattern*. The additional presence of punctate, peripheral, echogenic foci within the cyst wall is a very specific sign for an endometrioma (Fig. 23.8).

Endometriomas can also have a more complex multiloculated appearance, with fluid-debris levels, or, less commonly, thick internal septa. They are more frequently multiple, and their appearance is more stable over time when compared with hemorrhagic cysts. The presence of irregular walls or vascular nodularity should raise concern, because clear cell or endometroid carcinomas rarely may develop within endometriomas. Follow-up imaging is useful for differentiating endometriomas from pathologic entities such as hemorrhagic ovarian cysts, which resolve, and malignancies, which progress.

ADNEXAL TORSION

Ovarian or adnexal (ovary and fallopian tube) torsion is a surgical emergency that requires prompt diagnosis and treatment. There is increased risk during pregnancy. Enlargement of the ovary secondary to a corpus luteal cyst or incidental benign ovarian neoplasm, most commonly a mature cystic teratoma or cystadenoma, also can predispose to ovarian torsion. Ovarian torsion rarely occurs in the presence of ovarian carcinoma or endometriosis because of fixation of the ovaries to adjacent structures by adhesions.

Ovarian torsion is the result of partial or complete rotation of the ovarian pedicle on its axis, which results initially

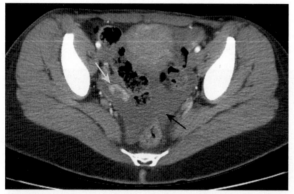

Fig. 23.7 Ruptured hemorrhagic cyst in the right ovary with enhancing irregular wall (*yellow arrow*) and hemoperitoneum (*black arrow*).

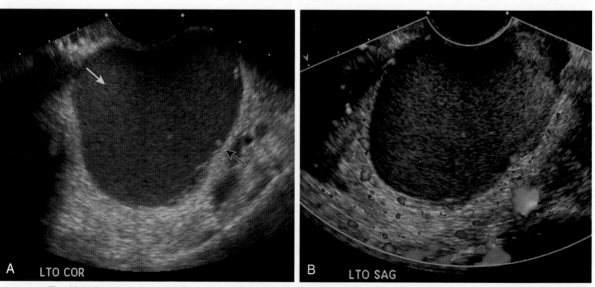

Fig. 23.8 Endometrioma. (A) Cyst with diffuse, low-level internal echoes in a "ground glass" pattern (*yellow arrow*). Punctate peripheral echogenic foci (*black arrow*). (B) No blood flow in the cyst.

in impaired lymphatic and venous drainage and eventual loss of arterial perfusion. It can be difficult to diagnose clinically because the presenting symptoms, including pain, nausea, and vomiting, are nonspecific and similar to many causes of acute abdomen. Because ovarian enlargement of more than 6 cm predisposes to ovarian torsion, women who undergo ovulation induction have the highest incidence because of the development of numerous theca lutein cysts, which can massively enlarge the ovaries.

The US appearance of ovarian torsion varies depending on the degree of ischemia and infarction and the time course. The ovary is typically enlarged. Numerous small follicles are often seen at the periphery of the

ovary. The central ovarian stroma becomes heterogeneous with areas of increased echogenicity, which represent hemorrhage, and more hypoechoic areas, which represent edema. With frank infarction, cystic, clotted areas may be observed. Free fluid within the pelvis or adjacent to the ovary also can be seen (Fig. 23.9).

Although the range of grayscale features varies, the ovary rarely has a completely normal appearance. Classically, Doppler interrogation demonstrates the absence of arterial flow. It is important, however, to remember that early in the process there may be obstruction of lymphatic and venous flow with preservation of arterial perfusion. Occasionally, only diastolic or venous flow is lost early. Because the ovary has a dual arterial supply, in early torsion, only one may be occluded. In a patient who presents with acute pain and an ovary that demonstrates real-time findings consistent with ovarian torsion, the diagnosis should be suggested even in the presence of documented arterial blood flow.

When color Doppler imaging and pulsed Doppler sampling do not demonstrate arterial flow within the ovarian parenchyma, the diagnosis is more easily made (Fig. 23.10). All Doppler parameters must be set carefully to maximize detection of slow flow to avoid a false-positive diagnosis caused by technical factors. Sampling error also may cause false-positive diagnoses. The twisted vascular pedicle (whirlpool sign) also can be seen on color Doppler sonography. Adnexal torsion that is diagnosed before tissue infarction is managed with laparoscopic "detorsion" surgery, followed by progesterone

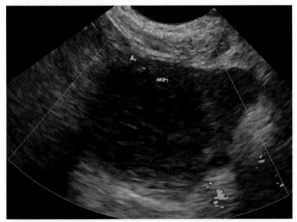

Fig. 23.9 Ovarian torsion. Heterogeneous enlarged ovary with minimal to absent blood flow by power Doppler.

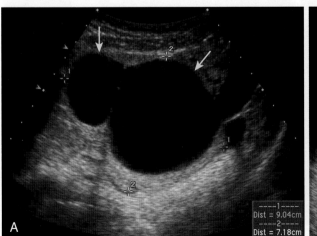 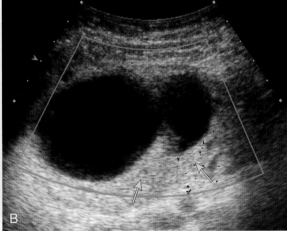

Fig. 23.10 Ovarian torsion. (A) Enlarged ovary with large simple cysts (*yellow arrows*). (B) Color Doppler evaluation demonstrates no blood flow in the ovarian parenchyma surrounding the cysts (*yellow arrows*).

replacement if the corpus luteum is removed. If tissue infarction and necrosis have occurred, then laparotomy with salpingo-oophorectomy is usually required to prevent peritonitis, and masses spontaneously resolve several months after delivery.

PELVIC INFLAMMATORY DISEASE

Pelvic inflammatory disease (PID) refers to a spectrum of infectious processes in the pelvis, typically ascending from cervicitis to involve the upper reproductive organs: the uterus (endometritis), fallopian tubes (salpingitis), and, ultimately, the ovaries. Most cases are caused by *Chlamydia trachomatis* and *Neisseria gonorrhoeae*. However, there is a high incidence of coinfection with other organisms, such as *Streptococcus* species, *Escherichia coli,* and *Bacteroides* species. If left untreated, the infection can progress to form pyosalpinx and tubo-ovarian abscess. The initial diagnosis of PID is usually made on clinical grounds in patients with pelvic pain and cervical motion tenderness on physical examination. Patients may also have fever and leukocytosis, although symptoms are often vague, and the extent of disease is often not evident clinically.

For this reason, imaging can play a crucial role in both the diagnosis and subsequent management of the patient's medical condition. Sonographic findings of early-stage PID in patients without pyosalpinx or tubo-ovarian abscess are usually very subtle and not easily detectable with ultrasonography: enlargement of the uterus and ovaries, indistinct soft tissue margins, thickening of the broad ligament and tubes, and fluid within the endometrial cavity or cul-de-sac.

As the disease progresses and involvement of the fallopian tubes persists, tubal sonographic findings are some of the most specific hallmarks of PID. Dilated, fluid-filled, folded, and tubular structures in the adnexae are the key findings in hydro/pyosalpinx. The luminal fluid may be purely anechoic or complex with floating echoes. The walls of the tubes become thickened and hyperemic and in cross-section can adopt a "cog wheel" appearance due to the thickened endosalpingeal folds. The inflamed ovary can acquire a reactive polycystic appearance and eventually become adherent to the tube, often situated posteriorly and inferiorly in the region of the cul-de-sac. This is termed a *tubo-ovarian complex.* Persistent untreated disease leads to disruption of the normal adnexal and ovarian architecture, with leakage of pus from the tube and the formation of a tubo-ovarian abscess (TOA), which appears as a complex, mixed solid and cystic mass in the pelvis (Fig. 23.11).

Treatment for advanced PID involves the use of broad-spectrum antibiotics. Abscesses are drained using image guidance, either ultrasonography or computed tomography (CT), with catheters placed via a transgluteal, transvaginal, or transrectal route.

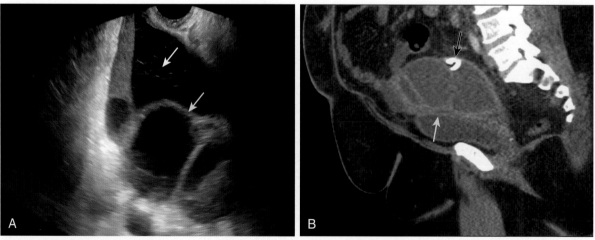

Fig. 23.11 TOA. (A) Complex cystic left adnexal mass with septations (yellow arrow) and echoes (*white arrow*). (B) Sagittal CT image demonstrating complex cystic mass (*yellow arrow*) with a pigtail drainage catheter in place (*black arrow*).

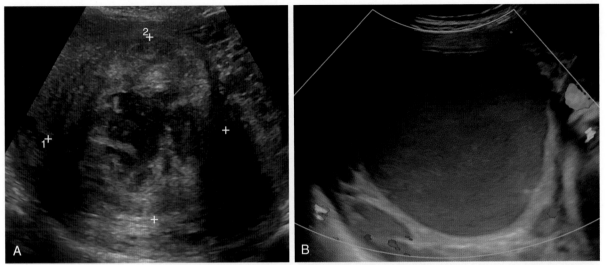

Fig. 23.12 (A) Grayscale image of a heterogeneous fibroid before the patient was pregnant. (B) Same patient presenting with complete cystic degeneration of the fibroid during pregnancy.

ACUTE FIBROID COMPLICATIONS

Red Degeneration

Leiomyomata (fibroids) are the most common gynecologic neoplasm, occurring in 20% to 40% of all women. They are associated with a variety of symptoms, including menorrhagia, dysmenorrhea, urinary frequency, pain, pressure, and infertility. Acute pain is usually due to acute fibroid degeneration that occurs when a leiomyoma enlarges and outgrows its blood supply. Degeneration can be of various types, including hyaline or myxoid, calcific, cystic, and hemorrhagic. Local pain may be accompanied by systemic symptoms, such as low-grade fever and leukocytosis. Fibroids are hormonally responsive and can increase rapidly in size during pregnancy, predisposing them to hemorrhagic or "red degeneration."

US is usually diagnostic in detecting fibroids, with magnetic resonance imaging (MRI) used for further characterization if clinically necessary. The most common sonographic appearance of a fibroid is a well-defined, hypoechoic mass. However, they can be heterogeneous, hyperechoic, or calcified with acoustic shadowing. Anechoic, irregular spaces may be seen in necrotic fibroids that have undergone degeneration (Fig. 23.12). Occasionally, it may be difficult to distinguish a pedunculated fibroid from a solid ovarian neoplasm, and MRI can be useful in further characterization.

Torsion of Subserosal Fibroid

Acute torsion of a subserosal uterine leiomyoma is rare. The differential diagnosis includes ovarian torsion, ovarian tumor, large leiomyoma with massive necrotic infarction, or uterine torsion. With visualization of normal ovaries, ovarian torsion or an ovarian tumor can be eliminated. It may be difficult to identify a twisted pedicle of a subserosal leiomyoma at radiologic imaging because a twisted pedicle of subserosal leiomyoma torsion is thin compared with that of ovarian torsion. Regardless of utilization of many imaging modalities, torsion of subserosal leiomyoma is a rare condition and is seldom diagnosed preoperatively.

UTERINE ARTERIOVENOUS MALFORMATIONS

Arteriovenous malformations (AVMs) are classified as congenital and acquired. In the uterus, they may appear after curettage, cesarean delivery, and myomectomy, among others. Their clinical feature is usually vaginal bleeding, which may be severe if curettage is performed in unrecognized cases.

Sonographically on two-dimensional grayscale US scanning, the AVM appears as irregular, anechoic, tortuous, tubular structures that show evidence of increased vascularity when color Doppler is applied (Fig. 23.13).

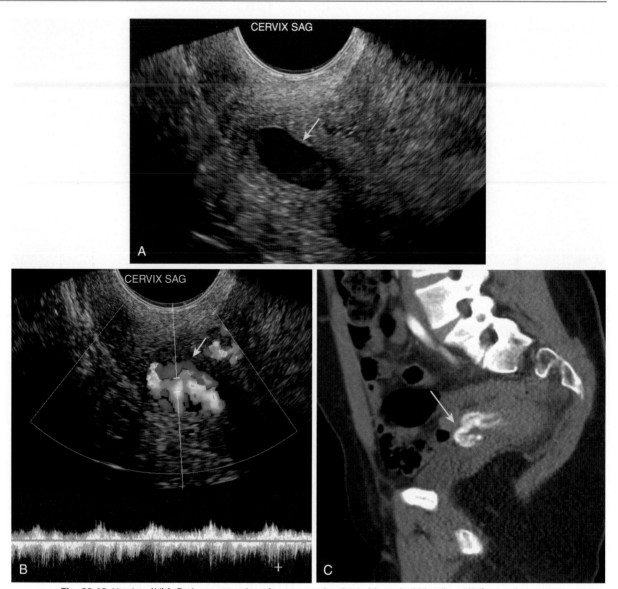

Fig. 23.13 Uterine AVM. Patient presenting after recent abortion with vaginal bleeding. (A) Grayscale image of the lower uterine segment (LUS)/cervix shows hypoechoic ovoid lesion (*yellow arrow*). (B) Doppler evaluation of the lesion shows turbulent blood flow (*yellow arrow*). (C) Sagittal image from CT angiogram shows tangle of vessels in the LUS (*yellow arrow*) with early venous opacification consistent with AVM.

Most of the time they resolve spontaneously; however, if left untreated, they may require involved treatments such as uterine artery embolization or hysterectomy.

In the past, uterine artery angiography was the gold standard for diagnosis; however, US scanning has diagnosed successfully and helped in the clinical management.

COMPLICATIONS RELATED TO INTRAUTERINE DEVICES

Intrauterine device (IUD) placement is commonly performed for the purpose of contraception. On US, it appears as a well-defined and hyperechoic T-shaped device. The stem of a properly placed IUD is straight and is entirely within the endometrial cavity, with the arms of the IUD

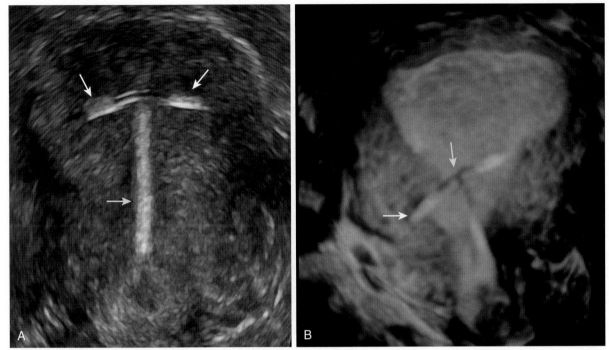

Fig. 23.14 (A) 3D ultrasound image shows appropriately placed IUD. The stem is straight within the endometrial cavity (*yellow arrow*), and the arms extend laterally at the uterine fundus (*white arrows*). (B) 3D ultrasound image shows an inferiorly displaced IUD with the arms in the lower uterus (*yellow arrow*) and the right arm embedded in the myometrium (*white arrow*).

extending laterally at the uterine fundus. Three-dimensional US is often crucial for determining the location of the arms of the IUD with respect to the uterine cavity.

Uterine expulsion of the IUD is a relatively common complication. When the IUD is not seen at US and expulsion is suspected, the fact that the IUD is not within the peritoneal cavity must be confirmed with abdominopelvic radiography.

Another commonly encountered problem with intrauterine contraception is displacement of the IUD within the uterine cavity. The greater the displacement of the IUD from its proper position in the uterine fundus, the less effective it is for contraception (Fig. 23.14).

Rarely, perforation may occur as a complication of IUD placement. IUD perforation is variable in extent and symptomatology, ranging from embedment in the myometrium to complete transuterine perforation, with migration of the IUD into the peritoneal cavity. US is the modality of choice for initial imaging in patients with suspected perforation. Three-dimensional US in particular has been shown to be helpful in identifying malpositioned and embedded IUDs in symptomatic patients (Fig. 23.15).

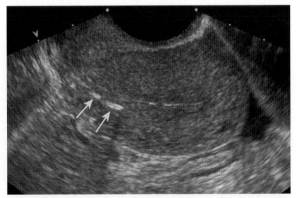

Fig. 23.15 Grayscale sagittal image of the uterus shows an IUD completely embedded in the myometrium (*yellow arrows*).

Complete uterine perforation is a more serious complication because the IUD has perforated through all three layers of the uterus and is either partially or completely within the peritoneal cavity. It can cause adhesion formation, which can lead to infertility, chronic pain, and intestinal obstruction. Rarely, an intraperitoneal IUD can perforate adjacent structures, leading to peritonitis,

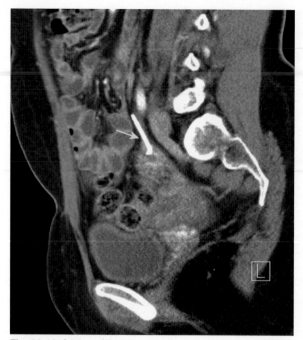

Fig. 23.16 Sagittal CT image shows complete uterine perforation and IUD in the peritoneal cavity abutting the bowel (*yellow arrow*).

fistulas, or hemorrhage. Pelvic US should be the initial imaging study. In some patients, US is followed with abdominopelvic radiography. A definite diagnosis of complete perforation can be made by CT (Fig. 23.16).

OVARIAN HYPERSTIMULATION SYNDROME

Ovarian hyperstimulation syndrome (OHSS) is a potentially dangerous iatrogenic complication of pharmacologic ovulation induction for the treatment of infertility. It occurs in the setting of abnormally high levels of beta-human chorionic gonadotropin (b-hCG). It is more severe in patients who become pregnant after ovulation induction. The spectrum of clinical presentation ranges from nausea, vomiting, and abdominal pain to massive ascites, acute respiratory distress syndrome, and hypotension.

US is the most accurate method of detecting ovarian enlargement. On US, multiple large, thin-walled cysts are identified. Acute pain may be caused by hemorrhage into a cyst, cyst rupture, or ovarian torsion. US examination may demonstrate ascites or pleural fluid, the criteria used in determining whether hospitalization is necessary (Fig. 23.17).

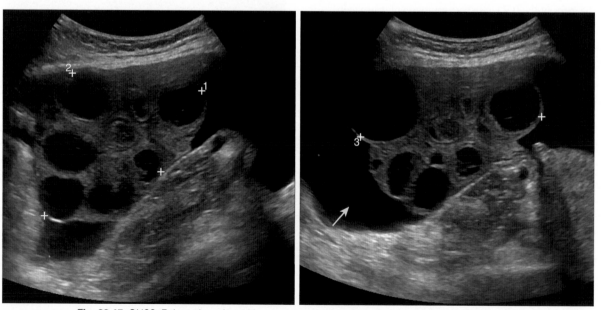

Fig. 23.17 OHSS. Enlarged ovaries with numerous cysts and surrounding ascites (*yellow arrow*).

POSTPARTUM COMPLICATIONS

Imaging in the postpartum period is only performed if the patient has symptoms such as unexplained fever or pelvic pain. The primary concern in this setting is for endometritis or retained products of conception. Ovarian vein thrombosis (OVT) is another important cause of pelvic pain and fever in the postpartum setting.

Endometritis

Endometritis is the most common cause of postpartum fever. The diagnosis is usually based on the clinical findings. Imaging is often not helpful because of the overlap in findings between endometritis and the normal postpartum state. Both may appear as an enlarged uterus with a small amount of blood or fluid. The presence of gas is not diagnostic either, because a small amount of gas may be seen by US and CT in the endometrial cavity in up to 21% of healthy postpartum women several weeks after delivery.

Imaging is usually reserved for patients who are nonresponsive to treatment. The uterus may appear normal or may show nonspecific findings that overlap with retained products of conception, including a thickened heterogeneous endometrium and intrauterine fluid with or without internal echoes representing blood, retained products of conception, or gas. Similar findings are seen on CT. CT has the added advantages over US of better demonstrating associated inflammation of the parametrial soft tissues and identifying potential extrauterine abscesses.

Ovarian Vein Thrombosis

OVT is an uncommon yet potentially fatal disorder because of the risk for pulmonary embolism. It occurs most often in the early postpartum period. Doppler US has been used to diagnose this condition and may demonstrate an enlarged ovary with a dilated, noncompressible ovarian vein showing little or no flow. In 80% to 90% of cases, the right ovarian vein is involved. The vein should be followed cephalad to look for extension

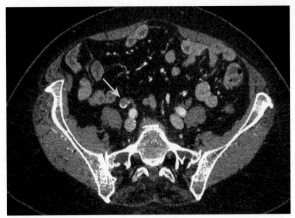

Fig. 23.18 OVT. Axial CT image shows filling defect (*yellow arrow*) in the right ovarian vein consistent with a thrombus.

into the inferior vena cava. Contrast-enhanced CT and MRI have shown greater sensitivity and specificity than Doppler US in the detection of OVT (Fig. 23.18).

BIBLIOGRAPHY

Boortz HE. Migration of intrauterine devices: radiologic findings and implications for patient care. *RadioGraphics*. 2012;32:335–352.

Chang HC. Pearls and pitfalls in diagnosis of ovarian torsion. *Radiographics*. 2008;28:1355–1368.

Dupuis CS. Ultrasonography of adnexal causes of acute pelvic pain in pre-menopausal non-pregnant women. *Ultrasonography*. 2015;34:258–267.

Iraha Y. CT and MR imaging of gynecologic emergencies. *RadioGraphics*. 2017;37:1569–1586.

Potter AW. US and CT evaluation of acute pelvic pain of gynecologic origin in nonpregnant premenopausal patients. *Radiographics*. 2008;28:1645–1659.

Timor-Tritsch IE. Ultrasound diagnosis and management of acquired uterine enhanced myometrial vascularity/arteriovenous malformations. *Am J Obstet Gynecol*. 2016;214:731.e1–e10.

Vandermeer FQ. Imaging of acute pelvic pain. *Best Pract Res Clin Obstet Gynaecol*. 2009;52(1):2–20.

Webb EM. Adnexal mass with pelvic pain. *Radiol Clin N Am*. 2004;42:329–348.

24

Female Pelvis, Pregnant: First Trimester

Simran Sekhon

NORMAL FIRST-TRIMESTER ULTRASOUND APPEARANCE

Pelvic ultrasound is the key imaging modality in the diagnosis of early pregnancy and its associated complications. Both transabdominal and transvaginal sonography (TVS) techniques are used.

Gestational Sac

Intradecidual Sign. The intradecidual sign refers to an eccentric, extraluminal, rounded, cystic structure located within the endometrium. It is the earliest imaging sign of an intrauterine pregnancy (IUP) on TVS and is observed as early as 4½ weeks of menstrual age.

Double Decidual Sac Sign. The hyperechogenic peripheral decidua vera and the inner decidua capsularis with intervening anechoic endometrial lumen is seen on TVS at about 5 menstrual weeks (Fig. 24.1).

The gestational sac (GS) is composed of anechoic amniotic fluid and chorionic extraembryonic coelom, which may contain low-level echoes.

Yolk Sac

With TVS, the yolk sac (YS) is usually visualized within the extraembryonic coelom at approximately 5½ weeks or 8-mm mean sac diameter (MSD). It appears as a thin-walled, circular structure with an anechoic center. A normal YS measures less than 5.6 mm internal diameter between 5 and 10 weeks and starts to regress by 11 weeks. The YS is no longer seen after the amniotic cavity expands to obliterate the chorionic cavity by 14 to 16 weeks.

Embryo

The embryo is first visible at approximately 6 weeks of gestational age as a 1- to 2-mm structure at the periphery of the YS. The length of the embryo is measured from the head (crown) to the buttocks (rump), hence the term *crown–rump length (CRL),* which is the most accurate measurement of gestational age through the first 12 weeks of pregnancy. The embryo should be visualized when the MSD is at least 25 mm (Fig. 24.2).

The embryo resides within the amniotic cavity. It is possible to observe cardiac activity in embryos as small as 1 to 2 mm. However, absence of cardiac activity in embryos smaller than 4 mm may also be normal. The embryonic heart rate accelerates over the first 6 to 8 weeks of gestation, with the lower limit of normality near 100 beats per minute at 6.2 weeks of gestation and 120 beats per minute at 6.3 to 7.0 weeks of gestation.

Embryonic morphology is rather featureless until 7 to 8 weeks, when the spine can be visualized. At approximately 8 weeks of gestation, the head curvature can be separated from the body and the four limb buds become apparent. The rhombencephalon, which is the developing hindbrain, is a prominent landmark at 8 to 10 weeks of gestation, appearing as an anechoic, round structure within the head.

Twin Pregnancy

It is important to determine the number of fetuses and their chorionicity and amnionicity in the first trimester, when it is easiest.

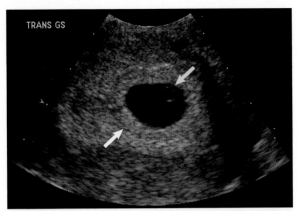

Fig. 24.1 Normal IUP. Gestational sac with double decidual sign (*white arrow*) containing a yolk sac (*yellow arrow*).

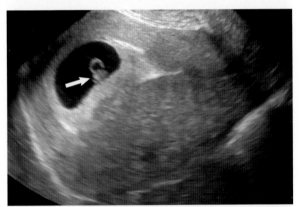

Fig. 24.2 Normal IUP. Gestational sac containing a yolk sac and an embryo (*arrow*).

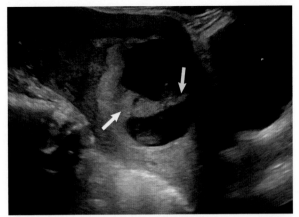

Fig. 24.3 Diamniotic dichorionic gestation. Thick intertwin membrane (*yellow arrow*) and twin peak sign (*white arrow*).

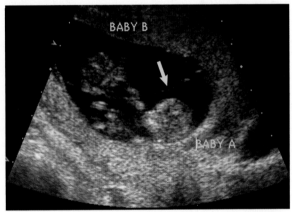

Fig. 24.4 Diamniotic monochorionic gestation. Thin intertwin membrane (*arrow*).

Dichorionic diamniotic: The twin peak sign is reliable evidence of dichorionicity. Both the amnions and the chorions reflect away from the placental surface, creating a potential space into which villi can grow. There is a thick intertwin membrane (Fig. 24.3).

Monochorionic diamniotic: A single layer of continuous chorion limiting villous growth. There is a thin intertwin membrane separating the two amniotic cavities (Fig. 24.4).

Monochorionic monoamniotic: No intertwin membrane (Fig. 24.5).

CHORIONIC BUMP

The chorionic bump is a focal solid or complex protuberance from the choriodecidual region bulging into the GS (Fig. 24.6). Harris et al. identified this sign in 0.7%

of 2178 early obstetrical sonograms and noted that 50% of these pregnancies aborted—a pregnancy failure rate four times that of the general population control group.

Based on the sonographic evolution of the chorionic bump on follow-up studies and pathologic investigation of abortuses, the chorionic bump likely represents a small subchorionic bleed.

SUBCHORIONIC HEMORRHAGE

Intrauterine hematomas, a common ultrasound finding associated with first-trimester bleeding, have a reported incidence between 4% and 22%. Subchorionic hemorrhage is the most common type of intrauterine chorionic bleed and is thought to result from partial detachment of the trophoblast from the uterine wall, with blood dissecting

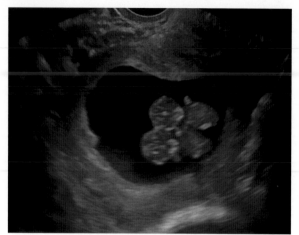

Fig. 24.5 Monoamniotic monochorionic gestation. No intertwin membrane.

between the chorion and the decidual layer of endometrium. When the hematoma dissects into the endometrial cavity, the patient can present with vaginal bleeding.

Subchorionic bleeds are graded into small, medium, and large according to their sizes relative to GS circumference. One large retrospective review reported a rate of pregnancy loss of 7.7% for small hematomas (less than one-third the circumference of the GS), 9.2% for medium hematomas (encompassing one-third to one-half the circumference of the GS), and 18.8% for large hematomas (encompassing at least two-thirds the circumference of the GS).

Subchorionic hemorrhage has a worse prognosis when associated with advanced maternal age or early gestational age. A subchorionic hemorrhage may progress into an abruption when the bleed extends behind the placenta.

Subchorionic hemorrhage can be crescentic, ovoid, linear, or curvilinear, and its echogenicity is dependent on the stage of the hemorrhage. It is echo-poor in the hyperacute setting, transitioning to hyperechogenic as the hematoma organizes and subsequently decreasing in echogenicity as the hematoma undergoes hemolysis and liquefaction (Fig. 24.7).

Due to its variable appearance, a first-trimester subchorionic hematoma can be confused with normal first-trimester incomplete chorioamniotic fusion, an intrauterine mass, a vanishing twin, or slow flow within perigestational veins. The latter condition may be recognized by detection of slow-moving particles on grayscale or color Doppler imaging.

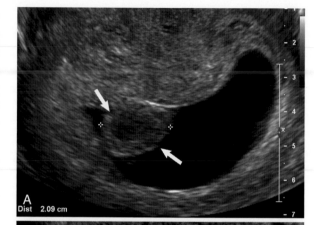

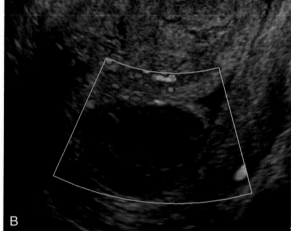

Fig. 24.6 (A) Chorionic bump. A focal solid protuberance bulging into the GS (*arrows*). (B) No flow detected within the chorionic bump with color Doppler.

The majority of subchorionic hematomas are small, regress spontaneously, and do not result in pregnancy loss. Larger or persistent hemorrhages tend to have worse prognoses.

MISCARRIAGE

The sonographic appearance of a normal IUP follows a predictable pattern during the 5- to 7-week period. Any substantial deviation from this pattern raises concern that the pregnancy has already, or will soon, fail. An important aspect of ultrasound in early pregnancy is distinguishing between the abnormal sonographic findings that are definitive for pregnancy failure and those that are suspicious but not definitive, requiring follow-up testing to establish a definitive diagnosis.

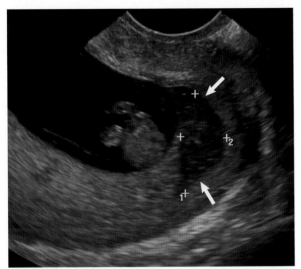

Fig. 24.7 Subchorionic hematoma. Crescentic hypoechoic hematoma (*arrows*) surrounding less than one-third the circumference of the GS.

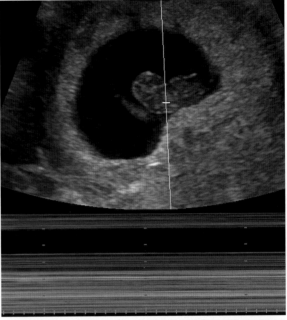

Fig. 24.8 Embryonic demise. No cardiac activity in this embryo with a CRL of 22 mm.

Current criteria for definitive pregnancy failure on transvaginal ultrasound are the following:
- Nonvisualization of cardiac activity in an embryo whose CRL is at least 7 mm (Fig. 24.8)
- Nonvisualization of an embryo in a GS whose MSD is at least 25 mm
- Nonvisualization of an embryo at least 2 weeks after a scan that showed a GS without a YS
- Nonvisualization of an embryo at least 11 days after a scan that showed a GS with a YS

Findings that are suspicious but not diagnostic of pregnancy failure include:
- Failure to visualize cardiac activity in an embryo whose CRL is less than 7 mm
- Failure to visualize an embryo in a GS whose MSD is 16 to 24 mm
- Enlarged YS >7 mm (Fig. 24.9)
- Empty amnion
- Small GS relative to embryo
- No embryo 7 to 13 days after a GS is seen by ultrasound
- No embryo 6 weeks after last menstrual period (LMP)

RETAINED PRODUCTS OF CONCEPTION

Retained products of conception (RPOC) can be seen in 1% of all pregnancies after an abortion or postpartum. Persistent vaginal bleeding after an abortion may be due to retained trophoblastic tissue, but these women may also present with symptoms of infection, including pain and fever. Normal to mildly elevated beta-human chorionic gonadotropin (b-hCG) is common.

Sonography is the preferred modality to diagnose retained products. Sonographic findings that are suspicious for RPOC include thickened endometrium (>80% sensitive and 20% specific), presence of an endometrial mass (sensitivity 29%, positive predictive value [PPV] >80%), and internal Doppler flow, with internal vascularity and thickened endometrium being associated with a PPV ≈96% for RPOC (Fig. 24.10). RPOC can be excluded with a high degree of confidence in the absence of these sonographic findings. The caveat is that color or power Doppler examination is not 100% sensitive for RPOC, so follow-up may be required in cases of intrauterine content without demonstrated vessels, because hypovascular or avascular (necrotic) RPOC may still be present.

ECTOPIC PREGNANCY

Ectopic pregnancy (EP) is defined as a pregnancy that occurs outside the uterine cavity. It is still the leading cause of maternal deaths in first-trimester pregnancies in the United States. These affect 1% to 2% of pregnancies but increase to 2% to 5% of pregnancies achieved from assisted reproductive technology. Predisposing factors for EP include previous pelvic inflammatory

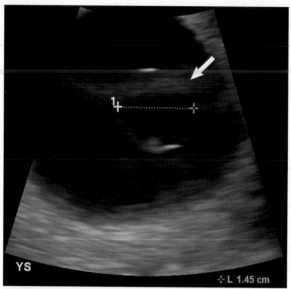

Fig. 24.9 Abnormally large yolk sac (*arrow*).

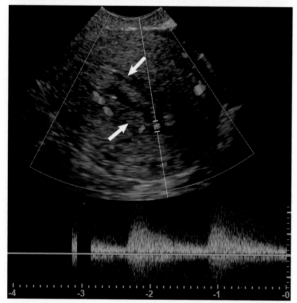

Fig. 24.10 RPOC. Heterogeneous endometrium (*arrows*) with arterial flow.

disease, tubal surgery, previous EP, intrauterine contraceptive device use, and endometriosis.

The classical clinical triad seen is pain, abnormal vaginal bleeding, and a palpable adnexal mass; however, this is seen in only 45% of patients with EP. Correlation with ultrasound and serum quantitative b-hCG is important. EPs can be classified by location.

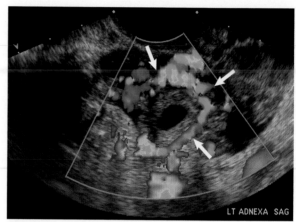

Fig. 24.11 Left adnexal tubal ectopic pregnancy demonstrating the "ring of fire" sign (*arrows*).

Tubal Ectopic Pregnancy

On ultrasound, tubal EP most commonly manifests as an extraovarian heterogeneous mass, usually representative of a hematoma at the site of ectopic implantation. The mass may demonstrate various degrees of echogenicity, depending on the age of the blood products. Tubal EP can also be seen as an echogenic ring in the adnexa surrounding an unruptured EP, which is known as the *tubal ring sign*. This is the second most common sign of EP and has a 95% PPV. Color Doppler often shows a ring of circumferential vascularity (Fig. 24.11). Visualization of an extrauterine GS with an embryo directly confirms an EP, but this finding is rarely observed (Fig. 24.12).

When there is uncertainty about whether an adnexal mass is intraovarian (representing a corpus luteum) (Fig. 24.13) or extraovarian (representing an EP), the distinction can be made by observing whether the mass moves together or separately from the ovary when pressure is applied via the transvaginal probe. The PPV of a mobile adnexal mass separate from the ovary in a symptomatic patient with a positive hCG and no IUP is over 90%.

Although free fluid is a nonspecific finding that can be seen both physiologically and in other pathologies, a moderate or large volume of free fluid greater than expected for a physiologic volume and complexity of the free fluid, with floating debris, blood products, and/or organized blood clots, are suspicious features for EP.

A so-called *pseudogestational sac* represents a small amount of intrauterine fluid, which can be

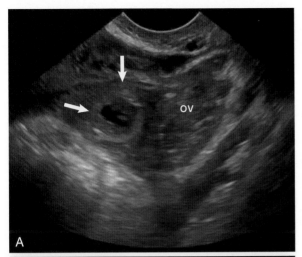

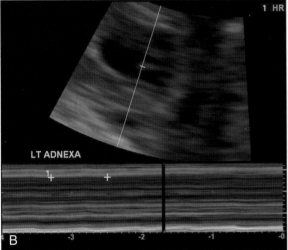

Fig. 24.12 Tubal ectopic pregnancy. (A) Left adnexal mass (*arrows*) adjacent to the left ovary (OV). (B) Embryonic cardiac activity is noted within the ectopic gestation in the left adnexa.

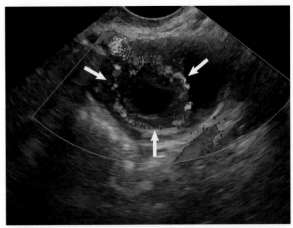

Fig. 24.13 Left ovary corpus luteum cyst demonstrating "ring of fire" sign (*arrows*).

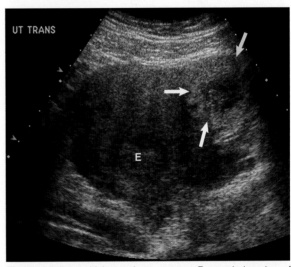

Fig. 24.14 Interstitial ectopic pregnancy. Eccentric location of the GS (*white arrows*) with virtually no overlying myometrium and a bulged contour (*yellow arrow*). Endometrium (*E*).

misinterpreted as a true GS in cases of EP. It is estimated to be seen in 10% of patients with EPs. Real-time observation of this phenomenon will often show a shifting of the fluid as the examination progresses, unlike the fixed position of a true intrauterine GS.

Interstitial Ectopic Pregnancy

Interstitial EP accounts for 2% to 4% of all EPs and involves the implantation of the GS in the portion of the fallopian tube traversing the muscular wall of the uterine cornu, at the junction with the fallopian tube. It can be especially dangerous due to a high risk of profuse hemorrhage resulting from its propensity for delayed rupture at a larger size

and its proximity to the intramyometrial arcuate vasculature. It can be difficult to distinguish on ultrasound from a normal IUP that is eccentrically positioned.

Classic sonographic findings associated with interstitial EP include eccentric location of the GS within the uterine cavity, with virtually no overlying myometrium, and a bulged contour of the superolateral aspect of the uterus (Fig. 24.14). When the two-dimensional grayscale images are equivocal about whether a pregnancy is located normally or interstitially, three-dimensional coronal reconstruction is often useful to confirm the location of the GS. The interstitial line sign

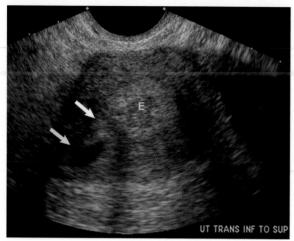

Fig. 24.15 Interstitial line sign. Echogenic line (*white arrow*) extending from the endometrium (*E*) to the ectopic gestational sac (*yellow arrow*).

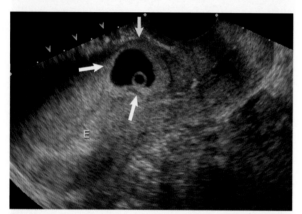

Fig. 24.16 Cesarean section scar ectopic pregnancy. A low-lying GS (*white arrows*) within the anterior lower uterine segment at the site of a prior cesarean section scar. Complete absence of overlying myometrium (*yellow arrow*). Endometrium (*E*).

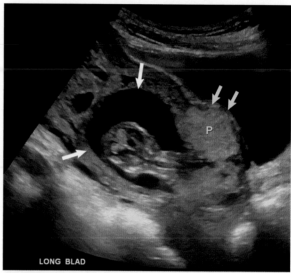

Fig. 24.17 Cesarean section scar ectopic pregnancy with placenta percreta. Lower uterine segment gestation (*white arrows*) with placenta (*P*) invading into the bladder wall (*yellow arrows*).

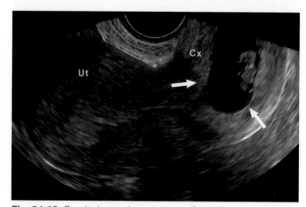

Fig. 24.18 Cervical ectopic pregnancy. Gestational sac containing an embryo (*arrows*) in the cervix (*Cx*) resulting in the hourglass shape of the uterus (*Ut*).

is an echogenic line extending from the endometrium to the interstitial ectopic GS, and is also helpful in diagnosis (Fig. 24.15).

Cesarean Section Scar Ectopic Pregnancy

Scar EPs account for fewer than 1% of EPs. A GS is found within the myometrium of the anterior lower uterine segment at the site of a prior cesarean section scar. Severe myometrial thinning or complete absence of the myometrium between the GS and the bladder will often be seen (Figs. 24.16 and 24.17). Scar EPs pose a significantly increased risk for uterine rupture.

Cervical Ectopic Pregnancy

Cervical EP occurs in fewer than 1% of EPs. It is diagnosed when a GS is visualized within the cervical stroma, usually in an eccentric position. The resulting cervical distention results in an hourglass-shaped uterus. It is important to note that cervical EP can closely resemble a miscarriage in progress, because the latter may be located within the cervix at the time of the sonogram.

A cervical EP appears on ultrasound as a nonmobile, well-formed GS (with or without a heartbeat) in the cervix (Fig. 24.18). A miscarriage in progress, on the other

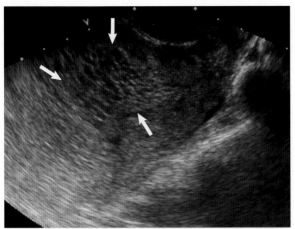

Fig. 24.19 Complete hydatidiform mole. Distended endometrium with "Swiss cheese" appearance (*arrows*).

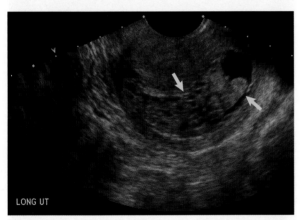

Fig. 24.20 Complete hydatidiform mole. Heterogeneous, echogenic endometrial mass (*arrows*) with multiple variable-sized cysts.

hand, generally appears as a flattened, often irregular, GS in the cervix that contains no heartbeat and may move when pressure is applied with a transvaginal probe. When the distinction between these two diagnoses based on ultrasound findings is uncertain and the patient is hemodynamically stable, a follow-up scan performed in 24 hours is helpful. If the GS is still seen within the cervix, the likely diagnosis is cervical EP, whereas disappearance of the sac would favor a miscarriage in progress.

Ovarian Ectopic Pregnancy

An ovarian EP refers to the intraovarian implantation of a GS and may account for up to 3% of EPs. However, an anechoic or even complex ovarian mass is much more

likely to be a corpus luteum cyst, because ovarian EPs are rare. The diagnosis of ovarian pregnancy is often very difficult to make sonographically, and most cases are diagnosed intraoperatively.

Abdominal/Peritoneal Ectopic Pregnancy

An EP within the peritoneal cavity constitutes approximately 1% of EPs. It is most often located in the pouch of Douglas (rectouterine space), but it can be anywhere within the peritoneal cavity. Transvaginal and abdominal sonographies are used to diagnose abdominal EPs. Findings that suggest an abdominal EP on ultrasound include an empty uterus, intraperitoneal GS likely surrounded by bowel, placenta outside the confines of the uterus, and absence of more common tubal or cesarean scar implantations.

Heterotopic Pregnancy

This is a rare condition with two concurrent pregnancies: a normal IUP and another pregnancy in an ectopic location. The most common form is a combination of an IUP with a tubal EP. Heterotopic pregnancy has a significantly higher incidence among patients receiving in vitro fertilization (IVF), at close to 1%, compared with a trivial incidence among patients who conceive naturally, at 1:30,000. Timely diagnosis and treatment may be critical not only for reducing maternal morbidity and mortality but also for preserving the IUP.

GESTATIONAL TROPHOBLASTIC DISEASE

Trophoblastic disease is a spectrum of medical conditions, including hydatidiform mole, invasive mole, and choriocarcinoma. First-trimester bleeding is one of the most common clinical presentations for this group of disorders. Other clinical signs and symptoms include rapid uterine enlargement, excessive uterine size for gestational date, and hyperemesis gravidarum or preeclampsia that occurs before 24 weeks. The common feature for this group of disorders is the abnormal proliferation of trophoblastic tissue with excessive production of b-hCG.

Hydatidiform Mole

Hydatidiform mole is a complication with malignant potential occurring in 1 out of every 1000 to 2000 pregnancies. There are two types: complete and partial molar

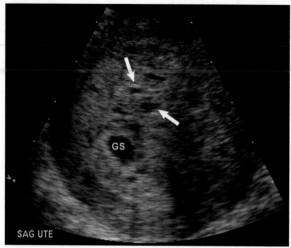

Fig. 24.21 Partial mole. Single GS surrounded by multiple cysts (*arrows*).

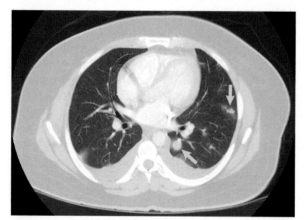

Fig. 24.22 Choriocarcinoma metastasis. Multiple lung nodules (*arrows*).

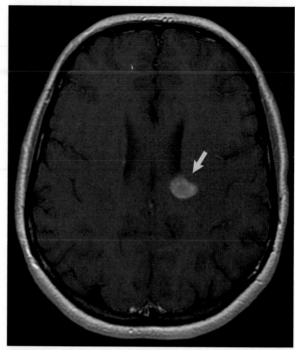

Fig. 24.23 Choriocarcinoma metastasis to the brain. Enhancing lesion (*arrow*).

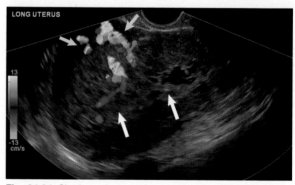

Fig. 24.24 Choriocarcinoma. Heterogeneous, echogenic endometrial mass with cysts (*white arrows*) demonstrating blood flow and invading into the anterior myometrium (*yellow arrows*).

pregnancy. The complete hydatidiform mole (CHM) is the most common gestational trophoblastic disease.

The sonographic appearance of a CHM is usually described as a heterogeneous, echogenic endometrial mass with multiple variable-sized cysts ("Swiss cheese" or "snowstorm" endometrium) and no visible embryo. Doppler examination of a CHM reveals increased uterine vascularity (Figs. 24.19 and 24.20).

Theca lutein cysts are present in 50% of CHM cases and are caused by hyperstimulation of the ovaries due to excessive production of b-hCG by abnormal trophoblastic tissue. These appear as bilateral enlarged ovaries with multiple cysts.

The sonographic appearance of a partial mole demonstrates an enlarged placenta with focal areas of multiple cysts. The fetus has multiple congenital anomalies and growth retardation (Fig. 24.21).

Invasive Mole and Choriocarcinoma

Invasive moles present deep growth into the myometrium and beyond, sometimes with penetration into the peritoneum and parametria. These tumors are locally invasive but very rarely metastasize.

Choriocarcinoma typically presents with extensive metastasis to the lung and other organs (Figs. 24.22 and 24.23). Half of the tumors arise after a molar pregnancy, 25% after abortion, and 25% after an apparently normal pregnancy. Diagnosis is made when the gonadotropin levels remain elevated after the evacuation of pregnancy.

Sonography can demonstrate the presence of a uterine mass identical to a CHM and sometimes the myometrial or adnexal invasion (Fig. 24.24).

Computed tomography (CT) is useful to detect distant metastasis to the lung (75%) and pelvis (50%). Magnetic resonance imaging (MRI) can better demonstrate myometrial and vaginal invasion.

BIBLIOGRAPHY

Bennett GL, Bromley B, Lieberman E, Benacerraf BR. Subchorionic hemorrhage in first-trimester pregnancies: prediction of pregnancy outcome with sonography. *Radiology*. 1996;200(3):803–806.

Dighe M, Cuevas C, Moshiri M, Dubinsky T, Dogra VS. Sonography in first trimester bleeding. *J Clin Ultrasound*. 2008;36(6):352–366.

Doubilet PM. Ultrasound evaluation of the first trimester. *Radiol Clin North Am*. 2014;52(6):1191–1199.

Doubilet PM, Benson CB, Bourne T, et al. Diagnostic criteria for nonviable pregnancy early in the first trimester. *N Engl J Med*. 2013;369(15):1443–1451.

Harris RD, Couto C, Karpovsky C, Porter MM, Ouhilal S. The chorionic bump: a first-trimester pregnancy sonographic finding associated with a guarded prognosis. *J Ultrasound Med*. 2006;25(6):757–763.

Lee R, Dupuis C, Chen B, Smith A, Kim YH. Diagnosing ectopic pregnancy in the emergency setting. *Ultrasonography*. 2018;37(1):78–87.

Mazzariol FS, Roberts J, Oh SK, Ricci Z, Koenigsberg M, Stein MW. Pearls and pitfalls in first-trimester obstetric sonography. *Clin Imaging*. 2015;39(2):176–185.

Nyberg DA, Hughes MP, Mack LA, Wang KY. Extrauterine findings of ectopic pregnancy of transvaginal US: importance of echogenic fluid. *Radiology*. 1991;178(3):823–826.

Phillips CH, Wortman JR, Ginsburg ES, Sodickson AD, Doubilet PM, Khurana B. First-trimester emergencies: a radiologist's perspective. *Emerg Radiol*. 2018;25(1):61–72.

Rodgers SK, Chang C, DeBardeleben JT, Horrow MM. Normal and abnormal US findings in early first-trimester pregnancy: review of the society of radiologists in ultrasound 2012 consensus panel recommendations. *Radiographics*. 2015;35(7):2135–2148.

Shaaban AM, Rezvani M, Haroun RR, et al. Gestational trophoblastic disease: clinical and imaging features. *Radiographics*. 2017;37(2):681–700.

Trop I. The twin peak sign. *Radiology*. 2001;220(1):68–69.

Zucchini S, Marra E. Diagnosis of emergencies/urgencies in gynecology and during the first trimester of pregnancy. *J Ultrasound*. 2014;17(1):41–46.

25

Female Pelvis, Pregnant: Second and Third Trimesters

John P. McGahan

ANATOMY

This chapter is different from other chapters, in that there may be a variety of causes and different anatomic regions may be the etiology of pain in later pregnancy. As for anatomic considerations, the main focus of this chapter will be on obstetrical etiologies of pain and/or bleeding. Much of the focus will be on the placenta, cervix, umbilical cord, and amniotic fluid. During the second and third trimesters of pregnancy, the fetus continues to grow with concomitant changes in the placenta that connects the fetus to the uterus. The placenta develops from the chorion frondosum that has developed from the blastocyst of the embryo. It is attached to the uterus via the decidua basalis (from the maternal placenta). The placenta is the connection between the maternal circulation and the fetal circulation and allows for exchange of oxygen and nutrients between mother and fetus. The location of the placenta and its relationship to the cervix are important and will be discussed in more detail. The cervical is closed during pregnancy and effaces and shortens before birth. Premature opening of the cervix, placental abnormalities, and the relationship of the placenta to the cervix will be discussed in more detail in this chapter.

The umbilical cord is composed of one vein flowing toward the fetus and two arteries flowing from the fetus to the placenta. Normally, the umbilical cord should insert in the more central portion of the placenta. If the cord inserts on the placenta edge or is the presenting part during delivery, this can have devastating consequences on the pregnancy.

Amniotic fluid volume is dependent on the balance between the production and removal of amniotic fluid. In the second and third trimesters of pregnancy, the major source of fluid is production of urine by the fetal kidneys. In late pregnancy, amniotic fluid is reabsorbed into the gastrointestinal tract after fetal swallowing. Amniotic fluid is important for the well-being of the fetus.

ULTRASOUND TECHNIQUES/FINDINGS

Placenta

The placenta appears uniform in echotexture and thickness between the eighth and twentieth weeks of pregnancy. At that time the placenta measures up to 3 cm in thickness. Later in pregnancy the placenta usually measures less than 4 cm in thickness. However, there may be myometrial contractions in which the placenta may appear artificially thickened. Later in pregnancy hypoechoic regions may develop within the placenta, as "placental lakes." There may be other hypoechoic regions within the placenta, most of which are benign in etiology.

The placenta is usually attached in the mid-to-fundal portion of the uterus. Identification of the location of the placenta and its relationship to the cervix is of utmost importance. Overdistention of the urinary bladder and/or focal uterine contractions may give the false impression of a placenta previa by compressing the lower portion of the uterus.

The placenta is separated from the myometrium by a subplacental venous complex called the *decidua basalis*.

This is a few millimeters in thickness and has different appearances depending on the location of the placenta. The decidua basalis is important to visualize because, with placenta accreta, placental tissue invades through this region into the myometrium.

Umbilical Cord

The placenta can be scanned and color flow may be utilized to identify the insertion of the cord into the placenta. Routine visualization of the location of the cord into the placenta is essentially the diagnosis of marginal and velamentous insertion of the umbilical cord. Color flow imaging is helpful in this identification and following the very circuitous course of the umbilical cord. Also important in the third trimester of pregnancy is to examine the cervix with color to make sure the umbilical cord does not overlay the cervical os.

Cervix

The appearance of the cervix is important when evaluating a patient with pain or bleeding in the second or third trimester of the pregnancy. Abdominal ultrasound examination of the cervix often may be difficult because of myometrial contractions or fetal parts overlying the lower portion of the uterus/cervix. In these cases translabial or transvaginal techniques may be helpful to image the cervix when the transabdominal approach is unsuccessful. Translabial scanning is performed with the patient's bladder empty. A sterile glove or cover is placed over the probe using this approach. The translabial approach is useful to exclude placenta previa. Endovaginal scanning with the bladder partially full may be helpful when evaluating for such abnormalities as placenta previa or placenta accreta. These entities will be discussed in more detail later in the chapter. Cervical incompetence, shortening of the cervix, mild dilatation of the endocervical canal, or bulging of the amniotic membranes may be diagnosed with the transabdominal technique, but in many cases translabial and/or endovaginal scanning may be needed.

Amniotic Fluid

Amniotic fluid volume can be assessed quantitatively or qualitatively by ultrasound. Subjective assessment of amniotic fluid by an experienced examiner is usually as good as quantitative measurements of amniotic fluid volume. Quantitative measurements for amniotic fluid include an amniotic fluid index (AFI). The AFI is obtained by assessing the four quadrants of the uterus for the deepest vertical pocket in centimeters and adding the sum of these four measurements. AFI measurements are approximately 12 cm throughout pregnancy. The upper limits of normal is 24 cm, and the lower limits of normal are from 5 to 8 cm. A second method of quantitative detection of amniotic fluid is by the single deepest pocket method, called *maximum vertical pocket (MVP)*. The single deepest pocket is considered too small if less than 2 cm and too large if greater than 8 cm.

ABDOMINAL PAIN IN PREGNANCY

In many situations, pain in later pregnancy may be secondary to relatively harmless etiologies such as Braxton-Hicks contractions, round ligament pain, or constipation. However, there are more serious gynecologic and nongynecologic causes of abdominal pain in pregnancy. The nongynecologic causes of pain in pregnancy will be briefly discussed. However, these causes are discussed in more detail in specific anatomic chapters 16-19. Pain in pregnancy is problematic, as there are two patients. In all pregnant patients with abdominal pain there should always be careful maternal and fetal monitoring, including checking the fetal heart rate. As there are concerns about radiation to the fetus, in most situations, ultrasound is the first imaging study performed on these patients. The nongynecologic etiologies of pain in the third trimester of pregnancy can include acute appendicitis, acute cholecystitis, obstructive renal calculi, bowel obstruction, ovarian torsion, and, rarely, pancreatitis. Right lower quadrant pain may be secondary to acute appendicitis or renal colic. In pregnancy, the appendix may be difficult to image. Typical findings include a blind-ending, noncompressible, tubular structure greater than 6 mm in diameter. There may be mesenteric standing, free fluid, and a possible appendicolith. If there is strong suspicion of appendicitis and the ultrasound is nondiagnostic, magnetic resonance imaging (MRI) would be the next imaging choice.

For pregnant patients with renal colic, the stones may be difficult to identify, but ultrasound may be used to identify the accompanying hydronephrosis. Color flow of the bladder may be useful to look for ureteral jets. This is discussed in more detail in Chapter 19, on the kidney. In critical situations low-dose, noncontrast computed tomography (CT) may be utilized.

Suspected acute cholecystitis is imaged by ultrasound. Findings have been previously discussed in

Chapter 17, on the gallbladder and biliary tract. Other suspected nongynecologic causes of pain in pregnancy are rarer. These are discussed in other chapters. In some situations, low-dose CT may be needed to determine the etiology of pain.

Patients in the third trimester who have preeclampsia may develop hemolysis, elevated liver enzymes, and low platelets called the *HELLP syndrome*. These patients may present with vague symptoms such as nausea, vomiting, headache, and malaise. Diagnosis is made on clinical presentation and laboratory values showing hemolysis, low platelet count, and elevated biliary enzymes. Very rarely, these patients can develop hepatic hemorrhage and ruptures. Liver ultrasound findings include hypoechoic-to-heterogeneous intraparenchymal and perihepatic hematomas. CT may be used in these cases. The syndrome usually resolves with delivery of the fetus.

OBSTETRIC CAUSES OF PAIN OR BLEEDING IN LATE PREGNANCY

Many of the obstetric etiologies of pain or bleeding in pregnancy are emergencies, which may require prompt action and special expertise. Some causes, such as ovarian torsion, are more frequent in the first trimester of pregnancy. These etiologies will be discussed in Chapters 23 and 24 . Pain or bleeding in later pregnancy may be due to a number of different etiologies. Many women have discomfort during later pregnancy due to fairly harmless etiologies. This was previously discussed and can include discomfort or pain due to Braxton-Hicks contractions, round ligament stretching, back pain, or constipation. Obviously, identification of the etiology of abdominal pain or bleeding in the third trimester is of utmost urgency. In all situations both maternal and fetal monitoring are important. Training modules have advocated obtaining fetal heart rate, fetal head position, and estimated gestational age on an emergent ultrasound examination in later pregnancy. The examination must then be tailored for each clinical situation. More severe causes of pain or bleeding in the second or third trimester of pregnancy can include the following:

Placenta Previa

Placental localization is important throughout pregnancy, but it is especially important in the third trimester of pregnancy, particularly if the patient presents with pain, bleeding, or active labor. The distance from the edge of the placenta to the internal cervical os can be measured on transabdominal scan but is best evaluated on endovaginal scanning. There are different subtypes of placenta previa (Fig. 25.1). These include a low-lying placenta, where the lower margin of the placenta is within 2 cm of the internal cervical os. The term marginal placenta previa and partial placenta previa are no longer used. A complete placenta previa is where the placenta covers the internal os (Fig. 25.2, Videos 25.1 and 25.2). A central previa is where the placenta is implanted centrally, directly over the internal os. In evaluating placenta previa, one must remember that the placenta is not only anterior and posterior but may extend from the side close to and/or over the endocervical canal. If fetal parts obscure visualization of the cervix, translabial or endovaginal scanning may be helpful. There are several pitfalls in the diagnosis of placenta previa. Myometrial contractions in the lower uterine segment may mimic a placenta previa. Additionally, if the bladder is overdistended there may be a false-positive diagnosis of placenta previa. In cases where there is doubt about placenta previa, endovaginal scanning is very helpful (Fig. 25.3, Videos 25.3 and 25.4).

Placenta Accreta

Placenta accreta is a potentially life-threatening entity for both the fetus and the mother. It usually has associated risk factors. Some of these risk factors include previous cesarean section, with an increase in the risk of placenta accreta with each subsequent cesarean section. Placenta previa is an associated risk factor for placenta accreta. A patient with placenta previa and a prior cesarean section has approximately a 10% risk of placenta accreta. However, those with a placenta previa and two to three cesarean sections have increased risk of placenta accreta—between 40% and 60%. Other risk factors for accreta include advanced maternal age, vigorous curettage, or previous myomectomy.

The etiology for placenta accreta is thought to be a defect in the region of the decidua basalis. The chorionic villus from the fetus grows into the myometrium through the defect in the cesarean section scar. There are three subtypes of placenta accreta. These include *placenta accreta,* where the placenta attaches deep into the uterine wall but does not penetrate the uterine muscle. This occurs in approximately three-quarters of the cases. *Placenta increta* occurs

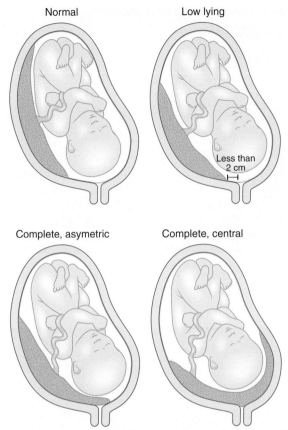

Fig. 25.1 Various classifications of placenta previa. *Normal*: Lower edge of the normal placenta is more than 2 cm from the cervical os. *Low lying*: The distance between the inferior edge of the placenta and the cervical os is less than 2 cm. *Complete, asymmetric*: The placenta asymmetrically covers the cervical os. *Complete, central*: The central portion of the placenta completely covers the cervix. (Redrawn from Hertzberg BS, Middleton WD. *Ultrasound: The Requisites*. 3rd ed. Philadelphia, PA: Elsevier; 2016:474.)

when the placenta attaches even deeper into the uterine wall but does not penetrate the uterine muscle. This occurs in approximately 20% of cases. Finally, *placenta percreta* is the most serious type of placenta accreta, in which the placenta penetrates through the uterine wall and attaches to another organ—most commonly the bladder. All forms of placenta accreta are potentially devastating to both the mother and the fetus. As the placenta attaches to the myometrium, any attempt to remove the placenta can result in potentially massive bleeding. In fact, if the placenta penetrates through the myometrium into the bladder, hysterectomy or even partial cystectomy may be needed.

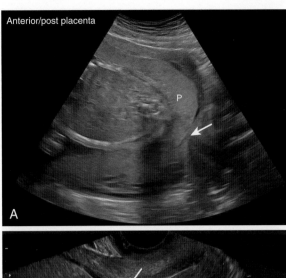
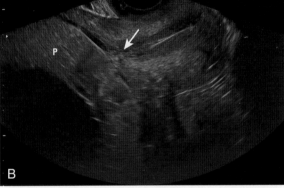

Fig. 25.2 Complete placenta previa. (A) On the transabdominal scan it appears that the placenta (*P*) lies centrally over the cervical os (*arrow*). (B) The endovaginal scan demonstrates that the placenta (*P*) does in fact lie centrally over the cervical os (*arrow*).

Ultrasound may be helpful in the diagnosis of placenta accreta. In normal situations, the retroplacental hypoechoic region of the decidua basalis is seen with ultrasound. However, there may be thinning in this region with placenta accreta. When there is deeper invasion of the placental tissue, the hyperechoic border between the uterine serosa and the bladder is lost. Other sonographic findings associated with placenta accreta include visualization of the vascular lacunae within the placenta. Visualization of these lacunae, or lakes, has one of the highest positive predictive values for diagnosis of placenta accreta. There may be thickening of the placenta in some cases of placenta accreta. When there is placenta percreta, there may be masslike tissue with echogenicity similar to that of the placenta protruding into the bladder (Fig. 25.4).

MRI can often be used to identify and diagnose placenta accreta. There may be focal thinning of the

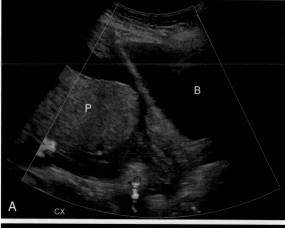

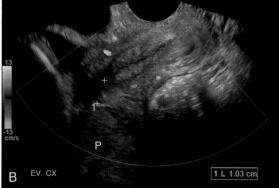

Fig. 25.3 Low-lying placenta. (A) On this transabdominal scan there is a posterior placenta (*P*), which appears to be a complete placenta previa. *B*, Bladder. (B) On the endovaginal scan the tip at the placenta (*P*) does not completely cover the cervical os but is less than 2 cm (*calipers*) from the internal cervical os.

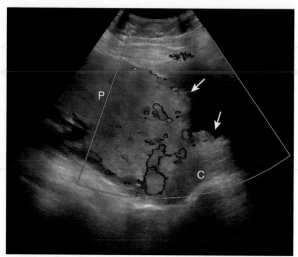

Fig. 25.4 Placenta percreta. Parasagittal ultrasound demonstrates complete placenta previa. Also note thickening of the placenta (*P*) with vascular lacunae in color (*blue*). There is also bulging of the placenta into the bladder (*arrows*). *C*, Cervix.

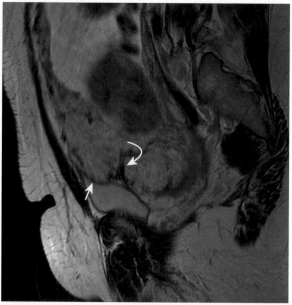

Fig. 25.5 MRI of placenta percreta. Sagittal T2-weighted MRI demonstrated a complete placenta previa. The placenta was thickened with dark bands (*curved arrow*). There is also bulging of the placenta into the anterior portion of the bladder (*arrow*). Note the dark border of the bladder is disrupted at the site of placenta invasion.

myometrium with disruption of the junctional zone, with bulging of the placenta in that region. Often, the placenta is heterogeneous. T2 dark bands are often seen in cases of placenta accreta (Fig. 25.5). When there is deeper invasion, as with placenta percreta, there may be a masslike protrusion of the placenta into the bladder.

Placental Abruption

Placental abruption may have devastating consequences for both the fetus and the mother but may be a difficult sonographic diagnosis. Placental abruption refers to the premature separation of the placenta from the uterine wall. Risk factors include maternal hypertension, smoking, substance abuse, and trauma, but in many cases no etiology is found. Traumatic abruption is discussed in Chapter 15, on the FAST scan. It may be very difficult to identify hemorrhage from placental abruption on sonography. Subchorionic

hemorrhage occurs on the edge of the placenta and may be secondary to rupture of the uteroplacental veins. The hemorrhage can dissect under the subchorionic membranes and appear as a subchorionic hematoma. Retroplacental

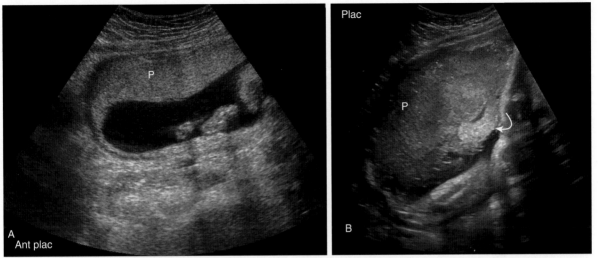

Fig. 25.6 Placenta abruption. (A) Transabdominal ultrasound obtained at 24 weeks demonstrates a homogeneous texture and normal thickness to the placenta (*P*). (B) Sagittal and transverse images of the placenta (*P*) later in pregnancy after trauma. The placenta has changed appearance and now appears thickened and heterogeneous. There is a more echogenic region (*curved arrow*) representing a hematoma.

hemorrhage is thought to be due to rupture of a spiral artery. This will result in bleeding that separates the placenta from the uterine wall. These women may present with tenderness over the uterus. Unfortunately, the hematoma may be the same echogenicity as that of the placenta. In some cases, the hemorrhage may cause placental thickening. There may be subtle sonographic changes, such as a more heterogeneous appearance to portions of the placenta, due to hemorrhage (Fig. 25.6). Echogenic debris thought to be due to hemorrhage can be seen in the amniotic fluid. Even fluid/fluid layers due to the amniotic fluid–blood interface have been seen in some cases. The diagnosis of placenta abruption is very difficult. MRI has been useful in cases when the patient is stable. Although a discussion of MRI features of placental hemorrhage is beyond the scope of this chapter, MRI is very helpful to show areas of hemorrhage. Areas of hemorrhage have different T1 or T2 signal, depending of the acuity of the hemorrhage. These regions can be distinguished from the adjacent placenta on MRI. In any pregnant patient, maternal and fetal monitoring and M-mode ultrasound should always be performed.

Vasa Previa

Vasa previa is a condition in which fetal blood vessels cross or run near the cervical os. This is a rare entity, which occurs between 1 in 3000 and 1 in 4000 deliveries.

If the diagnosis is missed, there is a 60% to 80% fetal mortality rate. Vasa previa is usually an incidental finding that is identified in a search for vaginal bleeding. The etiologies of vasa previa are usually twofold. Velamentous cord insertion is an entity where the umbilical cord inserts at the periphery of the placenta. When there is a low-lying placenta with a very peripheral cord, the cord and/or membranes containing the cord may lie over the cervical os. This can be difficult to visualize. Endovaginal ultrasound with color flow is helpful to make this diagnosis (Fig. 25.7). Another etiology of vasa previa is a succenturiate lobe. In this entity there are two portions of the placenta, with one portion being smaller than the other. Bridging vessels between the two placentas traverse the cervical os. If vasa previa is diagnosed, the patient is usually placed on bed rest awaiting cesarean section.

Incompetent Cervix/Bulging Membranes

During normal scanning the endocervical canal appears as an echogenic line, or at times with a hypoechoic line representing the mucous plug. In most situations, 3 cm is felt to be the lower limits of normal for the cervical length. Although cervical length can be measured on transabdominal scanning, endovaginal scanning usually provides more accurate information. On transabdominal scanning, overdistention of the urinary bladder

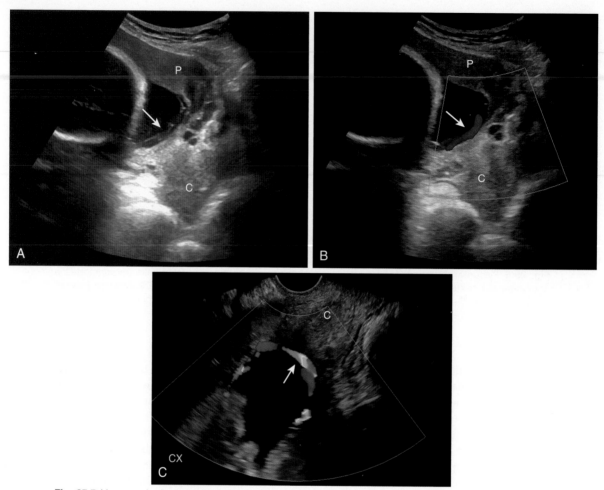

Fig. 25.7 Vasa previa due to velamentous cord insertion. (A) Transabdominal real-time ultrasound demonstrates low-lying anterior placenta (*P*). Also note subtle membrane (*arrow*) overlying the region of the cervical os (*C*). (B) When color Doppler ultrasound is performed, the subtle membrane in fact represents velamentous insertion of the cord (*arrow*) lying over the cervical os (*C*). *P*, Placenta. (C) Endovaginal ultrasound demonstrates the velamentous insertion of the cord (*arrow*), which completely covers the cervical os (*C*), representing vasa previa.

can give the impression of an erroneous elongation of the cervix. In situations where there is a short cervix or fetal parts obscure visualization of the cervix on transabdominal scanning, endovaginal scanning should be performed. This will give a more accurate measurement of cervical length or demonstrate unsuspected findings, such as an open endocervical canal, with bulging membranes (Fig. 25.8, Videos 25.5 and 25.6). These membranes bulge into the vagina and have been termed *"hourglass"* membranes. When severe, these bulging

membranes can be seen on transabdominal scanning (Fig. 25.9). In this situation, it is important to make this diagnosis, as there may be a precipitous delivery once there are bulging membranes.

Funic Cord Presentation

If the umbilical cord is the presenting part during pregnancy, this is called a funic cord presentation. In this situation the umbilical cord lies over the internal cervical os in the lower uterine segment. This may be

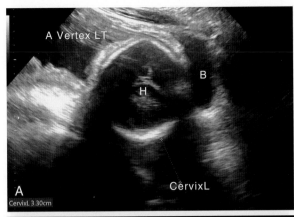

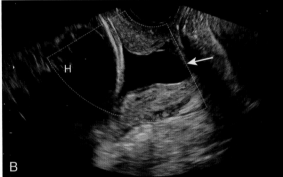

Fig. 25.8 Bulging membranes. (A) Transabdominal parasagittal ultrasound demonstrates the fetal head (*H*) overlying the region of the cervix, which was measured with calipers. *B*, Bladder. (B) However, endovaginal ultrasound with color flow demonstrates that the internal os was open with bulging membranes (*arrow*). There was no prolapse of the umbilical cord. *H*, Head.

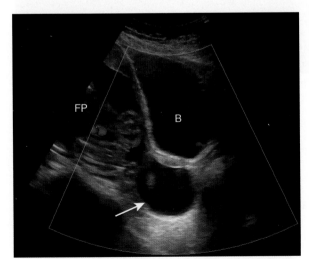

Fig. 25.9 Bulging "hourglass" membranes. Transabdominal parasagittal ultrasound demonstrates bulging of the membranes (*arrow*) through the open cervix. *B*, Bladder; *FP*, fetal parts.

a transient phenomenon and is usually considered insignificant until the third trimester of pregnancy. If this occurs later in pregnancy, this is concerning, and a search for an underlying etiology for a funic cord presentation may be needed. Such things as a marginal cord insertion, where the cord is low lying and may lie over the cervical os during delivery, should be excluded. In these situations color Doppler ultrasound should be used to locate the cord and its relationship to the cervical os. If the transabdominal scan fails to demonstrate the cord location, endovaginal ultrasound with color flow may be needed. In most situations the placenta insertion is in a normal site, unlike cases of vasa previa, in which there is a low-lying placenta with a peripheral cord insertion over the endocervical canal. A funic cord may be a dangerous situation in the third trimester of pregnancy, especially when there is premature labor and bulging membranes. In some situations, only translabial or endovaginal scanning can reliably detect the presenting part (Fig. 25.10, Videos 25.7 and 25.8).

Prolapse of the Umbilical Cord

Prolapse of the umbilical cord usually occurs when there has been premature rupture of the membranes. When this occurs, the cord may prolapse through the endocervical canal and can even prolapse into the vagina. Obviously, it is very important to make this diagnosis because if vaginal delivery does occur, it will compress on the umbilical cord. If there is premature rupture of the membranes and any suspicion of umbilical cord prolapse, usually a translabial scan is first performed, followed by an endovaginal scan depending on the findings. With a translabial scan, color flow must be utilized to demonstrate the prolapse of the umbilical cord (Fig. 25.11). If there is prolapse of the umbilical cord, the patient must be placed in the knee–chest position and emergently taken to labor and delivery for potential cesarean section.

Oligohydramnios and Premature Rupture of Membranes

In the third trimester of pregnancy patients may present with possible leaking of amniotic fluid. Premature rupture of membranes may be assessed by visual inspection during a speculum examination, nitrazine testing, the fern test with microscopy, or, more

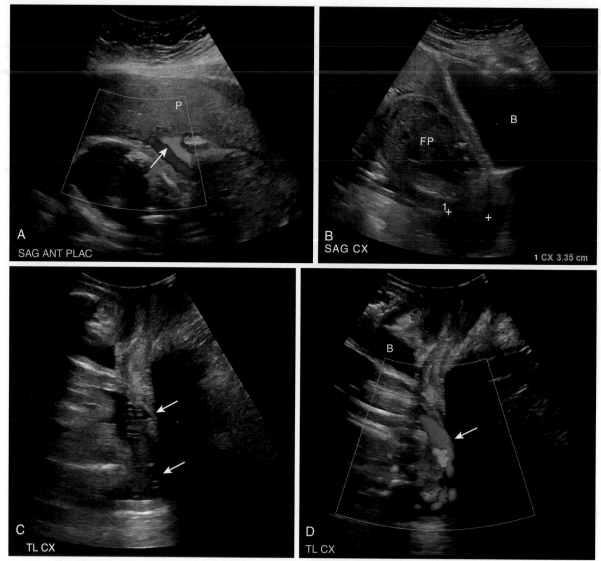

Fig. 25.10 Funic umbilical cord presentation. (A) Real-time transabdominal ultrasound examination shows an anterior placenta (*P*) with the umbilical cord (*arrow*) inserting into the central portion of the placenta. (B) Real-time transabdominal ultrasound with calipers over what is thought to represent the cervix. The fetal parts (*FP*) prevent complete visualization of the cervix. *B*, bladder. (C) Translabial ultrasound demonstrates fluid and membranes bulging though the open cervix (*arrow*). (D) Translabial ultrasound with color flow demonstrates that the umbilical cord (*arrow*) is the presenting part in the open cervix.

recently, use of biomarkers of amniotic fluid. Sonography may be helpful to detect premature rupture of membranes by noting decreased AFI. Lower limits of AFI are between 5 and 8 cm, an MVP than 2 cm, and/or subjective assessment of amniotic fluid to be low. In this situation comparison with prior ultrasound examinations is important to ensure there are no other etiologies of oligohydramnios, such as chromosomal abnormalities, renal agenesis, or intrauterine growth retardation. Careful fetal monitoring of the fetal heart should always be performed.

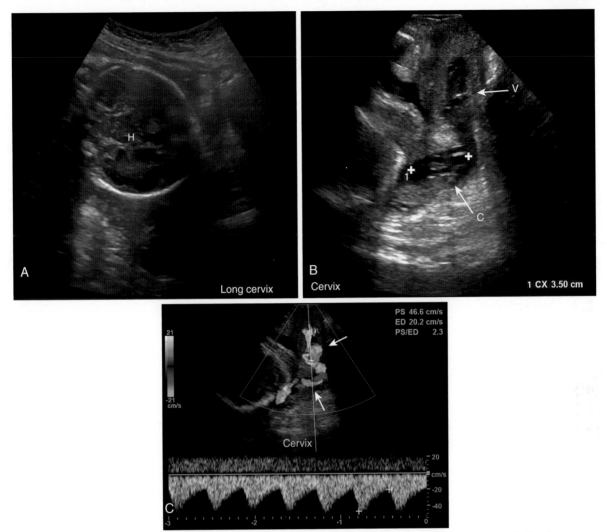

Fig. 25.11 Prolapse of the umbilical cord. (A) Transabdominal parasagittal ultrasound demonstrates the head (H) overlying the region of the cervix, preventing visualization of the cervical os. (B) Translabial scan was performed with measurement of the cervix (calipers). Note the linear echoes in the cervical canal (C) and the vagina (V). (C) Translabial scan with color Doppler ultrasound demonstrated that the cord had prolapsed through the cervix (arrow) and into the vagina (arrow).

BIBLIOGRAPHY

McDermott A. Abdominal pain during pregnancy: is it gas pain or something else? 2017. https://www.healthline.com/health/pregnancy/gas-pain-during-pregnancy.

Fadl S, Moshiri M, Fligner CL, Katz DS, Dighe M. Placental imaging: normal appearance with review of pathologic findings. *Radiographics.* 2017;37:979–998.

Hasegawa J, Farina A, Nakamura M, et al. Analysis of the ultrasonographic findings predictive of vasa previa. *Prenat Diagn.* 2010;30:1121–1125.

Mar WA, Berggruen S, Atueyi U, et al. Ultrasound imaging of placenta accreta with MR correlation. *Ultrasound Q.* 2015;31:23–33.

McGahan JP, Hanson F. Prolapsing amniotic membranes: detection, sonographic appearance, and management. *J Perinatol.* 1987;7:204–209.

McGahan JP, Phillips HE, Bowen MS. Prolapse of the amniotic sac ("hourglass membranes"): ultrasound appearance. *Radiology.* 1981;140:463–466.

McGahan JP, Phillips HE, Reid MH. The anechoic retroplacental area: a pitfall in diagnosis of placental-endometrial abnormalities during pregnancy. *Radiology*. 1980;134: 475–478.

McGahan JP, Phillips HE, Reid MH, Oi RH. Sonographic spectrum of retroplacental hemorrhage. *Radiology*. 1982;142:481–485.

Nunes JO, Turner MA, Fulcher AS. Abdominal imaging features of HELLP syndrome: a 10-year retrospective review. *AJR Am J Roentgenol*. 2005;185:1205–1210.

Shah S, Adedipe A, Ruffatto B, et al. BE-SAFE: bedside sonography for assessment of the fetus in emergencies: educational intervention for late-pregnancy obstetric ultrasound. *West J Emerg Med*. 2014;15:636–640.

Zaidi SF, Moshiri M, Osman S, et al. Comprehensive imaging review of abnormalities of the placenta. *Ultrasound Q*. 2016;32:25–42.

Extremity Ultrasound

26

Peripheral Veins and Arteries

William C. Pevec, Deborah S. Kim

PERIPHERAL ARTERY DISEASE

Patients may present with acute or chronic lower extremity arterial insufficiency. Chronic lower extremity arterial insufficiency is typically secondary to atherosclerosis. Atherosclerosis is a gradual, degenerative disease where plaque accumulates in the wall of the artery and typically causes gradual, progressive clinical manifestations. However, plaques may become unstable and result in acute ischemic symptoms as well. The two primary risk factors for chronic lower extremity arterial occlusive disease are tobacco use and diabetes mellitus. Tobacco use leads to plaque formation in the aortoiliac, femoral-popliteal, and infrapopliteal arterial segments; significant aortoiliac atherosclerosis is uncommon without a history of tobacco use. Diabetes leads to plaque formation in the femoral-popliteal and infrapopliteal arterial segments, frequently with severe involvement of the tibial and pedal arteries. Other less common causes of chronic lower extremity arterial insufficiency include popliteal artery entrapment syndrome, cystic adventitial disease, thrombosed femoral and popliteal aneurysms, and chronic aortic dissection.

Chronic lower extremity arterial occlusive disease may be asymptomatic, particularly in sedentary patients who have well-developed collateral arterial networks.

The mildest symptom of chronic lower extremity arterial occlusive disease is claudication, which is pain in the large muscle groups (gluteus, thigh, and/or calf) with walking. In claudication, the arterial supply is adequate to meet the resting demands of the lower extremity tissues but inadequate to meet the increased metabolic demands of the exercising muscle. The pain is manifested in any or all of the large muscle groups distal to the culprit arterial stenosis or occlusion. The pain typically is reproducible every time the patient walks a given distance at a given gait; the pain may occur earlier and/or be more severe if the patient walks up an incline or at a faster pace. The pain should rapidly resolve with rest.

The next level of symptomatic presentation of chronic lower extremity arterial occlusive disease is ischemic rest pain. With ischemic rest pain, the arterial supply is inadequate to meet even the minimal resting metabolic demands of the lower extremity nerves. The pain is located in the feet, particularly the toes and forefoot. It is worsened with elevation and improved with dependency. It is severe and unrelenting.

The most severe symptom of chronic lower extremity arterial occlusive disease is ischemic tissue loss, either ulceration or gangrene. With ischemic tissue loss, the arterial supply is inadequate to maintain viability of the skin. The tissue loss is frequently on the toes, which are at the distal limits of the arterial tree, or on areas subject to friction and pressure, including the skin over the metatarsal heads and heel (Fig. 26.1).

Ischemic rest pain and tissue loss are considered *critical limb ischemia*, as progression to major amputation is likely without arterial reconstruction. Claudication is a relative indication for arterial reconstruction; critical limb ischemia is an absolute indication to arterial reconstruction.

Acute lower extremity arterial insufficiency most commonly is secondary to thromboembolization, with the heart being the most common source. Conditions

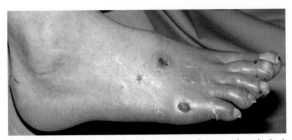

Fig. 26.1 Skin ulcers of the foot, secondary to chronic ischemia. Note the dry, scaly skin; rubor (red discoloration of the forefoot); and the well-demarcated, dry ulcers.

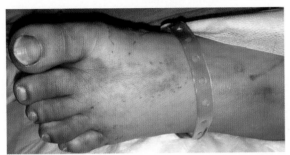

Fig. 26.2 Acutely ischemic foot. Note the mottling of the dorsal forefoot and the dusky toes.

that may predispose to formation of thrombus in the heart include atrial fibrillation; acute transmural myocardial infarction; and ventricular wall hypokinesis, akinesis, or dyskinesis. The thoracic aorta may also be a source of arterial thromboemboli. Other conditions that may result in acute lower extremity ischemia include acute aortic dissection, traumatic injury, disruption of atherosclerotic plaque, and thrombosis of femoral or popliteal aneurysms.

Clinical manifestations of acute lower extremity arterial insufficiency include pain, pallor, paresthesia, paralysis, and cold temperature (Fig. 26.2). Temperature demarcation is typically at one segment distal to the arterial occlusion: occlusion of the popliteal artery bifurcation leads to a cold forefoot; occlusion of the femoral artery bifurcation leads to a cold distal calf and foot; and occlusion of the iliac artery bifurcation leads to a cold distal thigh, calf, and foot. Numbness and motor dysfunction are ominous signs; without prompt revascularization, permanent pain and paralysis or major amputation is likely.

Pseudoaneurysms occur when there is disruption of the wall of an artery, with contained but persistent blood flow into the soft tissues surrounding the artery. Most pseudoaneurysms are traumatic, with iatrogenic trauma being a more common etiology than violent trauma. Anastomotic pseudoaneurysms develop when an arterial anastomosis breaks down, most typically due to the sutures pulling through the wall of the artery. Pseudoaneurysms may cause pain from irritation of local nerves, swelling from compression of adjacent veins, thrombosis of the parent artery, or pressure necrosis of the overlying skin and fat.

Arteriovenous fistulae may be congenital or acquired. Congenital fistulae are frequently complex, with multiple connections between the artery and vein. Acquired fistulae are secondary to trauma, either iatrogenic or violent. Acquired fistulae typically involve a single connection between the vein and artery. Arteriovenous fistulae are usually asymptomatic, but may cause swelling of the affected extremity, ischemia of the affected extremity, or high-output heart failure.

Normal Anatomy

The abdominal aorta bifurcates into the common iliac arteries at about the level of the umbilicus. In the midpelvis, the common iliac artery bifurcates into the internal and external iliac arteries. The internal iliac artery gives blood supply to the gluteal muscles, the organs of the pelvis, and the adductor muscles of the thigh. The external iliac artery provides flow to the lower extremity.

As it crosses deep to the inguinal ligament, the external iliac artery becomes the common femoral artery. The common femoral artery bifurcates into the deep and superficial femoral arteries. The deep femoral artery dives deep to the adductor longus muscle, medial to the femur; it supplies blood to the remaining muscles of the thigh. The superficial femoral artery courses deep to the sartorius muscle and through the adductor canal of the adductor magnus muscle. The superficial femoral artery is the conduit carrying blood to the leg.

After the superficial femoral artery exits the adductor canal, it becomes the popliteal artery. The popliteal artery passes posterior to the knee, between the heads of the gastrocnemius muscle. The popliteal artery bifurcates into the anterior tibial and tibioperoneal (posterior tibial) arteries at the distal edge of the popliteus muscle. The anterior tibial artery crosses the interosseous ligament and travels through the anterior compartment of the

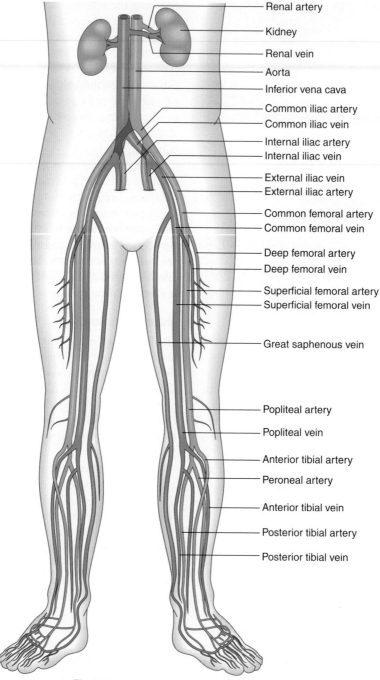

Fig. 26.3 Arterial anatomy of the lower extremity.

leg and, as it crosses the ankle, becomes the dorsal pedal artery on the medial dorsum of the foot. The tibioperoneal (posterior tibial) artery bifurcates in the midleg into the peroneal and posterior tibial arteries, both of which are located in the deep posterior compartment of the leg. The peroneal artery is more lateral, running along the fibula, and ends in the distal leg. The posterior tibial artery runs more medially, crosses posterior to the medial malleolus, and terminates in the plantar foot as the lateral and medial plantar arteries (Fig. 26.3).

Imaging

Duplex ultrasound is accurate in the analysis of the lower extremity arteries. Color flow imaging is helpful to identify the arteries quickly and to identify segments of occlusion and reconstituted flow. Transducer frequencies of 2 to 3 MHz are ideal to evaluate the aorta and iliac arteries, and of 5 MHz for the lower extremity arteries. A Doppler angle of 60 degrees is optimal. B-mode images and spectral analysis of pulsed Doppler data should be obtained at all levels.

Imaging of the aorta and iliac arteries may be limited by overlying bowel gas; ideally, the patient should fast 8 to 12 hours before evaluating the arteries of the abdomen and pelvis.

With the patient supine, the aorta is imaged from just inferior to the xyphoid to the umbilicus, with a 2- to 3-MHz transducer, in a longitudinal plane. The aortic bifurcation is evaluated with the transducer angulated obliquely on the left side of the umbilicus. The distal common iliac and proximal external iliac arteries are visualized with the transducer angled medially at the level of the iliac crests.

A 5-MHz transducer pointed cephalad at the groin is used to evaluate the distal external iliac artery, and then the transducer is moved distally along the thigh to evaluate the common, deep, and superficial femoral arteries. The distal superficial femoral and popliteal arteries may need to be evaluated with the transducer on the posterior thigh and popliteal fossa; this may be accomplished by flexing the patient's knee or placing the patient in the prone position.

The anterior tibial artery is located at the dorsum of the ankle and then followed up the anterolateral leg. The posterior tibial artery is identified posterior to the medial malleolus and then followed up the medial leg. The peroneal artery is located posterior to the lateral malleolus and then followed up the posterolateral leg.

Pathology

Chronic Lower Extremity Atherosclerosis. The diagnosis of chronic lower extremity atherosclerosis is typically made on the basis of the history (claudication, rest pain, foot ulceration, or gangrene) and physical examination (pulse deficits, bruits, skin changes, etc.). In the presence of diagnostic uncertainty, measurement of the blood pressure at the ankle and/or toes and/or calculating an ankle–brachial index is typically sufficient to confirm or exclude the diagnosis of chronic lower extremity atherosclerosis. Duplex ultrasound is rarely needed in the diagnosis. Duplex ultrasound is indicated when a more precise assessment of the arterial anatomy is needed, such as treatment planning or surveillance after prior treatment.

A normal arterial Doppler signal in a lower extremity artery will have a triphasic signal with a brisk systolic upstroke (Fig. 26.4A). The first phase, with antegrade acceleration and deceleration, is due to contraction of the left ventricle (Fig. 26.4B–E). The second phase, with retrograde flow, is due to reflection of the pressure wave off the distal resistance arteries. The third phase, with brief antegrade flow, is due to elastic recoil of the aortic root. As the aorta becomes stiffer with age, the third phase may be lost; a biphasic signal in an artery of the lower extremity may be normal in an elderly individual (Fig. 26.5).

The normal peak systolic velocity decreases from the proximal to the distal arteries of the lower extremity. The peak systolic velocity in the iliac arteries is typically about 120 cm/sec, and in the popliteal artery about 70 cm/sec, but the values vary substantially from patient to patient.

Stenosis is diagnosed primarily by an increase in the peak systolic velocity at the level of stenosis; a doubling or tripling of the peak systolic velocity usually correlates with a >50% diameter stenosis (Fig. 26.6). With a severe stenosis, peak systolic velocities may decrease and resistance increase proximal to the stenosis (Fig. 26.7). Turbulence is commonly seen immediately distal to the stenosis, and the distal waveforms may become monophasic (Fig. 26.8). Plaque in the wall and luminal narrowing may be seen on B-mode or color flow imaging (Fig. 26.9), but peak systolic velocity elevation is the most reliable criterion to diagnose stenosis.

Occlusion is diagnosed by the absence of flow in the artery; waveforms distal to the occlusion typically are monophasic with low peak systolic velocity (Fig. 26.10). Heavy calcification of the arterial wall, commonly seen in patients with diabetes and/or renal failure, may limit the ability of the ultrasound waves to penetrate the arterial wall and may lead to an erroneous diagnosis of arterial occlusion (Fig. 26.11).

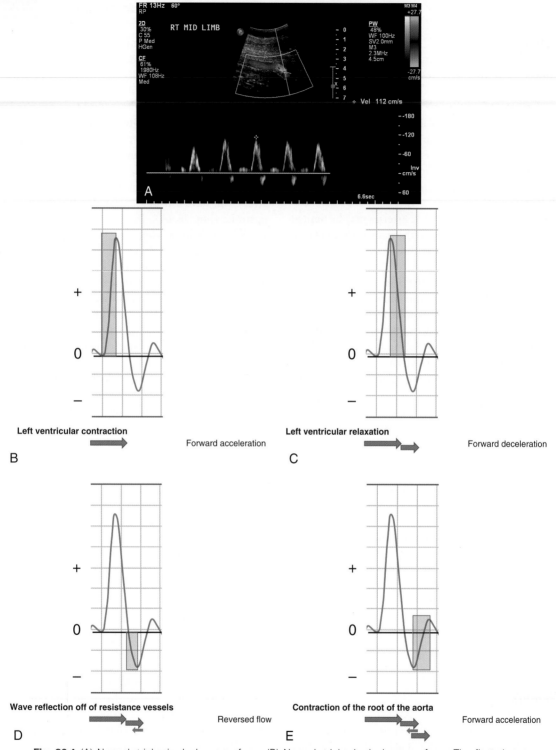

Fig. 26.4 (A) Normal, triphasic duplex waveform. (B) Normal, triphasic duplex waveform. The first phase starts with forward acceleration of the blood, secondary to contraction of the left ventricle. (C) Normal, triphasic duplex waveform. The first phase finishes with continued forward flow that decelerates as the left ventricle relaxes. (D) Normal, triphasic duplex waveform. In the second phase, flow is reversed, as the arterial pressure wave is reflected off the resistance vessels. (E) Normal, triphasic duplex waveform. In the third phase, flow is again in the forward direction, as the aortic root recoils and propels the blood forward.

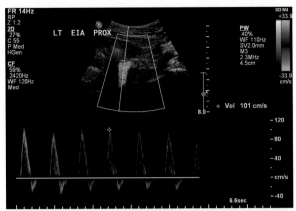

Fig. 26.5 Near-normal, biphasic duplex arterial waveform.

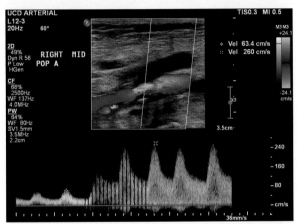

Fig. 26.6 Greater than 50% stenosis of the popliteal artery, with quadrupling of the peak systolic velocity and turbulent flow.

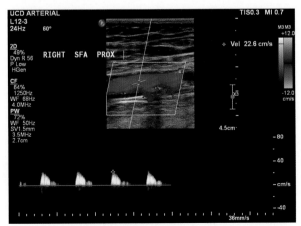

Fig. 26.7 Low-velocity, high-resistance arterial waveforms proximal to a severe stenosis of the superficial femoral artery.

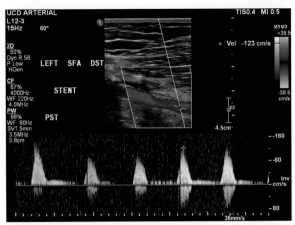

Fig. 26.8 Turbulent, monophasic waveforms distal to a significant stenosis of the superficial femoral artery.

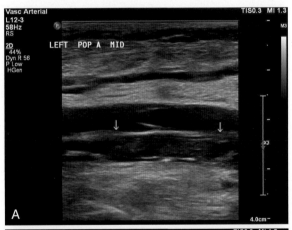

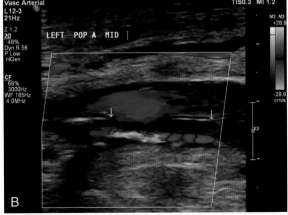

Fig. 26.9 B-mode (A) and color flow (B) images of calcified plaque and a narrow lumen of the popliteal artery.

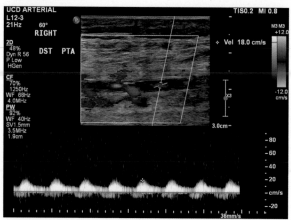

Fig. 26.10 Monophasic, low-velocity flow in the posterior tibial artery, distal to an occlusion.

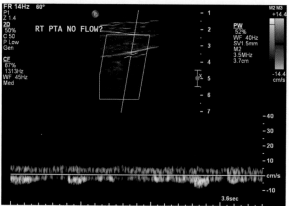

Fig. 26.11 Severe calcification of a posterior tibial artery. Due to poor penetration of ultrasound through the calcium, the artery may appear to be occluded when there is flow present.

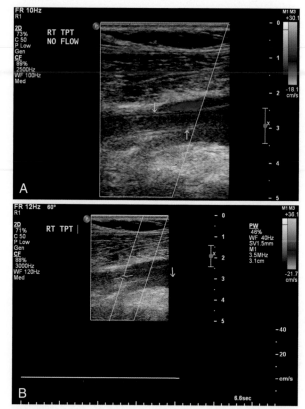

Fig. 26.12 The tibioperoneal artery is filled with echolucent thrombus that is not visible on the B-mode image (A), where the artery is between the *white arrows*. The absence of flow is documented with color Doppler and spectral analysis (B).

Arterial Thrombus. Acute thrombus typically results in occlusion of the artery. The thrombus may be echolucent or mildly hyperechoic (Fig. 26.12). With fresh thrombus, some movement may be detected at the proximal end of the thrombus. Flow distal to an occluding thrombus is typically monophasic with a low peak systolic velocity.

Popliteal Entrapment. Popliteal entrapment occurs when the popliteal artery is compressed by the medial head of the gastrocnemius muscle or by the popliteus muscle. It results in calf claudication, typically in healthy, young individuals.

The diagnosis is suggested by a normal pedal pulse at rest that disappears with passive dorsiflexion or active plantarflexion of the ankle. Duplex ultrasound shows compression of the popliteal artery with calf muscle contraction.

Cystic Adventitial Disease. The popliteal is the most common artery affected by cystic adventitial disease, a condition where gelatinous cysts are present in the adventitia, leading to compression of the arterial lumen. The typical presentation is a man in his 30s with a relatively acute onset of claudication.

Duplex ultrasound will show cysts in the wall of the popliteal artery, with a pulsating hyperechoic line between the cyst and the lumen. Elevated velocities are noted in the lumen (Fig. 26.13). Diagnosis with ultrasound is more difficult if the arterial lumen is occluded.

Aneurysms of the Femoral and Popliteal Arteries. An aneurysm is a focal dilatation of the artery. The most common location for an aneurysm in the lower

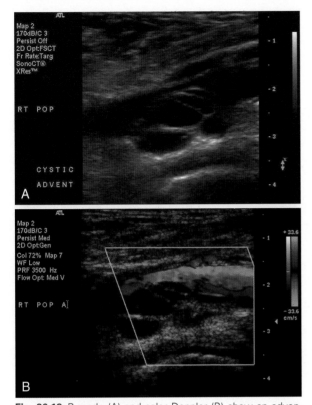

Fig. 26.13 B-mode (A) and color Doppler (B) show an adventitial cyst of the popliteal artery, with narrowing of the arterial lumen.

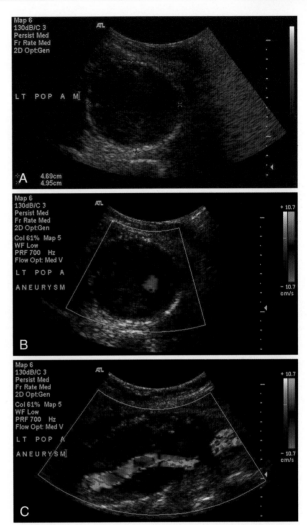

Fig. 26.14 An aneurysm of the popliteal artery, with mural thrombus, is shown with B-mode image in the transverse plane (A) and with color Doppler in the transverse plane (B) and sagittal plane (C).

extremity is the popliteal artery; the femoral artery is a less common site.

Popliteal artery aneurysms are of clinical concern because they commonly contain mural thrombus, which can embolize distally or lead to acute thrombosis of the aneurysm; either of these conditions may result in limb loss. Popliteal artery aneurysms may also cause limb swelling due to compression of the adjacent popliteal veins, or pain due to compression of the adjacent tibial nerve; rupture may occur but is uncommon. The natural history of femoral artery aneurysms is less well understood, but femoral artery aneurysms may also be a source of emboli, thrombus, and rupture.

B-mode imaging is used to evaluate for peripheral artery aneurysms. The maximum diameter of the aneurysm should be recorded, taking care to place the transducer perpendicular to the long axis of the artery to avoid measuring a tangent rather than the true diameter. The diameters of the unaffected arteries proximal and distal to the aneurysm are routinely recorded. The presence or absence of mural thrombus should be noted (Fig. 26.14). Spectral analysis of the pulsed Doppler data should be performed to assess for patency and any associated stenosis.

Pseudoaneurysms. The most commonly encountered pseudoaneurysms are iatrogenic, secondary to puncture or catheterization of an artery for a diagnostic or therapeutic intervention, or unintentional puncture of

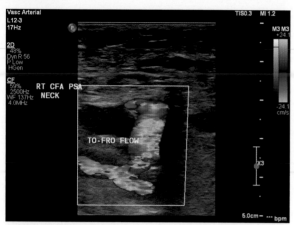

Fig. 26.15 Color flow image of an iatrogenic pseudoaneurysm of the common femoral artery.

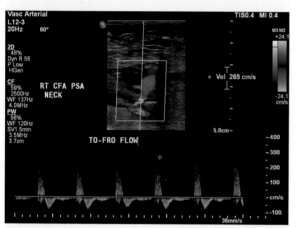

Fig. 26.16 Bidirectional flow is demonstrated in the "neck" of an iatrogenic pseudoaneurysm of the common femoral artery.

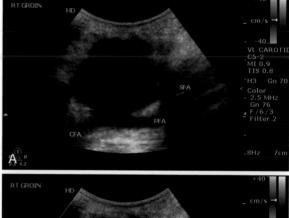

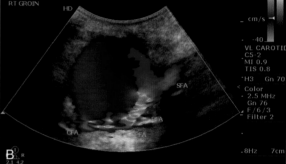

Fig. 26.17 An anastomotic pseudoaneurysm of the common femoral artery is demonstrated with B-mode (A) and color Doppler (B) ultrasound.

an artery during a venous procedure. Color flow imaging is helpful to detect blood flow outside the lumen of the artery (Fig. 26.15). Pulsed Doppler will show bidirectional flow at the connection between the artery and the pseudoaneurysm cavity (Fig. 26.16). Pseudoaneurysms should be differentiated from hematomas, which present as fluid collections adjacent to the artery with the absence of flow in the fluid collection.

An anastomotic pseudoaneurysm will present as a dilated cavity with arterial flow at the level of an arterial anastomosis (Fig. 26.17).

Arteriovenous Fistula. A continuous bruit throughout systole and diastole will be detected on auscultation over an arteriovenous fistula. Duplex interrogation of the artery proximal to the fistula will show low resistance with antegrade flow throughout diastole; flow velocities will be elevated if the volume of flow in the fistula is high. Distal to the fistula, the artery will have a normal, high-resistance waveform (Fig. 26.18). A turbulent, high-velocity jet may be detected at the site of the connection between the artery and the vein (Fig. 26.19). The vein cephalad to the fistula will have high velocity, pulsatile waveforms, and may be dilated (Fig. 26.20).

ACUTE AND CHRONIC DEEP VENOUS THROMBOSIS

Clinical Correlation

Venous thromboembolism (VTE) is a complex, multifactorial disease of heritable and acquired risk factors. The prevalence of all types of VTE in the United States is not truly known, but the incidence is increasing, recurrence is high, and deep venous thrombosis (DVT) can

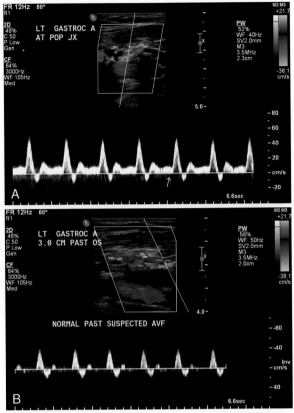

Fig. 26.18 Arterial waveforms proximal to a small arteriovenous fistula have abnormal, low-resistance flow throughout diastole (A). Waveforms distal to the fistula resume the normal, high-resistance flow pattern seen in arteries supplying skeletal muscle (B).

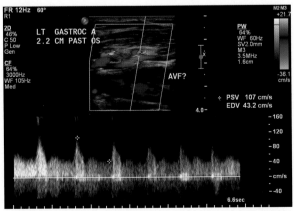

Fig. 26.19 Turbulent, high flow at the site of the fistula between the artery and the vein.

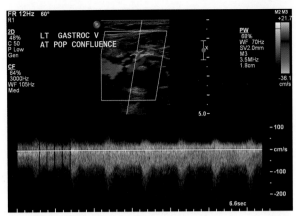

Fig. 26.20 High-velocity, pulsatile flow in the vein cephalad to the arteriovenous fistula.

lead to progression of its critical complication, pulmonary embolism (PE). In the United States, DVT may have a prevalence of about 20% in symptomatic outpatients and a 9.6% to 12% incidence among intensive care unit (ICU) patients despite VTE prophylaxis. Progression from DVT to PE is estimated to range anywhere between 10% and 50%. This highly morbid, often silent, disease is critical to diagnose, and the ultrasound evaluation of the deep vasculature has become one of the most useful examinations for emergency and critical care physicians.

An ultrasound vascular examination for lower extremity DVT is indicated whenever a patient presents with lower extremity swelling or pain, a PE is highly suspected but the patient cannot undergo other testing modalities, and in a pulseless electrical activity (PEA) cardiac arrest when PE is a possible treatable cause.

Most cases of DVT occur in the lower extremities and can be spontaneous. In contrast, most cases of upper extremity DVT are secondary from obvious inciting causes, such as the existence of a central catheter or other foreign body. Primary upper extremity DVT is rare, and ultrasound examination of the deep veins of the upper extremity is not covered here.

The distribution of lower extremity DVT is overwhelmingly concentrated in the popliteal and femoral confluences. As much as 90% of lower extremity DVTs are found at these confluences, with only 5% falling between the two regions (i.e., along the length of the femoral vein). Testing for VTE in the calf and distal lower extremity as well as the deep venous system is still a topic of some debate, as more than 50% of these distal thrombi are thought to spontaneously resolve and the risks of anticoagulation are not insignificant. Ultrasound imaging of the calf has comparably lower accuracy than of the thigh and also results in a higher incidence of nondiagnostic examinations.

The two-region compression ultrasound technique discussed here therefore focuses on imaging the leg from the femoral triangle to the popliteal fossa of the knee and checking compressibility to rule out the presence of thrombus.

Normal Anatomy

The common femoral vein (CFV) is the most proximally visualizable deep vein of the lower extremity outside of the abdomen. It enters the pelvis to become one of the external iliac veins, which is most often imaged transabdominally. Before entering the pelvis, the CFV can be visualized along the groin alongside the common femoral artery until its most proximal tributary, the great saphenous vein (GSV), joins. Distal to this confluence, as we follow these vessels down the thigh, the CFV is split into two parts: the femoral vein (FV) and deep femoral vein (DFV). As we follow the FV distally, it becomes the popliteal vein and is most easily imaged from the popliteal fossa. Here, the anterior tibial vein, posterior tibial vein, and peroneal vein join, creating a trifurcation that meets the popliteal vein (Fig. 26.21).

Imaging

For optimal visualization, a high-frequency (4–10 MHz) linear array transducer is preferred. The narrow, flat footprint of the linear array aids in the application of direct and even pressure to the vessel(s) of interest during the examination. Higher frequencies of ultrasound provide superior detail over short distances, and most of the study will examine 2 to 8 cm of tissue depth. Larger, lower-frequency curvilinear probes can be used for obese patients requiring deeper visualization.

Most modern ultrasound machines have available B-mode imaging settings for vascular or superficial soft tissue studies. If available, these are the ideal settings to use for this examination. Doppler and color flow modalities can also be used to help identify vein versus artery, but the presence of Doppler sound/pulse wave and color flow cannot be used in isolation without compression to rule out thrombus.

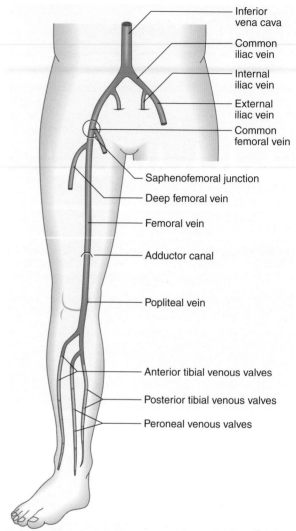

Fig. 26.21 Lower extremity venous anatomy of the deep venous system of the leg from the common iliac vein down to the popliteal trifurcation.

Two regions of the lower extremity (femoral and popliteal) need to be interrogated to complete an ultrasound examination for DVT.

The patient should be positioned to optimize the visualization of each region (Figs. 26.22 and 26.23). Gel is applied, and then each region should be scanned until the deep vessel of interest is identified. Compression is then applied with the transducer until the visualized vessel collapses completely to form a thin line. This complete collapse of the vessel rules out the presence of thrombus. When in doubt, apply enough

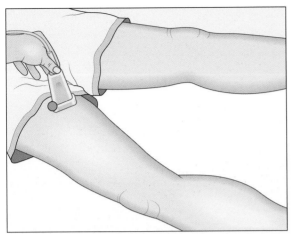

Fig. 26.22 Femoral scanning position of patient lying supine with the patient's right hip slightly externally rotated and the patient's left lower extremity straight and draped from the groin. A linear ultrasound transducer is applied to the hip crease of the right leg, with the transducer marker to the patient's right.

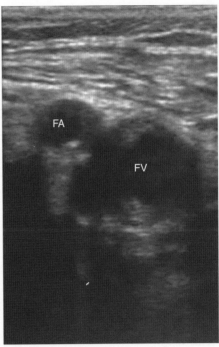

Fig. 26.24 Ultrasound image of the femoral artery (*FA*) and vein (*FV*).

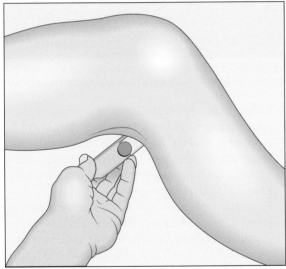

Fig. 26.23 Popliteal scanning position of patient lying supine with the right knee flexed and the left lower extremity straight and draped from the groin. A linear ultrasound transducer is applied behind the knee, with the transducer marker to the patient's right.

pressure to completely collapse any nearby arterial vessels that may be present on the same screen. If the vein of interest does not collapse when the artery does, the scan is considered positive for thrombus (Figs. 26.24–26.26).

The femoral examination begins as proximally as possible on the thigh, just inferior to the inguinal ligament. The CFV should be seen in cross-section, paired with the common femoral artery. Moving distally, the GSV should also appear and separate from the CFV, moving medially away from the CFV. Distally, the CFV can be seen until it bifurcates into the DFV and the FV. This entire region can represent as little as 6 to 12 cm of thigh on an average adult. Along the scan, stop to compress the FV and GSV completely at regular intervals. Compress every 1 to 2 centimeters along the region, or a distance about the width of the transducer (Figs. 26.27–26.30).

Some authors advocate continuing to follow the CFV distally as it becomes the FV during the ultrasound examination, compressing the FV regularly along the thigh until the knee is reached. This additional interrogation can identify isolated less common thrombi along the FV and increase the sensitivity of your total examination.

The popliteal examination begins at the proximal popliteal fossa. Identify the popliteal vein, which is usually directly superficial to the popliteal artery (which can

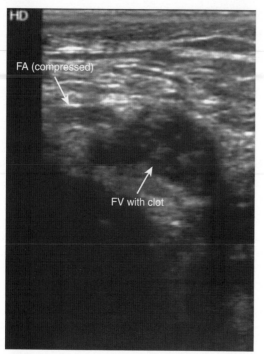

Fig. 26.25 Ultrasound image of the same femoral artery (*FA*) and femoral vein (*FV*) in Fig. 26.30, with compression. Note that the femoral artery is partially compressed, but the femoral vein reveals a clot of mixed echogenicity.

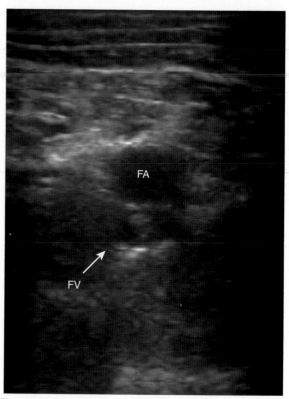

Fig. 26.26 Femoral artery (*FA*) with the femoral vein (*FV*) directly below, which contains a floating echogenic clot (*arrow*).

be remembered with the mnemonic "Pop on Top"). The fossa of the knee is interrogated distally until the anterior tibial, posterior tibial, and peroneal veins join the popliteal vein to form a trifurcation, seen as three vessels coming together. Along the scan, stop to compress the popliteal vein completely at regular intervals (Figs. 26.31 and 26.32).

As with any imaging skill, avoiding false positives and negatives in vascular ultrasound is a matter of practice and familiarity with the most common mistakes.

Image acquisition pitfalls include:

- Failing to be truly perpendicular to the vessel, therefore sliding away off the vessel, not achieving full compression, or compressing unevenly.
- Patient obesity, soft tissue edema, scar tissue, or poor positioning compromising visualization.
- Patients with duplicate femoral veins only undergoing imaging of the nonthrombosed limb of the vessel.
- Mistaking a lymph node, baker's cyst, or aneurysm for a vessel or clot.

- Failing to remember the limits of this technique—if your clinical suspicion is high, or if the patient has a positive D-dimer, the use of a clinical risk score/algorithm or alternative test (repeat examination in 1 week, contrast venography, magnetic resonance imaging [MRI]) is appropriate.
- Failing to remember that regional lower extremity vessel ultrasound cannot visualize iliofemoral clots (consider abdominal ultrasound) and may miss segmental FV or calf vein clots (consider extending your compression tests along the FV and into the calf).

Pathology

Distinguishing acute from chronic thrombus can be challenging with ultrasound alone, especially if no previous studies are available for comparison. Signs that suggest chronic clot include increased thrombus echogenicity, irregularly thickened vessel walls, small vessel lumens, and the presence of multiple collateral vessels.

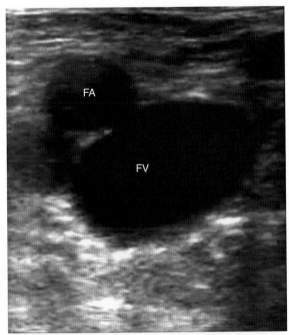

Fig. 26.27 Ultrasound image of the proximal femoral artery (*FA*) and femoral vein (*FV*).

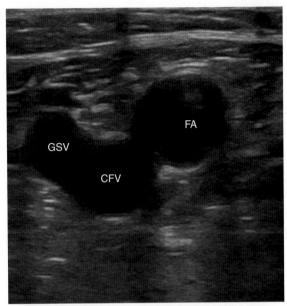

Fig. 26.29 Ultrasound image of the femoral anatomy (*FA*), with the great saphenous vein (*GSV*) joining the common femoral vein (*CFV*).

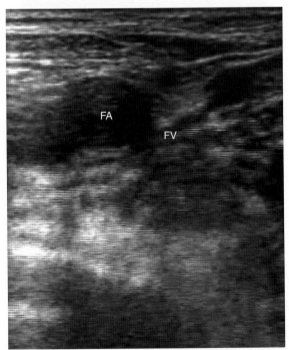

Fig. 26.28 Ultrasound image of the same proximal femoral artery (*FA*) and femoral vein (*FV*), with compression. Note the femoral vein becomes a nearly invisible, thin, echogenic line.

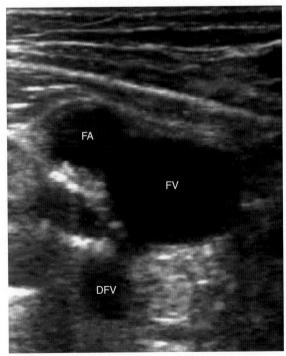

Fig. 26.30 Ultrasound image of the femoral artery (*FA*), with the deep femoral vein (*DFV*) joining the femoral vein (*FV*).

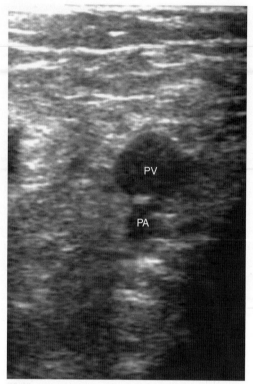

Fig. 26.31 Ultrasound image of the popliteal artery (*PA*) and vein (*PV*).

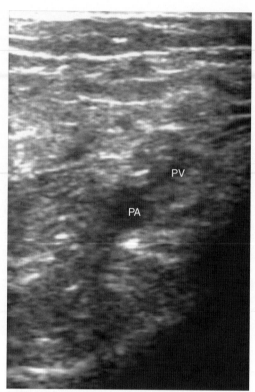

Fig. 26.32 Ultrasound image of the same popliteal artery (*PA*) and vein (*PV*) in Fig. 26.31, with compression. Note the popliteal vein becomes a nearly invisible, thin, hypoechoic line.

TABLE 26.1 **Acute vs. Chronic Thrombus Characteristics on Ultrasound Imaging**

Acute Thrombus	Chronic Thrombus
Homogenous, anechoic or hypoechoic	Heterogenous, brightly echoic
Free floating, poorly attached to vessel walls	Well attached to vessel walls
Large-diameter vein with thin walls	Small contracted vein, irregularly thickened vessel walls
Small or no collateral vessels	Large or multiple collateral vessels
Soft, often deformable	Rigid, irregular in shape

Repeat ultrasound examination after treatment or use of other imaging modalities (MRI, contrast venography) may be indicated (Table 26.1).

BIBLIOGRAPHY

Adhikari S, et al. Isolated deep venous thrombosis: implications for 2-point compression ultrasonography of the lower extremity. *Ann Emerg Med.* 2015;66(3):262–266.

Anderson FA. Physician practices in the prevention of venous thromboembolism. *Ann Intern Med.* 1991;115(8):591.

Bernardi E. Serial 2-point ultrasonography plus D-Dimer vs. whole-leg color-coded Doppler ultrasonography for diagnosing suspected symptomatic deep vein thrombosis. *JAMA.* 2008;300(14):1653.

Burns GA, et al. Prospective ultrasound evaluation of venous thrombosis in high-risk trauma patients. *J Trauma.* 1993;35(3):405–408.

Crafts RC. *A Textbook of Human Anatomy.* 2nd ed. New York: John Wiley and Sons; 1979:450–453.

Cronenwett JL, Johnston KW, eds. *Rutherford's Vascular Surgery.* 8th ed. Philadelphia: Elsevier Saunders; 2014:1808–1814.

Cronenwett JL, Johnston KW, eds. *Rutherford's Vascular Surgery.* 8th ed. Philadelphia: Elsevier Saunders; 2014:1801–1805.

Cronenwett JL, Johnston KW, eds. *Rutherford's Vascular Surgery*. 8th ed. Philadelphia: Elsevier Saunders; 2014:66–77.

Gottlieb RH, Widjaja J, Tian L, et al. Calf sonography for detecting deep venous thrombosis in symptomatic patients: experience and review of the literature. *J Clin Ultrasound*. 1999;27:415–420.

Heit JA. Epidemiology of venous thromboembolism. *Nat Rev Cardiol*. 2015;12(8):464–474.

Hirsch DR. Prevalence of deep venous thrombosis among patients in medical intensive care. *JAMA*. 1995;274(4):335.

Joffe Hv. Upper-extremity deep vein thrombosis. *Circulation*. 2002;106(14):1874–1880.

Marik PE, et al. The incidence of deep venous thrombosis in ICU patients. *Chest*. 1997;111(3):661–664.

Zierler RE, Dawson DL, Kluver Wolters, eds. *Standness's Duplex Scanning in Vascular Disorders*. 5th ed. New York; 2016:151–163.

Soft Tissue and Musculoskeletal Ultrasound

27

Soft Tissue

Sarah Medeiros

CLINICAL CONSIDERATIONS

Ultrasound is an ideal modality to supplement evaluation of the soft tissue. The high–frequency linear transducer produces a detailed image of the area in question. By adding dynamic interrogation, such as manual compression or color flow, we can further characterize the findings to help confirm or rule out many common diagnoses.

Soft tissue infections, including cellulitis and abscess, are extremely prevalent, and becoming more so, with emergency department (ED) visits for these conditions more than doubling in recent years. Clinically, these infections present as areas of erythema, edema, induration, warmth, and sometimes with fluctuance. It can be challenging to differentiate between cellulitis and abscess based on physical examination alone, but the distinction is important, as they require different management. Point-of-care ultrasound (POCUS) has been shown to reliably diagnose an abscess with sensitivity of 96% and specificity of 83%. When an abscess is identified, POCUS can then be used to guide incision and drainage (I&D), reducing treatment failures.

POCUS is also useful for localizing and removing foreign bodies. In the ED and outpatient settings, foreign bodies are most commonly lodged in the hand or foot. Missed foreign bodies can lead to increased infection rates, delayed healing, and pain. X-ray is at times unreliable for identifying and localizing foreign bodies. Some materials, such as metal, bullets, gravel, or glass, may be radio-opaque, but plastic and organic material, such as wood or thorns, and some types of glass, are radiolucent and difficult to identify with X-ray. POCUS identifies most foreign bodies and is also useful to guide removal.

ANATOMY

Soft tissue anatomy has a reliable appearance on ultrasound (Fig. 27.1). The most superficial layer is the skin, composed of epidermis and dermis, which generally appears on ultrasound as a thin, hyperechoic layer, closest to the probe. Below the skin is the subcutaneous tissue, or hypodermis, which varies in thickness and contains hyperechoic fat with hypoechoic septa, as well as blood vessels, nerves, and lymphatics. Vessels appears as tubular structures with a hyperechoic wall and anechoic center. Nerves have a honeycomb appearance in the short axis and appear striated in the long axis. Nerves exhibit anisotropy, appearing more hyperechoic or hypoechoic, depending on the angle of the transducer. Muscle may be superficial or deep to nerves and appear more hypoechoic with hyperechoic striations and fascial planes. Tendons, nerves, and blood vessels also run along the muscle layer. Tendons have a regular, striated appearance and, like nerves, are anisotropic. Bone underlies the muscles in most areas of the body and appears brightly hyperechoic with dark shadowing. Using color flow Doppler with and without compression can help identify vascular structures and differentiate these from other fluid collections (Fig. 27.2).

Cellulitis and abscesses develop in the skin and subcutaneous tissue and are commonly caused by *Streptococcus* species and *Staphylococcus aureus*. Abscesses can extend into deeper tissue, including muscle, even reaching bone. POCUS identifies the size and depth of soft tissue infections. In rare cases, necrotizing infections can develop in the muscle (necrotizing myositis) and fascial planes (necrotizing fasciitis) and may appear on ultrasound as gas with ring-down artifact. These infections

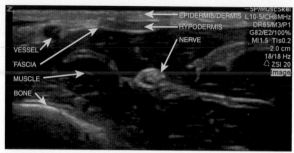

Fig. 27.1 Normal tissue: epidermis/dermis, hypodermis, muscle, fascia, and vessels.

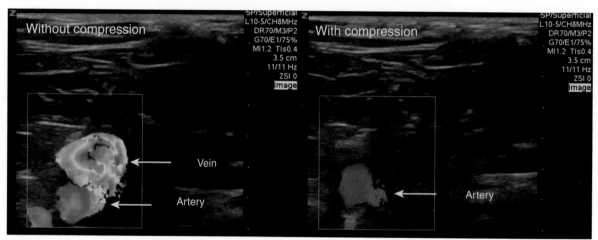

Fig. 27.2 Normal tissue: vessels visualized with color Doppler.

are often rapidly progressive and can be life threatening. Early identification with POCUS should prompt further workup, including emergent surgical consultation.

When evaluating foreign bodies, it is important to identify key anatomic structures in the area, including nerves, blood vessels, tendons, and lymph nodes, to avoid injuring these structures during foreign body removal. Hands and feet are commonly affected, and it may help to review the anatomy of the specific region of interest before removal.

SKIN AND SOFT TISSUE INFECTIONS

Preparation and Technique

1. *Select a transducer.* High-frequency ultrasound provides good resolution at shallow depths, up to about 6 to 8 cm. This is ideal for evaluating most soft tissue infections.
2. *Select a setting.* Most ultrasound machines will have a "soft tissue," "small parts," or similar setting.

3. *Apply gel.* Gel conducts the ultrasound waves, improving the image. For the hands and feet, consider using a water bath. Water is an excellent conductor of sonographic waves and provides very clear images, and the examination is essentially pain free for the patient (Fig. 27.3, Video 27.1). Hold the transducer perpendicular to the skin and keep it approximately 1 to 2 cm above the skin to maximize image quality. If a water bath is not available or feasible, you may choose to scan through a saline bag or a glove filled with water.
4. *Explore deep and shallow fields.* Whereas cellulitis is generally more superficial, abscesses can extend into deeper tissues. It is important to determine the depth of the fluid pocket and its relationship to structures underlying the skin.
5. *Evaluate in two orthogonal planes.* Generally, an area is imaged in both long (sagittal or coronal) and short (transverse) planes. This helps characterize the shape and size of the infection.

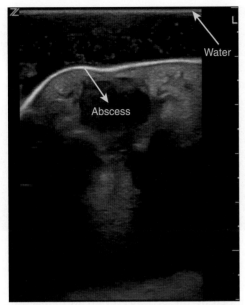

Fig. 27.3 Abscess visualized using a water bath.

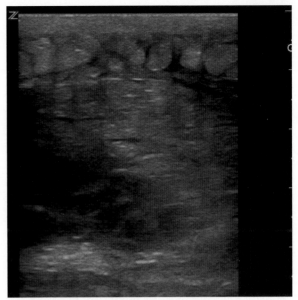

Fig. 27.4 "Cobblestoning" consistent with cellulitis.

6. *Follow the findings.* Trace the fluid collection in all directions to determine the size and extent of the infection.

7. *Identify surrounding anatomy.* This is important for procedural planning. Identify nearby bones, muscles, tendons, nerves, vessels, and lymph nodes. Use color Doppler as appropriate to clarify structures.

Ultrasound Findings

In a patient with cellulitis, the subcutaneous tissue takes on a characteristic "cobblestone" appearance (Fig. 27.4, Video 27.2). Hypoechoic edema in the tissue surrounds and delineates the hyperechoic fat lobules. Note that the fluid seen in cobblestoning thinly outlines the fat lobules, but does not form large pockets.

In contrast, an abscess generally appears as a predominantly anechoic pocket, sometimes with mixed internal echoes caused by fibrinous debris (Fig. 27.5, Video 27.3). These fluid pockets may be well contained with a distinct hyperechoic wall, or they may be more infiltrative, with loculations extending in several directions into the subcutaneous tissue. Adjust your depth to include the bottom of the fluid pocket, and slide the transducer along the skin in two orthogonal planes to visualize the entire abscess cavity. Use the depth markers on the right side of the screen to assess the depth of the fluid collection. Light compression of the

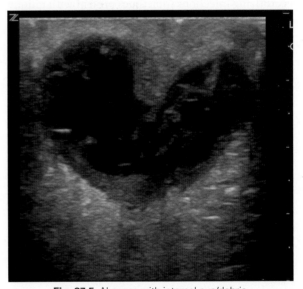

Fig. 27.5 Abscess with internal pus/debris.

abscess may result in a "swirl sign" caused by fibrinous debris moving in the fluid component of the abscess. Cobblestoning may or may not be present in the tissue surrounding the abscess. Abscesses on the hand or foot can be imaged utilizing a water bath (see Fig. 27.3).

Ultrasound is not the best imaging modality to rule in or out necrotizing infections. However,

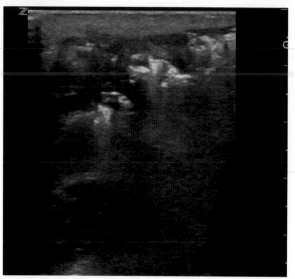

Fig. 27.6 Necrotizing infection suggested by the presence of gas within soft tissue. Note the hyperechoic air followed by ring-down artifact and dirty shadowing.

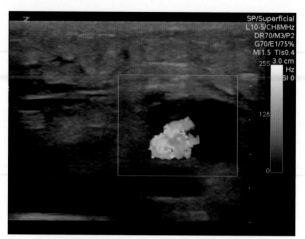

Fig. 27.7 Abscess adjacent to vasculature.

necrotizing infections sometimes present with unique sonographic findings, including gas in the subcutaneous tissue, muscle, or fascial planes (Fig. 27.6, Video 27.4). Small pockets of gas appear on ultrasound as hyperechoic areas with ring-down artifact, causing "dirty" shadowing that obscures the tissue behind the gas. Large accumulations of air may also create reverberation artifacts, with multiple linear hyperechoic repeating horizontal lines. In contrast, "clean" shadowing is seen behind dense structures, such as stones, bones, or calcifications, and has sharply demarcated borders. Fluid overlying the deep fascial layer (≥4 mm) may also suggest necrotizing fasciitis. The absence of these findings does not rule out a necrotizing infection.

Ultrasound-Guided Incision and Drainage

Once an abscess is identified with POCUS, ultrasound can then be used for procedural guidance. This can be done by determining the depth and extension of the fluid pocket using ultrasound, marking the area appropriately, and then proceeding with conventional I&D. Alternatively, the clinician can use a dynamic approach by positioning the probe over the abscess with one hand and making the incision with the other hand. Ultrasound can also be used throughout the procedure to identify loculations and ensure the

abscess has been completely drained, though this may be limited by the presence of air introduced during the procedure.

Pitfalls

Several conditions can mimic an abscess on physical examination, including inflamed lymph nodes, malignant mass, hernia, hemangioma, hematoma, and vascular structures. Color flow can help distinguish an abscess, which should not have flow inside the cavity, from pseudoaneurysm, which may exhibit pulsatile or turbulent flow, and from vascularized structures such as mass or hemangioma (Fig. 27.7, Video 27.5). Inflamed lymph nodes are often tender with overlying erythema and are common abscess mimics. Unlike abscesses, which have an anechoic center, lymph nodes generally have a relatively hyperechoic core and slightly hypoechoic outer cortex, resembling small kidneys (Fig. 27.8, Video 27.6). Finally, interstitial edema associated with cellulitis can be confused with abscess. Cellulitis is not definitively differentiated from fasciitis by ultrasound. POCUS is useful for identifying these before incising the skin.

FOREIGN BODY IDENTIFICATION

Preparation and Technique

The techniques involved in identifying foreign bodies are similar to those described earlier for soft tissue infections. Most foreign bodies are very superficial (less than 2 cm from the surface), so the linear probe

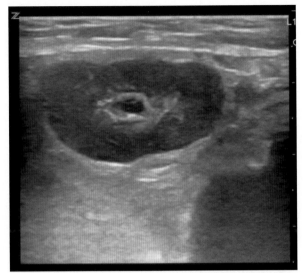

Fig. 27.8 Lymph node: a common abscess mimic. Resembles a small kidney on ultrasound.

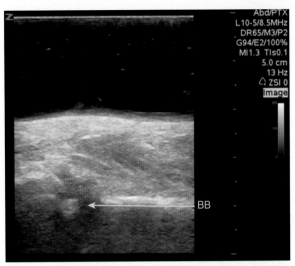

Fig. 27.9 Foreign body: BB in foot with surrounding edema/hematoma.

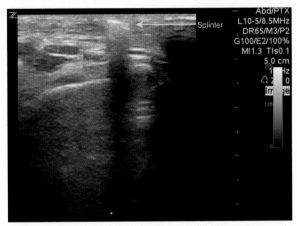

Fig. 27.10 Foreign body: superficial splinter. This image could be improved with the use of a water bath.

is again the transducer of choice. Water baths are especially helpful for imaging the hands and feet, especially when the foreign body is close to the surface (Fig. 27.9, Video 27.7).

Attempt to identify surrounding structures, including bone, tendon, muscle, nerves, and vessels. For extremities, it can be helpful to image the contralateral side for comparison.

Ultrasound Findings

Foreign bodies, including wood, metal, plastic, and glass, appear hyperechoic on ultrasound, usually with clean shadowing (Figs. 27.9 and 27.11). Bones exhibit similar shadowing. Care must be taken not to confuse bone with foreign bodies. The foreign body may be surrounded by a hypoechoic or anechoic rim, representing edema or hematoma.

Ultrasound-Guided Removal

The first step in planning the removal of a foreign body is to identify important anatomy, including nerves, tendons, bone, and vessels. Color flow can enhance the differentiation of some structures. Position the probe over the area of interest, and keep one hand on the probe, maintaining visualization of the foreign body. With the other hand, insert a sterile needle in a long-axis plane and advance until it touches the foreign body. Use a

scalpel to incise along the guide needle, then insert a sterile hemostat in the same plane to grasp the foreign body and pull gently to remove it. If the foreign body moves, reposition the probe as needed.

Pitfalls

Detecting and removing a foreign body has some potential pitfalls. Very small foreign bodies may not be visualized due to limits of ultrasound resolution. Subcutaneous air, either from an open wound or necrotizing infection, can obscure a foreign body, as can overlying hyperechoic structures, such as bone. Hematomas, scar tissue, and sesamoid

TABLE 27.1 Summary of Important Findings

Condition	Common Findings
Cellulitis	Cobblestoning
Abscess	Anechoic pocket or mixed with debris, swirl sign
Foreign body	Hyperechoic, clean shadowing, usually <2 cm deep

bones may mimic other anatomic structures, making localization more challenging. Some anatomic locations, such as web spaces, are difficult to access, complicating both image acquisition and foreign body removal.

SUMMARY

POCUS is a useful bedside tool for identifying skin and soft tissue infections, localizing foreign bodies, and guiding procedures (Table 27.1). Abscess and cellulitis are differentiated, which guides therapy. Foreign bodies, even those that do not appear on X-ray, may be visualized with ultrasound. Procedural guidance with POCUS facilitates safe I&D of abscesses and foreign body removal.

BIBLIOGRAPHY

Barbic D, Chenkin J, Cho DD, Jelic T, Scheuermeyer FX. In patients presenting to the emergency department with skin and soft tissue infections what is the diagnostic accuracy of point-of-care ultrasonography for the diagnosis of abscess compared to the current standard of care? A systematic review and meta-analysis. *BMJ Open.* 2017;7(1):e013688. https://doi.org/10.1136/bmjopen-2016-013688. Review. Erratum in: BMJ Open. 2017;7(9):e013688corr1.

DeAngeles J, St James E, Lema PC. Diagnosis of hand infections in intravenous drug users by ultrasound and water bath: a case series. *Clin Pract Cases Emerg Med.* 2018;2(2):132–135. https://doi.org/10.5811/cpcem.2018.1.36283.

Farrell G, Berona L, Kang T. Point-of-care ultrasound in pyomyositis: a cose series. *Am J Emerg Med.* 2018;36(5):881–884. https://doi.org/10.1016/j.ajem.2017.09.008. Epub 2017 Sep 18.

Fernandez MW, Desai BK. Incision and drainage of peritonsillar abscess. In: Latha G, ed. *Atlas of Emergency Medicine Procedures.* New York: Springer; 2016:347–350.

Gaspari RJ, Sanseverino A, Gleeson T. Abscess incision and drainage with or without ultrasonography: a randomized controlled trial. *Ann Emerg Med.* pii: S0196-0644(18)30451–30457. https://doi.org/10.1016/j.annemergmed.2018.05.014. [Epub ahead of print].

Harris JH, Harris WH. *The Radiology of Emergency Medicine.* 4th ed. Philadelphia: Lippincott Williams & Wilkins; 2000.

Hollinshead WH. *Anatomy for Surgeons.* 3rd ed. Philadelphia: Harper & Row; 1982.

Jones LC, Shafer D. Head, Neck, and orofacial infections in pediatric patients. In: Hupp JR, ed. *Head, Neck, and Orofacial Infections: A Multidisciplinary Approach.* St. Louis, MO: Elsevier; 2016:395–405.

Lin MJ, Neuman M, Rempell R, Monuteaux M, Levy J. Point-of-care ultrasound is associated with decreased length of stay in children presenting to the emergency department with soft tissue infection. *J Emerg Med.* 2018;54(1):96–101. https://doi.org/10.1016/j.jemermed.2017.09.017. Epub 2017 Oct 27.

Ma OJ, Mateer JR. *Emergency Ultrasound.* New York, NY: McGraw-Hill; 2003.

Mapelli E, Sabhaney V. Stridor and drooling in infants and children. In: Tintinalli JE, ed. *Tintinalli's Emergency Medicine: A Comprehensive Study Guide.* New York: McGraw Hill Education; 2016:800–801.

Socransky S, Wiss R, Hall G. *Point-of-Care Ultrasound for Emergency Physicians: "The EDE Book".* Ontario, Canada: Th EDE 2 Course Inc; 2013.

Subramaniam S, Bober J, Chao J, Zehtabchi S. Point-of-care ultrasound for diagnosis of abscess in skin and soft tissue infections. *Acad Emerg Med.* 2016;23(11):1298–1306. https://doi.org/10.1111/acem.13049. Epub 2016 Nov 1. Review.

Varshney T, Kwan CW, Fischer JW, Abo A. Emergency point-of-care ultrasound diagnosis of retained soft tissue foreign bodies in the pediatric emergency department. *Pediatr Emerg Care.* 2017;33(6):434–436. https://doi.org/10.1097/PEC.0000000000001158.

28

Musculoskeletal

Jeremiah W. Ray, Jeffrey L. Tanji

INTRODUCTION

Musculoskeletal ultrasound has become increasingly common over the last two decades. The possibility of a real-time, dynamic imaging modality that is both low cost and safe are among the key driving forces making this an important component of patient care for orthopedic presentations. Ultrasound-guided diagnostic and therapeutic procedures have become the cornerstone of many nonoperative sports medicine practices, as ultrasound guidance increases the efficacy and safety of many bedside procedures. Musculoskeletal ultrasound can be used to diagnose disorders of bone, joints, ligaments, tendons, muscles, nerves, and vascular structures.

TENDINOPATHY VS. TENOSYNOVITIS

For decades, the condition now known as tendinopathy has been incorrectly called *tendinitis* or *tenosynovitis*. Tendinitis was often a "wastebasket" diagnosis, lumping together any injury to a tendon. Largely as a result of the work of Karim Khan, the two conditions have been identified separately as two distinct entities and are treated each in their own way. This distinction is critical to the musculoskeletal ultrasonographer, because each has its own image characteristics, which lead to a distinctly different treatment.

Tendinopathy describes noninflammatory degeneration of a tendon with structural changes more consistent with scar tissue rather than inflammation. At the cellular level, tendinopathy describes chronic, degenerative change to a tendon with eosinophilic infiltration, fibrillar degeneration, and loss of organization of the vascular structure with disorganized tendon structure. Tendinitis or tenosynovitis describes an acute inflammatory process with migration of white blood cells, edema surrounding the tendon, and mobilization of inflammatory mediators.

On musculoskeletal ultrasound imaging, a normal tendon appears as a well-organized linear structure, often described as fibrillar, with an even "copper wire" appearance or the appearance of neatly combed hair (Fig. 28.1).

Tendinopathy takes on the appearance of broken lines, with an uneven, disorganized tendon matrix, often with thickening of the tendon structure showing a hyperechoic signal. On Doppler enhancement, the images will show patchy uptake of circulation, which does not appear with normal tendon (Fig. 28.2).

Tenosynovitis shows a classical anechoic ring in the transverse image of the tendon, the "target sign" consistent with fluid, or edema. Longitudinal images show anechoic fluid surrounding the peroneus longus and peroneus brevis tendons (Fig. 28.3).

ACHILLES TENDON RUPTURE

Achilles tendon rupture is one of the most common and disabling tendon ruptures, typically affecting women and men between the ages of 30 and 50. It occurs when an acute tensile overload is applied to a tendon that has been weakened by chronic, repetitive overuse microtrauma. Tendon weakening is visualized on musculoskeletal ultrasound as anechoic cystic formations embedded in the normal fibrillar tendon appearance on both longitudinal and transverse views (Fig. 28.4). When the tendon has

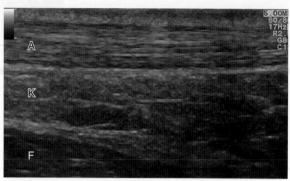

Fig. 28.1 Normal Achilles tendon with even, fibrillar appearance across the top of the figure. *A,* Achilles tendon; *F,* flexor hallucis longus muscle; *K,* Kager fat pad.

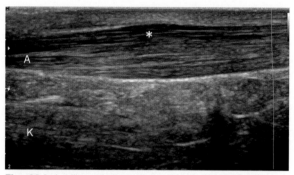

Fig. 28.2 Achilles tendinopathy with thickened tendon and patchy, uneven fibrillar appearance. *A,* Achilles tendon; *K,* Kager fat pad; (*) region of fusiform edema with loss of normal fibrillary appearance.

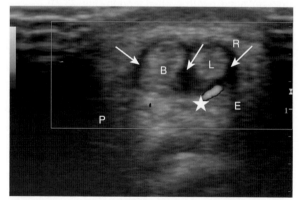

Fig. 28.3 The target sign of anechoic fluid surrounding the peroneus longus and peroneus brevis tendons in transverse view. *Arrows,* Anechoic fluid/edema; *B,* peroneus brevis tendon; *E,* edge artifact; *L,* peroneus longus tendon; *P,* posterior talofibular ligament; *R,* superior peroneal retinaculum; *star,* power angiography demonstrating neovessel formation.

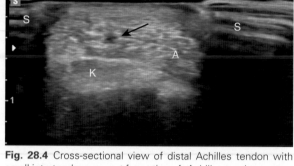

Fig. 28.4 Cross-sectional view of distal Achilles tendon with small intratendonous cyst formation. *A,* Achilles tendon; *arrow,* small anechoic cyst formation; *K,* Kager fat pad; *S,* acoustic standoff pad from ultrasound coupling gel.

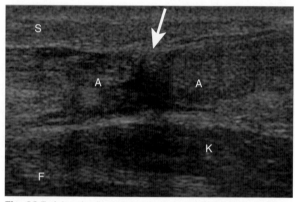

Fig. 28.5 A longitudinal view of a torn Achilles tendon with an anechoic gap. *A,* Two tendon edges of ruptured Achilles tendon; *arrow,* anechoic fluid gap interposed between ruptured Achilles tendon stumps; *F,* flexor hallucis longus tendon; *K,* Kager fat pad; *S,* superficial subcutaneous tissues.

completely or partially ruptured, an anechoic gap is visualized in the longitudinal view that interrupts the fibrillar tendon (Fig. 28.5). Image resolution of the Achilles tendon structure with static and dynamic images is superior to magnetic resonance imaging (MRI) in confirming this diagnosis and can be done in the examination room.

A dynamic Thompson test (squeezing the gastric-soleus muscle complex) will result in the loss of plantarflexion of the ankle on physical examination. This dynamic test can be replicated under real-time imaging of the Achilles tendon in longitudinal orientation, showing an increasing anechoic gap in the tendon structure with manual forced dorsiflexion. Dynamic testing of the Achilles tendon can decrease the false-negative rate of static imaging of a torn Achilles tendon.

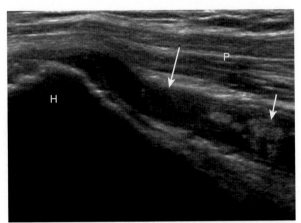

Fig. 28.6 A longitudinal ultrasound view of a proximal biceps tendon tear with anechoic gap. *H*, proximal humerus at level over tuberosities; *long arrow*, anechoic fluid where long head of biceps brachii tendon should lie; *P*, pectoralis muscle at myotendinous junction; *short arrow*, heterogenous clot formation due to tendon rupture.

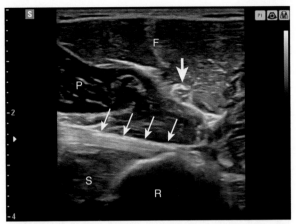

Fig. 28.7 Normal appearance of distal biceps brachii tendon as it inserts upon the radius. *F*, flexor carpi radialis muscle; *multiple thin arrows*, biceps brachii tendon; *P*, pronator teres muscle; *S*, supinator muscle; *single thick arrow*, median nerve.

PROXIMAL BICEPS TENDON RUPTURES

Both acute tensile overload and repetitive microtrauma result in biceps tendon tears. The proximal biceps tendon is the more common location for a tear of the long head of the biceps (97%) compared with distal tears (3%).

Longitudinal views of the long head of the biceps just inferior to the bicipital groove on the anterior humerus can visualize the musculotendinous junction of the biceps muscle and tendon and show the characteristic anechoic gap with a tear (Fig. 28.6). Dynamic testing of the long head of the biceps with internal and external rotation of the humerus often shows the absence of the long head of the biceps tendon within the bicipital groove, a characteristic finding with a complete tear.

DISTAL BICEPS TENDON RUPTURES

Tears of the distal long head of the biceps tendon are far less common than proximal tears but much more difficult to visualize. The Mayo Clinic "pronator window" approach by Jay Smith et al. is our favored diagnostic ultrasound imaging method, where visualization of the absent distal biceps tendon is performed while pronating and supinating the radius and ulna, showing the absence of the tendon. To perform this examination, place the high-frequency transducer on the medial aspect of the forearm over the pronator

muscle and direct the ultrasound beams toward the distal biceps tendon and proximal radius. The transducer is oriented along the long axis of the biceps brachii tendon (Fig. 28.7). As the patient is brought into supination, the insertion of the distal biceps brachii tendon is brought into view.

BAKER'S CYST

Baker's cyst (popliteal cyst) is a common condition affecting approximately 50% of the population above the age of 50. Clinically, it presents as fullness and often tightness and sometimes pain behind the knee with or without trauma. It represents fluid in the bursal sac of the knee that extends posteriorly into an open space. On musculoskeletal ultrasound imaging, it appears on both longitudinal and transverse views as an anechoic, round structure at the intersection of the distal, semimembranosus, and medial head of the gastrocnemius. It is best visualized with the patient in the prone position, with the transducer placed on the medial aspect of the popliteal fossa.

In the differential diagnosis of a popliteal cyst remain the possibilities of a vascular plexus, a ganglion cyst, or a hematoma. Doppler enhancement will generally visualize the vascular plexus, the ganglion cyst will have the classic grapelike appearance, and a hematoma will generally not have the stalk so often seen with a baker's cyst. Careful visualization with the probe both in longitudinal orientation to the leg and then in transverse

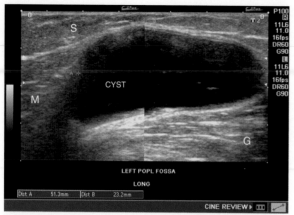

Fig. 28.8 Longitudinal view of baker's cyst in the popliteal fossa. *CYST,* Baker's cyst; *G,* proximal aspect of medial head of gastrocnemius; *M,* distal aspect of semimembranosus; *S,* superficial subcutaneous tissues.

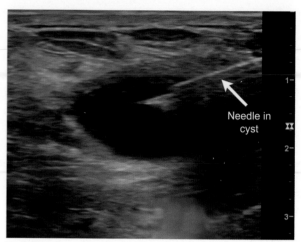

Fig. 28.9 Cyst aspiration. Ultrasound-guided aspiration of a baker's cyst in longitudinal orientation.

orientation will generally help to sort out these other possibilities.

If tender and of significant size (for example, 2–3 cm in diameter), it can be aspirated under ultrasound guidance. The rationale for using ultrasound guidance, besides visualization of the cyst for optimal aspiration, is to avoid reaching the popliteal artery, which can lie just below or adjacent to the cyst. The popliteal artery can be visualized as a pulsatile mass in standard view or enhanced using Doppler (Fig. 28.8).

There is approximately a 12.7% risk of recurrence after successful aspiration, which can be mitigated by a pressure dressing (Ace wrap or Coban). Some will recommend the use of a corticosteroid agent such as triamcinolone or dexamethasone, but there is not a lot of data to support the universal use of this concept.

Generally, a #16- or #18-gauge needle is used to aspirate a baker's cyst after local administration of lidocaine (Fig. 28.9).

JOINT EFFUSIONS

Two of the more common joints where diagnostic ultrasound imaging can be useful to visualize the presence of a moderate-to-large effusion are the knee and elbow. These effusions can be visualized rapidly and effectively compared with MRI imaging and at less cost. Further, if questionable by plain radiographs, the dynamic ultrasound allows movement of the joint to optimally visualize the presence of these effusions.

Knee effusions are best visualized using musculoskeletal ultrasound with the knee bent at about 30 degrees of flexion. The effusion is optimally seen, and loose bodies are also visualized when the knee is held at 30 degrees of flexion. Utilizing both longitudinal and transverse imaging of the joint yields the most accuracy (Fig. 28.10).

Elbow effusions (often an early clue for subtle fracture in children/adolescents) are best visualized with the elbow in 90 degrees of flexion. Place the transducer in a short-axis orientation to the distal aspect of the humerus posteriorly, over the distal triceps tendons. Fluid between the olecranon fossa and the posterior fat pad indicates the presence of an effusion. This visualization of an effusion in the absence of a fracture on plain radiographs is often suggestive of an occult condylar fracture. Elbow loose bodies can also be visualized by ultrasound imaging and are found in number only second to the knee (Fig. 28.11). Description of knee imaging is within the scope of this chapter.

FRACTURE IDENTIFICATION

High-resolution ultrasound possesses excellent sensitivity and negative predictive values for diagnosing short bone and long bone fractures. Ultrasound has proven to be a more sensitive diagnostic modality than plain film radiography in the setting of flat bone evaluation such as rib fractures and scapular fractures. It is important to note that ultrasound is best suited for areas of linear bone evaluation,

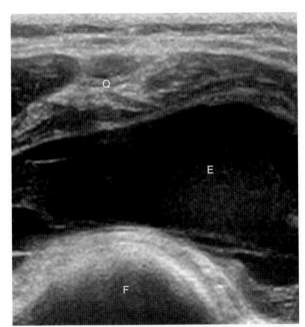

Fig. 28.10 Large knee effusion on ultrasound using the femoral condyle as a landmark. *E*, joint effusion; *F*, femoral condyle; *Q*, distal quadriceps.

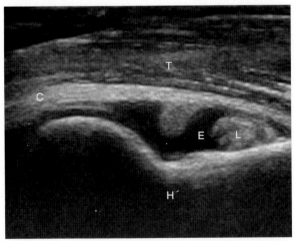

Fig. 28.11 Large elbow effusion by diagnostic ultrasound with loose bodies. *C*, joint capsule; *E*, effusion; *H*, distal aspect of humerus at the level of the olecranon fossa; *L*, loose bodies; *T*, triceps tendon.

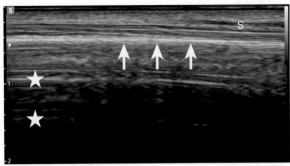

Fig. 28.12 Normal appearance of smooth, hyperechoic cortex with posterior acoustic shadowing and reverberation artifact. *bold arrows*, cortex; *S*, superficial soft tissue; *stars*, reverberation artifact lines.

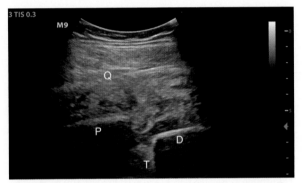

Fig. 28.13 Long-axis view of femur fracture demonstrating throughput artifact. *D*, Distal cortex; *P*, proximal cortex; *Q*, quadriceps muscle; *T*, throughput artifact.

Place the high-frequency linear transducer over the bony cortex where fracture is suspected and sweep in all planes to evaluate the entirety of the cortex.

A fracture appears as an abrupt disruption to the smooth, hyperechoic cortex, oftentimes with angulation of opposing cortices and a hypoechoic subperiosteal hematoma (Fig. 28.13). Outside of the setting of short bones, long bones, and flat bones, ultrasound loses much of its diagnostic accuracy due to incomplete evaluation of the cortical surfaces when neighboring bones block sound wave throughput. Thus a normal ultrasound of carpal bones and tarsal bones does not exclude fracture.

Because fracture identification depends on visualization of a cortical irregularity, ultrasound identifies stress fractures when the injured cortex is amenable to thorough scanning, such as the anterior aspect of the tibia or a metatarsal ray. Bone stress reactions are well visualized on ultrasound, with the development of a hypoechoic

such as diaphyseal and metaphyseal regions of short bones and long bones, and is not well suited for irregular bone evaluation. Normal bone appears as a smooth, hyperechoic, bright cortex with posterior acoustic shadowing and oftentimes with reverberation artifact (Fig. 28.12).

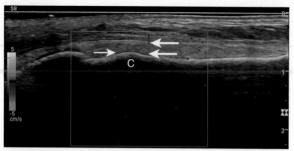

Fig. 28.14 Bone stress fracture showing periosteal thickening with hypoechoic stripe of periosteal edema and callus formation to the distal aspect of the fourth metatarsal diaphysis. *C*, Bony callus formation; *small arrow*, hypoechoic periosteal fluid; *thick arrow*, periosteal thickening.

stripe of periosteal edema, periosteal thickening, and callus formation (Fig. 28.14).

BIBLIOGRAPHY

Breidahl WH, Stafford Johnson DB, Newman JS, Adler RS. Power Doppler sonography in tenosynovitis. *J Ultrasound Med.* 1998;17:103–107.

Elias DA, McKinnon E. The role of ultrasound imaging in acute rupture of the Achilles tendon. *Ultrasound.* 2011;19:70–75.

Fukushima Y, Ray J, Kraus E, Syrop IP, Fredericson M. A Review and Proposed Rationale for the use of Ultrasonography as a Diagnostic Modality in the Identification of Bone Stress Injuries. *J Ultrasound Med.* 2018;37(10):2297–2307.

Herman AM, Marzo JM. Popliteal cysts: a current review. *Orthopedics.* 2014;37:c678–c684.

Hoffman DF, Adams E, Bianchi S. Ultrasonography of fractures in sports medicine. *Br J Sports Med.* 2015;49:152–160.

Hoksrud A, Ohberg L, Alfredson H, et al. Color Doppler ultrasound findings in patellar tendinopathy. *Am Jour Sports Med.* 2008;36:1813–1820.

Keyser R, Mehlfeld K, Heyde CE. Partial rupture of the proximal Achilles tendon: a differential diagnostic problem in ultrasound imaging. *Brit Jour of Sport Med.* 2005;39:878–892.

Khan KM, Cook JL, Taunton JE, Bonar F. Overuse tendinosis, not tendinitis. *Phys Sport Med.* 2000;28:44–49.

Korudin M, Calioglu M, Eris HN, Kayan M, et al. Ultrasound guided percutaneous treatment of Baker's Cyst in knee osteoarthritis. *Eur J Radiol.* 2012;81(11):3466–3471.

Savin DB, Watson J, Youdrian AR, Lee S, et al. Surgical management of distal biceps tendon rupture. *JBJS.* 2017;99:785–796.

Smith J, Finnoff JT, O'Driscoll SW, Lai JK. Sonographic evaluation of the distal biceps tendon using a medial approach. *J Ultrasound Med.* 2010;29:861–865.

Smith MK, Lesniak B, Baraga MC, Kaplan L, et al. Treatment of popliteal cysts with ultrasound guided aspiration. *Sports Health.* 2015;7(5):409–414.

Sunding K, Fahlstrom M, Werner S, Forssblad M, et al. Evaluation of achilles and patellar tendinopathy with grey scale ultrasound and colour doppler ultrasound: a four grade scale. *Knee Surg, Sports Traumatol Arthrosc.* 2016;24:1988–1996.

Thompson T. A test for rupture of the tendo achille. *Acta Orthop Scand.* 1962;32:461–465.

Turk F, Kurt AB, Saglam S. Evaluation by ultrasound of traumatic rib fractures missed by radiography. *Emerg Radiol.* 2010;17:473–477.

Waterbrook AL, Adhikari S, Stolz U, et al. The accuracy of point-of-care ultrasound to diagnose long bone fractures in the ED. *Am J Emerg Med.* 2013;31:1252–1356.

Interventional Techniques

29

Ultrasound-Guided Procedures

Viveta Lobo, Deborah Kimball, Kara M. Kuhn-Riordon

PERICARDIOCENTESIS

Introduction

Performing a pericardiocentesis in an unstable patient with cardiac tamponade is a lifesaving procedure. Pericardial fluid is a common finding on point-of-care echocardiography examination and can occur from many systemic disease processes or trauma. The normal pericardial space usually contains 15 to 50 mL of fluid, which acts as a lubricant between the visceral and parietal layers of the pericardium. An increase in fluid can easily be detected on point-of-care echocardiography and is often present before the onset of clinical symptoms. Clinical symptoms vary greatly and are dependent on the amount and rate of accumulation of the fluid. Cardiac tamponade occurs when cardiac filling is compromised due to compression of the heart by the pericardial fluid. This can occur with either small or large volumes. Signs of impending tamponade on point-of-care echocardiography often reflect the collapsing or "scalloping" thin-walled right atrium and ventricle. This will progress to complete collapse of the right ventricle during diastole, which is the definition of cardiac tamponade on point-of-care echocardiography. Pericardiocentesis removes excessive fluid from the pericardial sac, allowing the heart to fill. This procedure often will be followed by a pericardial window by a cardiac surgeon.

Indications

Patients with significant pericardial effusions with signs or symptoms of cardiac tamponade require emergent pericardiocentesis. Ultrasound guidance is used to increase success and decrease complications of pericardiocentesis and should be considered the standard of care.

Anatomy

The normal anatomy visualized on a subxiphoid point-of-care echocardiography view is seen in Video 29.1. This view will show all four chambers of the heart. Notice the circumferential bright white or hyperechoic pericardium that surrounds the heart. The pericardium is visualized on all four normal point-of-care echocardiography views.

Sonographic Findings

The most commonly used views when performing a pericardiocentesis is the subxiphoid view (Video 29.2) and the parasternal long-axis view (Video 29.3). However, optimal views and approach for the procedure will depend on the patient's position, habitus, and whether the primary operator has assistance while performing the procedure. Other views, like the apical four-chamber view or the parasternal short-axis view, may also be used if they are deemed most optimal.

Pathology

Early cardiac tamponade is seen on the subxiphoid view of the heart in Video 29.4. In early tamponade, the right ventricle free wall is struggling to contract and is noted to be "scalloping." This phenomenon will progress to become complete tamponade, as seen in Video 29.5. In this video of the subxiphoid view, the right ventricle is completely collapsed even during diastole.

Procedure and Technique

If able, appropriate consent should be obtained. The procedure should be explained to the patient and the patient made aware of potential risks that include puncture of the myocardium or coronary artery, pneumopericardium, pneumothorax, arrhythmias, cardiac arrest, infection, or puncture of surrounding structures.

When at all possible, pericardiocentesis should follow sterile conditions, with the operator wearing a gown, gloves, hat, and mask. The ultrasound probe should be draped in a sterile protective cover. Resuscitative equipment and drugs should be readily available at the bedside.

If possible, the patient should be lying with the head of the bed elevated at 30 to 40 degrees to help pool the pericardial fluid. However, if not possible, the patient should lie in the supine position. The chest wall is prepped and draped in sterile fashion. The ideal puncture site will be where the fluid has collected the most and is closest to the chest wall. It is recommended that multiple views be assessed before selecting the optimal site. For a subxiphoid approach, use a phased array probe (5–1 MHz) that is placed in a sterile probe cover and a 16- to 18-gauge needle as demonstrated in Fig. 29.1. Note the needle is parallel and adjacent to the probe and directed at a 45-degree angle toward the left scapula tip. The needle will appear on the screen as a hyperechoic structure with reverberation artifact as it is advanced toward the pericardium (Video 29.6). If using the parasternal long-axis approach, the position will look like Fig. 29.2. The needle should be inserted at a 45-degree angle in-plane to the probe on the anterior chest wall and directed down toward the effusion (Video 29.7). In any approach, make sure to aspirate every 1 to 2 mm as the needle is advanced and that the needle tip is visualized the entire time on the screen until fluid is obtained. To confirm placement, use the "activated saline technique." To do this, simply inject agitated saline through the needle, creating a "snowstorm appearance" within the pericardial effusion and confirming placement within the pericardial sac.

Complications

Complication rates for ultrasound-guided pericardiocentesis have reported to be between 1.2% and 4.7%. The parasternal long-axis view is considered advantageous over the subxiphoid approach, as it allows for visualization of the heart in the same plane as the needle, in addition to being in closer proximity to the effusion. It also avoids other vital structures like the lung and liver.

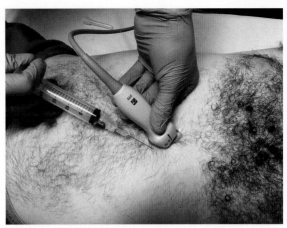

Fig. 29.1 Ultrasound probe and position of needle entry in subxiphoid approach. When using the subxiphoid approach to guide the pericardiocentesis procedure, the needle should be inserted parallel to the probe and directed at a 45-degree angle toward the left scapula tip.

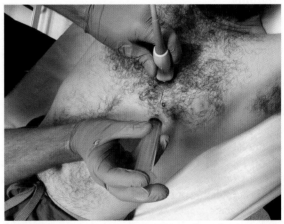

Fig. 29.2 Ultrasound probe and position of needle entry in the parasternal long-axis approach. When using the parasternal approach to guide the pericardiocentesis procedure, the needle should enter adjacent to the ultrasound probe and directed toward the effusion.

PARACENTESIS

Introduction

Ascites is accumulation of fluid in the peritoneum. Paracentesis involves aspirating ascitic fluid from the peritoneal cavity. This is done either for diagnostic or therapeutic purposes. Emergent diagnostic paracentesis involves removing a small amount of ascitic fluid to evaluate for spontaneous bacterial peritonitis (SBP). A therapeutic paracentesis involves removing a large volume of ascitic fluid, typically several liters, from a patient who is symptomatic due to the presence of the ascites.

Indications

A patient with ascites presenting with abdominal pain, fever, altered mental status, diarrhea, or any of a variety of other symptoms may have inflammation of the peritoneum, or peritonitis. Peritonitis is usually caused by a bacterial or fungal infection. When there is clinical concern for peritonitis, a diagnostic paracentesis should be performed and the fluid analyzed.

Patients can also accumulate a large volume of ascites that causes severe pain, respiratory compromise, and early satiety. This requires therapeutic paracentesis to relieve the patient's symptoms. If there is no concern for peritonitis, the fluid collected does not need to be analyzed.

Anatomy

To determine whether there is ascites, use the curvilinear probe (5–2 MHz). When there is no ascites in the abdomen, the peritoneal cavity is composed of gas-filled bowel. Video 29.8 shows a normal right upper quadrant of the abdomen without ascites.

Sonographic Findings

When simple ascites is present, anechoic fluid can be seen accumulating around peritoneal structures, forming a "pointed" or "triangular" shape. Video 29.9 demonstrates fluid surrounding the liver. Video 29.10 demonstrates fluid accumulating posterior to the bladder in the pelvis. Note the acute angles as the fluid accumulates around fixed structures. Video 29.11 demonstrates bowel floating in large-volume ascites.

Ultrasound guidance can improve the procedure by localizing the largest pocket of fluid available, identifying structures such as organs and vessels to avoid, or confirming a sufficient amount of ascitic fluid for a successful procedure. Ultrasound-guided paracentesis has been associated with fewer rates of adverse events, including postparacentesis infection, hematoma, and seroma.

Ultrasound can be used statically or dynamically during a paracentesis. With static use of ultrasound, the most accessible and deepest pocket of fluid is identified just before the procedure and marked on the patient. With dynamic use of ultrasound, the ultrasound is used during the procedure. Dynamic use of ultrasound requires more dexterity in holding the ultrasound probe with one hand while aspirating with the other. However, an assistant can also help by holding the ultrasound probe during the procedure. The preference for dynamic or static ultrasound guidance will be at the discretion of the clinician performing the procedure.

An ideal pocket of fluid identified on ultrasound will be at least 3 cm deep, measured from the peritoneal lining of the abdominal wall. As the curvilinear probe is used to identify the pocket of fluid for aspiration, continue to use this probe dynamically during the procedure. Decrease the depth so that the view is more superficial and so that it can be ascertained if there are abdominal wall structures such as blood vessels, especially the epigastric arteries that tend to course through this region, or other fluid collections that should be avoided. Some clinicians may prefer to identify the pocket of ascites with the curvilinear probe, then use the high-frequency linear probe dynamically (Video 29.12) with greater resolution to better visualize the needle and evaluate the abdominal wall to avoid puncturing blood vessels (Video 29.13).

Pathology

Distinguishing between SBP and large-volume ascites can be difficult clinically. Early paracentesis and treatment of SBP improves mortality. Diagnosis of SBP is made through laboratory analysis of the ascitic fluid aspirated during paracentesis. Fluid should be sent for cell count and differential, Gram stain, and culture. SBP is defined as having a polymorphonuclear count (PMN $\geq 250/m^3$) in ascitic fluid. Studies have shown high predictive value in the rapid diagnosis of SBP using a leukocyte esterase reagent strip test.

Procedure and Technique

Once the clinical concern for SBP exists, the only true contraindication to performing a paracentesis is a surgical cause of SBP. These cases need to be treated operatively. Although there is frequently cited clinical concern regarding the hypercoagulable state of the patient with ascites, large studies have demonstrated no significant procedure-related complications even with elevated international normalized ratio (INR) or thrombocytopenia.

Explain the procedure to the patient and obtain informed consent. Ask the patient to urinate immediately before the procedure to decompress the bladder. If the patient cannot spontaneously void, consider placing a urinary catheter before the procedure to decompress the bladder. If performing therapeutic paracentesis, place the patient on a monitor.

Gather supplies to perform a sterile technique. Paracentesis kits are commercially available. If these are not available, the supplies required are readily available in most emergency departments.

Place the patient in a position of comfort, typically supine or in a lateral decubitus position, depending on the optimal location for the paracentesis.

Assess the location of the liver, spleen, bowel, and bladder. Preferentially, it should be performed in the left or right lower quadrant 5 cm cephalad and medial to the anterior superior iliac spine (Fig. 29.3). Alternatively, the procedure can be done 2 cm below the umbilicus; however, the risk of iatrogenic bladder perforation is higher in this location (Fig. 29.4). Once the location for paracentesis has been identified, do not move the patient. If the patient is moved, repeat the ultrasound.

Cleanse and prep the skin in a sterile fashion. Cover the ultrasound probe with a sterile probe cover and again identify the pocket of fluid to aspirate. Create a wheal of anesthesia using a small 25- to 27-gauge needle, then exchange the needle for a larger 18- to 20-gauge and anesthetize down to the peritoneal layer. Pull the skin taut while inserting the large-bore needle perpendicular to the skin at the site of entry. Once the peritoneal lining has been penetrated, aspirate fluid into the syringe. Then release the taut skin. This will create a "Z"-tract down to the peritoneal layer, which will help to seal the tract after the procedure and decrease spontaneous leakage of peritoneal fluid. Next, exchange the syringe for a larger syringe for fluid collection. Remove the amount of ascites fluid desired. If performing a therapeutic paracentesis, consider using a larger blunt cannula housed over a hollow needle with side holes for the procedure after providing adequate anesthesia. However, if this is unavailable, using a larger needle with a stopcock is acceptable for therapeutic paracentesis. For therapeutic paracentesis, insert a stopcock into

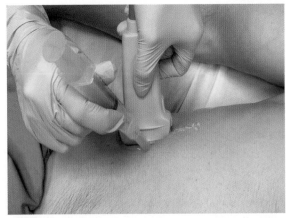

Fig. 29.3 Right and left lower quadrant approach to paracentesis under ultrasound guidance. The ultrasound probe is placed in the left or right lower quadrant 5 cm cephalad and medial to the anterior superior iliac spine.

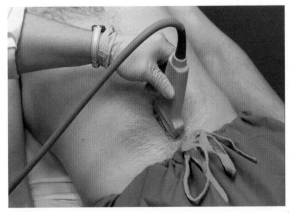

Fig. 29.4 Midline approach to paracentesis under ultrasound guidance. An alternative approach can be placing the probe 2 cm below the umbilicus; however, the risk of iatrogenic bladder perforation is higher in this location.

the cannula, connect to tubing, and hang to gravity. Use of a vacuum container can improve the rate of flow of the fluid. Remove the needle. Place a bandage over the puncture site. Assess the patient for immediate complications and again within 30 minutes for complications such as leakage.

Complications

Complications from a paracentesis are uncommon. They include hemorrhage, hematoma, persistent ascitic fluid leakage, peritonitis, perforation of bowel or bladder, liver or splenic puncture, epigastric artery pseudoaneurysm, and shearing of the catheter. Therapeutic paracentesis can cause hypotension or hyponatremia. Using sterile technique with ultrasound guidance will minimize these potential complications.

THORACENTESIS

Introduction

A pleural effusion is fluid that accumulates in the thoracic cavity between the parietal pleura, which abuts the chest wall, and the visceral pleura, which surrounds the lung parenchyma. This occurs most commonly from heart failure, malignancies, infections, or pulmonary embolism. Signs and symptoms of a pleural effusion include chest pain, shortness of breath, cough, tachypnea, and hypoxia. However, at times a pleural effusion may be asymptomatic. In these instances, appropriate diagnosis is still warranted. Thoracentesis involves aspirating pleural fluid from the thoracic cavity. This is done either for diagnostic or therapeutic purposes. The use of ultrasound to perform thoracentesis reduces costs and complications.

Indications

Diagnostic thoracentesis is performed on new accumulations of pleural fluid or for concern for infection of a pleural effusion. Therapeutic thoracentesis entails removing a larger volume of fluid for patient comfort. In the emergency department, this procedure can be lifesaving when performed for the patient with respiratory compromise.

Anatomy

Ultrasound imaging of the right or left upper quadrant in the oblique coronal view at the midaxillary line during the focused assessment with sonography for trauma (FAST) examination may reveal an anechoic or hypoechoic fluid collection above the echogenic diaphragm. Fig. 29.5 shows the normal anatomy at the right upper quadrant. Fig. 29.6 shows a pleural effusion in the thoracic cavity.

Sonographic Findings

Ultrasound has repeatedly been shown to be more sensitive in detecting pleural fluid than plain film radiography. Small quantities of pleural fluid that can more readily be seen with ultrasound may not be amenable to thoracentesis. As such, it is important to scan through

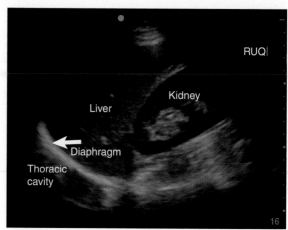

Fig. 29.5 Ultrasound of the normal right upper quadrant. In this image, the normal anatomy of the right upper quadrant can be identified. Be sure to avoid puncturing the diaphragm during thoracentesis.

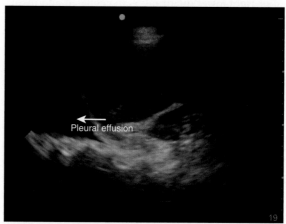

Fig. 29.6 Ultrasound of the left upper quadrant. A pleural effusion above the diaphragm can still be seen.

the entire thoracic cavity to delineate the extent of the pleural effusion. Ultrasound guidance is associated with a decreased number of attempts, which in turn reduces the rates of complications. Using a phased array (5–1 MHz) or curvilinear (5–2 MHz) probe, position the ultrasound probe perpendicular to the skin so as to avoid overestimating or underestimating distances, which can occur by angling the probe obliquely. Scan vertically from the inferior portion of the scapula to the upper lumbar region. Scan laterally from the paravertebral region to the posterior axillary line. An adequate pleural effusion appropriate for thoracentesis should measure at least 10 mm deep from the parietal pleura to the visceral pleura (Fig. 29.7, Video 29.14). Mark the extent of the effusion with ink. Evaluate the effusion with M-mode (Fig. 29.8), looking for a region where lung parenchyma is visualized at least 10 mm away from the parietal pleura during several respiratory cycles. With ink or a needle cap, mark the intercostal space for thoracentesis. One guide is to approach the effusion at least one intercostal space inferior to the most superior extent of the effusion for a diagnostic thoracentesis and two to three intercostal spaces for a therapeutic thoracentesis, always heeding caution to avoid the diaphragm.

Measure the depth from the surface to the parietal pleura, accounting for any potential compression of the subcutaneous tissue by the pressure of the ultrasound probe. Ensure that your equipment is long enough to penetrate through the tissue and into the thoracic cavity safely.

In the mechanically ventilated patient, due to the alteration in the intrathoracic pressures, some experts suggest only performing thoracentesis if the distance from the parietal to the visceral pleural is greater than 15 mm and the fluid is visible over at least three intercostal spaces.

Be sure to identify surrounding structures, including the diaphragm, spleen or liver, lung, chest wall, heart, and descending aorta, before any needle insertion. Document the presence of lung sliding or B-lines before the procedure (Fig. 29.9, Video 29.15). This will provide a postprocedural comparison when evaluating for lack of lung sliding due to pneumothorax.

Pathology

Up to 20 mL of pleural fluid can be found in the thoracic cavity to allow for free movement between the lung and the chest wall. Greater amounts can accumulate for aforementioned reasons. A pleural effusion is classified as transudative or exudative based upon a set of criteria. Transudative effusions typically require no further diagnostic evaluation. However, exudative effusions arise from diseases such as malignancies and infections and thus warrant further investigation.

A diagnostic thoracentesis involves aspirating a small volume of fluid to be sent for analysis, typically less than 50 mL. Common studies to obtain include cell count and differential, protein level, glucose level, lactate dehydrogenase (LDH) level, pH level, cytology, culture, and sensitivities. Simultaneously obtain serum samples for LDH and protein for comparison.

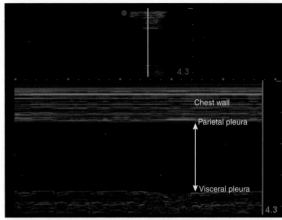

Fig. 29.7 Ultrasound of the effusion in M-mode. In this figure, M-mode is used to identify the distance between the parietal and visceral pleura to ensure adequate depth to perform thoracentesis.

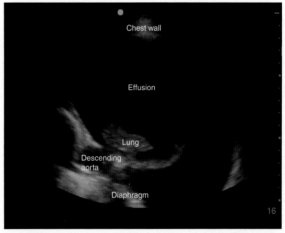

Fig. 29.8 Ultrasound of effusion with phased array probe. In this ultrasound, the extent of the pleural effusion and the nearby structures to avoid can be seen.

Procedure and Technique

As able, obtain informed consent from the patient. In the cooperative patient, have him or her sit upright, leaning forward over a bedside table. Approach approximately 5 to 10 cm lateral to the spine, ultimately guided by the location determined with the ultrasound as previously described (Fig. 29.10). If the patient cannot tolerate this position, you can perform the procedure with the patient lying supine or in the lateral decubitus position. If supine, approach at the midaxillary line with the patient's ipsilateral arm abducted, elbow flexed,

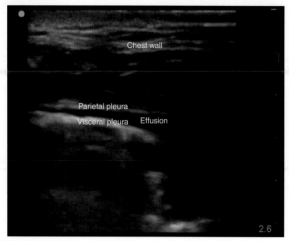

Fig. 29.9 Ultrasound with linear probe chest wall. Ultrasound of lung sliding and pleural effusion to rule out pneumothorax before thoracentesis.

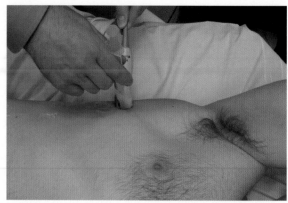

Fig. 29.11 Lateral decubitus position to thoracentesis using phased array probe. With the patient lying supine or in the lateral decubitus position, approach at the midaxillary line with the patient's ipsilateral arm abducted, elbow flexed, and hand behind the head.

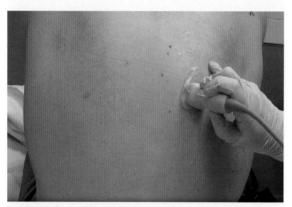

Fig. 29.10 Posterior approach to thoracentesis using a phased array probe. Approach approximately 5 to 10 cm lateral to the spine above the diaphragm to assess for the location and amount of pleural fluid.

and hand behind the head as if performing a tube thoracostomy (Fig. 29.11). If the lateral decubitus position is used, have the patient lie down on the side with the effusion and approach dorsally.

Perform the ultrasound immediately before the procedure. Ensure the patient does not move after the ultrasound is performed. More commonly, the ultrasound is used statically to identify the effusion. However, the ultrasound can be used intraprocedurally as well. Be sure to use sterile technique, including a sterile probe cover.

Identify the intercostal space for the thoracentesis. Use a 25-gauge needle to create a wheal of anesthesia

with lidocaine. Then exchange for a 21- or 22-gauge needle to anesthetize through the subcutaneous tissue to the rib. March along the superior aspect of the lower rib of the intercostal space to anesthetize the tissue, and avoid puncturing the neurovascular bundle on the inferior aspect of the rib. Aspirate as injecting and advancing. Once aspirating pleural fluid, stop advancing the needle and inject anesthesia to anesthetize the parietal pleura. Note the depth of the pleural cavity. Make a cut through the epidermis using an #11 blade scalpel to allow insertion of an 18-gauge, over-the-needle catheter attached to a syringe, commonly found in thoracentesis kits. Slowly advance over the superior aspect of the rib while aspirating continuously for negative pressure. Once pleural fluid is aspirated, stop advancing the needle and advance the catheter. Remove the needle and place a finger over the hub to prevent air entry. For diagnostic thoracentesis, attach a 60-mL syringe and aspirate. For therapeutic thoracentesis, attach a large syringe with stopcock closed to the outside and aspirate fluid for analysis as desired. Thoracentesis kits supply tubing to allow gravity drainage of the effusion. To avoid adverse intrathoracic pressures, place the drainage tubing and bag no more than 30 cm vertical distance from the catheter. When the desired volume of fluid has been removed, remove the catheter and syringe while the patient is holding their breath at end expiration. Cover the puncture site with an occlusive dressing. Evaluate for a pneumothorax using the ultrasound at multiple intercostal spaces.

Complications

The most common clinically significant complication is pneumothorax. Without the use of ultrasound, the rate of pneumothorax has been reported to occur up to 30% of the time, one-third of which generally require tube thoracostomy. However, with ultrasound performed by experienced operators, that rate drops to less than 3%. Other complications include pain, bleeding such as hematoma, hemothorax, hemoperitoneum, empyema, soft tissue infection; diaphragm, liver, or spleen puncture; vasovagal episode, shortness of breath, cough, and re-expansion pulmonary edema. One study showed a significant increase in rate of complications when volumes larger than 1.8 L are removed.

FOREIGN BODY REMOVAL

Introduction

Identification and removal of a superficial foreign body is a common and challenging chief complaint in the emergency department. Delay in identification or removal of foreign bodies has been shown to increase associated pain, infection, and inflammation. Injuries that have been left untreated will often require multiple physician visits, and possibly hospitalization with surgical intervention. Until the use of point-of-care ultrasonography, plain film radiography was the main mode of imaging to assess soft tissue foreign body injuries. Whereas metal and glass are radiopaque objects and promptly visualized on plain film radiography, wood and plastic are often radiolucent and will go undetected. Ultrasonography has been shown to be a reliable diagnostic mode when evaluating foreign body soft tissue injuries, as well as for guiding the removal of such objects. It has proven to be superior to plain film radiography and can detect radiopaque as well as radiolucent objects such as wood and plastic, with sensitivities as high as 94% to 98%. As with all ultrasound techniques, it is especially important to be able to first recognize normal soft tissue appearance on sonography before learning pathology. Most foreign bodies appear hyperechoic with specifically associated artifacts based on their composition and makeup. Refer to Chapter 27 for further reading on soft tissue ultrasound.

Indications

Patients with a history of retained foreign bodies should undergo point-of-care ultrasound evaluation to confirm and localize the reported structure. In addition,

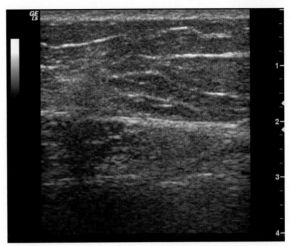

Fig. 29.12 Normal soft tissue appearance on sonography. Using the linear probe over the peripheral arm, notice the multiple distinct layers separated by hyperechoic fascial lines.

ultrasound should be used to assist in removal and verify a successful procedure.

Anatomy

Normal soft tissue appearance on sonography is shown in Fig. 29.12. Notice the clear distinction of multiple layers separated by hyperechoic fascia. Depending on location, it is also important to reliably recognize nearby normal structures, such as nerve bundles, vascular structures, muscle, or tendons. Changes in the tissue due to infection, inflammation, or abscess will alter this appearance (see Chapter 27).

Pathology

Sonographic appearance for soft tissue foreign bodies will vary depending on several factors, including composition, size, and length of time embedded. Material such as wood, glass, metal, plastic, and gravel often appears hyperechoic with posterior shadowing (Video 29.16). However, foreign bodies that have been retained for over one day may develop a hypoechoic "halo" due to surrounding inflammatory changes (Fig. 29.13, Video 29.17).

Procedure and Technique

Soft tissue ultrasound will often require a high-frequency (13–6 MHz) linear array probe. Given the superficial location of most foreign objects, a linear probe will likely be the optimal choice; however, alternative choices may be used for deeper objects. In addition, the examination

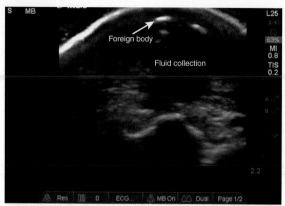

Fig. 29.13 Foreign bodies that have been retained for more than 1 day may develop a hypoechoic "halo" due to surrounding inflammatory changes.

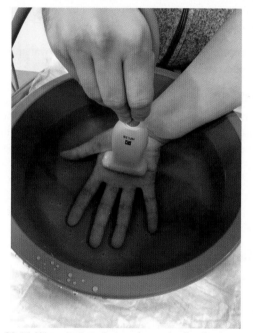

Fig. 29.14 Water bath technique for evaluating foreign bodies with point-of-care ultrasound. Submerging the injured extremity in water will eliminate the need for gel when performing the ultrasound and will create a high-resolution image for better evaluation.

can be performed in a water bath (Fig. 29.14). This technique replaces the need for ultrasound gel or contact between the ultrasound probe and the patient's skin, often eliminating any discomfort they may experience, and also leading to higher-resolution images (Video 29.18).

To assess for a foreign body, place the linear transducer over the injury or the assumed entrance site if visible. Once the foreign body is identified, evaluate it in both longitudinal and transverse axes, and measure its length and width, respectively. This will allow evaluation of its position and orientation, as well detection of any fragments alongside. Take note of any adjacent structures such as nerve bundles, vascular structures, muscle, or tendons, and their relative location to the foreign body. Next, identify the closest distance of the object in longitudinal axis from the skin's surface and mark the skin; this will be the entry point for removal. If an entry site is visible, irrigate the wound generously with water or saline if available. The skin is then disinfected using chlorhexidine or an alcohol swab. If a water bath is not being used, the transducer should be placed in a sterile sheath or glove. Apply gel to the skin surface and reidentify the object over the previously marked skin. If available, local anesthesia may be used under ultrasound guidance and directed close to the foreign body. Using a #11 blade scalpel, a small incision as wide as the width of the previously measured foreign body should be made over the skin marking. A large-bore needle can be used if the object is small. Using forceps and direct visualization, bluntly dissect a path toward the tip of the foreign body and grasp it. Next, gently retract the object to the skin surface, and once removed, confirm with ultrasound that the complete object, as well as any fragments or pieces, was removed. Video 29.19 demonstrates removal of a retained wooden piece under ultrasound guidance and a large-bore needle.

Irrigate the wound again and allow it to heal by secondary intention. Antibiotics may be considered based on the risk of infection, and a tetanus vaccination may be given. Patients should follow up within 1 week for wound recheck to their primary care provider.

Complications

The major limitation to point-of-care ultrasonography for foreign body detection is due to operator inexperience or error. Novice users may miss visualizing foreign bodies or incorrectly identify or measure them, setting them up for failure when attempting removal. Very shallow objects may also be hard to detect due to poor nearfield resolution; however, using the water bath technique as described may improve their successful identification. Subcutaneous air, either from an open wound or necrotizing infection, can obscure foreign bodies, as can overlying hyperechoic structures, such as bone. Hematomas, scar tissue, and sesamoid bones may mimic other anatomic structures, making localization more challenging. Some anatomic locations, such as web spaces, are difficult to access, complicating both image acquisition and foreign body removal.

NEONATAL PERIPHERALLY INSERTED CENTRAL CATHETER LINE

Clinical Correlation

Peripherally inserted central catheters (PICCs) are often placed in neonates in need of long-term access, especially those with a surgical abdomen or those too old for or with unsuccessful umbilical access. Ultrasound has been shown to be useful both during placement and after to identify tip position.

Normal Anatomy

PICCs are most commonly placed in the extremities but may also be placed in scalp veins when vascular access is limited. The ideal tip position is at the superior vena cava (SVC)–right atrial (RA) junction, or within the SVC for upper extremity or scalp PICCs. Lower extremity PICC tip position is ideally placed in the intraabdominal inferior vena cava (IVC) as far cephalad as the IVC–RA junction.

Imaging

PICC visualization with ultrasound can be difficult in neonates due to the small diameter of the catheters used. In the smallest of the catheters, the tip may appear as a hyperechoic dot separated from the hyperechoic parallel lines of the remainder of the catheter.

Ultrasound imaging is typically performed with a high-frequency microconvex transducer (5–10 MHz). For lower extremity PICCs, the patient is positioned supine and the probe is placed over the right upper quadrant and epigastric area. Sagittal and transverse views are utilized with the liver as an acoustic window to identify the IVC–RA junction and PICC tip position (Fig. 29.15). When examining upper extremity or scalp PICCs, parasternal, subcostal, and apical views may be utilized to identify the SVC–RA junction.

Careful attention should be paid to thermoregulation of the infant during the ultrasound study. Warm gel should be utilized, and warm blankets may be used to cover exposed areas as needed. Careful cleaning of the infant after the study to remove all gel is essential.

Pathology/Troubleshooting

Real-time scanning while moving the extremity from which the PICC originates can be useful for tip identification, especially in the smallest of catheters. Adduction of the arm and elbow flexion will move an upper extremity catheter into deeper position, and hip flexion can bring a lower extremity catheter into deeper position.

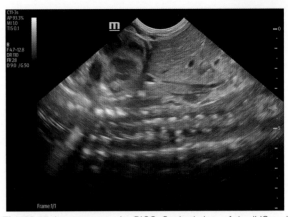

Fig. 29.15 Lower extremity PICC. Sagittal view of the IVC and heart with PICC visible as hyperechoic parallel lines terminating at the IVC–RA junction.

PICCs have many known complications, which increase with improper catheter tip position. PICC tips within the right atrium have caused arrhythmias, myocardial erosions, pericardial effusions, and tamponade. Other complications include pleural effusions, ascites, and thrombophlebitis. Noncentral PICCs also have a significantly higher rate of complications, especially infection, thrombus, and extravasation of infusing fluids or medications. Ultrasound can identify many of these complications, but clinical suspicion is essential.

NEONATAL UMBILICAL CATHETERS

Clinical Correlation

Very low birth weight and other critically ill neonates often require central venous access for parenteral nutrition, hypertonic medications or fluids, and blood sampling. Arterial access is also often necessary to obtain accurate blood gas measurements and arterial blood pressure monitoring. This access is most often accomplished via umbilical venous and arterial catheter placement. Umbilical venous and arterial catheters are placed under sterile conditions, and ultrasound may be utilized in real time during placement or after placement to interrogate tip position.

Normal Anatomy

Umbilical venous catheters (UVCs) enter the umbilical vein at the site of insertion, coursing cephalad and posteriorly in the midline to the left portal vein, through the ductus venosus to one of the hepatic veins and into the IVC, with the ideal tip location at the IVC–RA junction (Fig. 29.16).

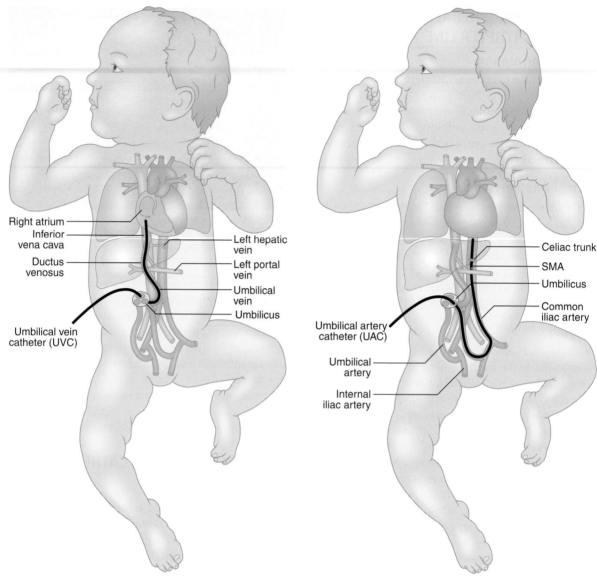

Fig. 29.16 UVC course.   **Fig. 29.17** UAC course.

Umbilical arterial catheters (UACs) enter the umbilical artery at the site of insertion, coursing caudally to the internal iliac artery, making a hairpin turn cephalad to the common iliac artery, and into the descending aorta (Fig. 29.17). The UAC tip should avoid major aortic branch takeoffs and may be in either high or low placement. The ideal tip location for high UAC placement is between the left subclavian artery and the celiac artery, which is traditionally identified by the T6–T10 vertebral levels on X-ray. Low UAC placement is between the renal arteries and the bifurcation of the aorta, at L3–L5 vertebral levels on X-ray.

Placement depth is estimated using one of several commonly accepted methods, including a regression equation using birth weight or shoulder-to-umbilicus distance. These estimations are frequently inaccurate, and many practitioners inserting lines intentionally place them deeper than the estimated distance, so the catheters may then be retracted to optimal positioning after imaging. There are several rare, but important, risks of deep insertion,

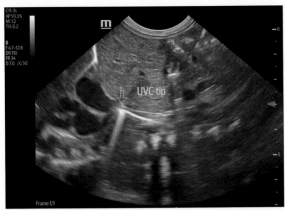

Fig. 29.18 Umbilical venous catheter. Sagittal view of the IVC and heart with UVC visible as hyperechoic parallel lines terminating at the IVC–RA junction.

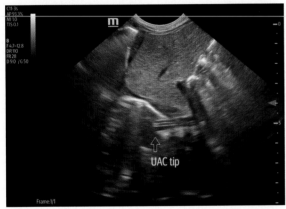

Fig. 29.19 Umbilical arterial catheter. Sagittal view of the thoracic aorta with the UAC visible in the descending thoracic aorta.

including arrhythmias, myocardial perforation, and pericardial tamponade. Additionally, UVCs placed deeply in the right atrium may pass across the patent foramen ovale into the left atrium and wedge into one of the pulmonary veins, which may contribute to acquired pulmonary vein stenosis.

Imaging

Historically, X-rays have been considered the gold standard for verifying umbilical catheter position, and vertebral levels have been used to guide tip location. Studies have shown that vertebral-level landmarks are not reliable, and a properly placed UVC tip may appear between T6 and T11 on X-ray. Ultrasound has been shown to be superior

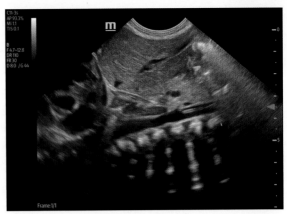

Fig. 29.20 Improperly positioned umbilical venous catheter. Sagittal view of the ductus venosus and IVC with UVC tip visible within the ductus venosus.

in both sensitivity and specificity for detecting umbilical catheter tips, particularly when they are malpositioned.

Ultrasound imaging is typically performed with a high-frequency microconvex transducer (5–10 MHz). The patient is positioned supine, and the probe is placed over the right upper quadrant and epigastric area using sagittal and transverse views, with the liver as an acoustic window to identify the IVC–RA junction, examining for UVC tip position. When examining high UACs, using an approach like that for UVC position can be useful; alternatively, sagittal views near the sternum can identify the descending thoracic aorta. Low UACs can be best visualized with coronal views via the flank, revealing the retroperitoneal aorta and avoiding bowel gas that often makes imaging difficult from ventral approaches.

Catheters appear as parallel, echogenic double lines when visualized in longitudinal/long-axis views and as an echogenic dot in transverse/short-axis views (Figs. 29.18 and 29.19). If unable to visualize tip position, a sterile saline flush may be utilized to create turbulent flow, which is easily seen with ultrasound. Additionally, flexion of the neonate's hips and knees can move the catheter tip into a deeper location, making visualization easier in real-time scanning.

Pathology/Troubleshooting

A UVC tip not identified in the IVC or IVC–RA junction may not have passed through the ductus venosus (Fig. 29.20) and may reside in the portal venous system, hepatic veins, and sometimes the splenic or superior mesenteric vein.

A UAC tip not identified in the abdominal or thoracic aorta may have coiled on itself in the common iliac artery or may have traversed into the ipsilateral femoral artery.

Of note, UVC placement may introduce a small amount of air into the portal venous system, which could be visualized as tiny, hyperechoic foci/bubbles within the portal venous system. This should not be confused with a diagnosis of necrotizing enterocolitis, as there will be no evidence of pneumatosis intestinalis secondary to UVC placement.

Thrombi may form along the course of the catheters and would be visible on ultrasound.

BIBLIOGRAPHY

Blaivas M, Lyon M, Brannam L, Duggal S, Sierzenski P. Water bath evaluation technique for emergency ultrasound of painful superficial structures. *Am J Emerg Med.* 2004;22(7):589–593.

Fleming SE, Kim JH. Ultrasound-guided umbilical catheter insertion in neonates. *J Perinatol.* 2011;31(5):344–349.

Goldwasser B, Baia C, Kim M, Taragin BH, Angert RM. Non-central peripherally inserted central catheters in neonatal intensive care: complication rates and longevity of catheters relative to tip position. *Pediatr Radiol.* 2017;47(12):1676–1681.

Graham DD. Ultrasound in the emergency department: detection of wooden foreign bodies in the soft tissues. *J Emerg Med.* 2002;22(1):75–79.

Jain A, McNamara PJ, Ng E, El-Khuffash A. The use of targeted neonatal echocardiography to confirm placement of peripherally inserted central catheters in neonates. *Am J Perinatol.* 2012;29(2):101–106.

Karber BC, Nielsen JC, Balsam D, Messina C, Davidson D. Optimal radiologic position of an umbilical venous catheter tip as determined by echocardiography in very low birth weight newborns. *J Neonatal Perinatal Med.* 2017;10(1):55–61.

Lichtenstein D, Hulot JS, Rabiller A, Tostivint I, Mezière G. Feasibility and safety of ultrasound-aided thoracentesis in mechanically ventilated patients. *Intensive Care Med.* 1999;25(9):955–958.

Light R. *Pleural Effusion - Pulmonary Disorders.* 2018. Merck Manuals Professional Edition. http://www.merckmanuals.com/professional/pulmonary-disorders/mediastinal-and-pleural-disorders/pleural-effusion. Accessed 2 February 2018.

Michel F, Brevaut-Malaty V, Pasquali R, et al. Comparison of ultrasound and X-ray in determining the position of umbilical venous catheters. *Resuscitation.* 2012;83(6):705–709.

Ohki Y, Tabata M, Kuwashima M, et al. Ultrasonographic detection of very thin percutaneous central venous catheter in neonates. *Acta Paediatr.* 2000;89(11):1381–1384.

Oppenheimer DA, Carroll BA, Garth KE, Parker BR. Sonographic localization of neonatal umbilical catheters. *AJR Am J Roentgenol.* 1982;138(6):1025–1032.

Osranek M, Bursi F, O'Leary PW. Hand-carried ultrasound–guided pericardiocentesis and thoracentesis. *J Am Soc Echocardiogr.* 2003;16(5):480–484.

Patel PA, Ernst FR, Gunnarsson CL. Ultrasonography guidance reduces complications and costs associated with thoracentesis procedures. *J Clin Ultrasound.* 2012;40(3):135–141.

Pezzati M, Filippi L, Chiti G, Dani C, Rossi S, et al. Central venous catheters and cardiac tamponade in preterm infants. *Intensive Care Med.* 2004;30(12):2253–2256.

Raptopoulos V, Davis LM, Lee G, Umali C, Lew R, Irwin RS. Factors affecting the development of pneumothorax associated with thoracentesis. *AJR Am J Roentgenol.* 1991;156(5):917–920.

Saul D, Ajayi S, Schutzman DL, Horrow MM. Sonography for complete evaluation of neonatal intensive care unit central support devices: a pilot study. *J Ultrasound Med.* 2016;35(7):1465–1473.

Schlesinger AE, Braverman RM, DiPietro MA. Pictorial essay neonates and umbilical venous catheters: normal appearance, anomalous positions, complications, and potential aid to diagnosis. *AJR Am J Roentgenol.* 2003;180(4):1147–1153.

Seneff MG, Corwin RW, Gold LH, Irwin RS. Complications associated with thoracocentesis. *Chest.* 1986;90(1):97–100.

Shrestha D, Sharma UK, Mohammad R, Dhoju D. The role of ultrasonography in detection and localization of radiolucent foreign body in soft tissues of extremities. *JNMA.* 48(173):5–9.

Smyrnios NA, Jederlinic PJ, Irtvin RS. Pleural effusion in an asymptomatic patient. *Chest.* 1990;97(1):192–196.

Soni NJ, Franco R, Velez MI, et al. Ultrasound in the diagnosis and management of pleural effusions. *J Hosp Med.* 2015;10(12):811–816.

Tayal VS, Kline JA. Emergency echocardiography to detect pericardial effusion in patients in PEA and near-PEA states. *Resuscitation.* 2003;59(3):315–318.

Tibbles CD, Porcaro W. Procedural applications of ultrasound. *Emerg Med Clin North Am.* 2004;22(3):797–815.

30

Venous Access

Leslie Palmerlee, Christopher M. Beck

INTRODUCTION

Since 2001 the Agency for Healthcare Research and Quality (AHRQ) and the American College of Emergency Physicians (ACEP) have recommended the use of ultrasound guidance for the placement of central venous catheters. The superiority of ultrasound guidance over traditional landmark-based approaches is well established in the emergency medicine literature and is a skill that all acute care practitioners should master. Ultrasound is utilized to improve the success of central line placement in the internal jugular (IJ), subclavian, and femoral veins, as well as placement of peripheral intravenous (IV) catheters. Understanding probe orientation and image display is critical for accurate interpretation and identification of the vascular structures of interest when performing vessel cannulation. Ultrasound guidance for vascular cannulation is most effectively utilized in real time, allowing visualization of the anatomic structures during actual needle placement, rather than static scanning, which visualizes structures before performing a landmark-based approach. Real-time scanning allows for faster cannulation with fewer needle attempts over static ultrasound imaging. Ultrasound-guided vascular access requires significant dexterity and multitasking for simultaneous probe direction and needle manipulation.

The first step in ultrasound-guided venous cannulation is prescanning, which includes visualization of the target vein and surrounding anatomy and locating the optimal position for cannulation. This should occur before the practitioner dresses in sterile attire and applies the sterile transducer cover. Linear, high-frequency transducers (5–13 MHz) are preferred for all venous access, as they provide better resolution of superficial structures.

Positioning

Correct positioning is key to the success of ultrasound-guided central line placement. The ultrasound machine should be placed directly in line with the operator's line of vision so that the physician minimizes movement when alternating their focus from the needle to the screen. Conventional probe positioning places the indicator to the patient's right or cephalad. For cannulation of the IJ vein and the supraclavicular approach to the subclavian vein, the operator will be located at the head of the bed facing the patient's feet (Fig. 30.1). In this position, the indicator should be directed toward the patient's feet or left side. Movement of the probe will then correspond to movement on the screen rather than presenting a mirror image, which can be confusing when attempting to align the needle and the vessel. The target vessel should always be centered on the screen, and the depth should be decreased to the most superficial setting in which the target vessel and surrounding structures can still be visualized.

Distinguishing Vein from Artery

Differentiating arteries from veins is crucial for proper placement of central lines and is easily accomplished with an understanding of anatomy and bedside ultrasound interrogation of vessel shape, pulsatility, compressibility, and respiratory variation. Veins are generally thin walled

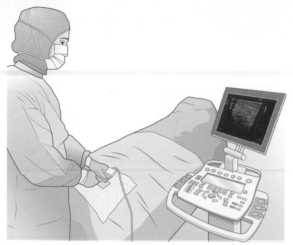

Fig. 30.1 Positioning of physician and ultrasound machine while performing IJ and supraclavicular cannulation.

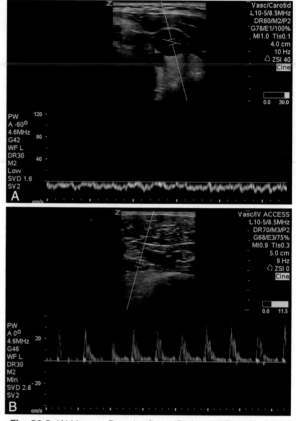

Fig. 30.2 (A) Venous Doppler flow. (B) Arterial Doppler flow.

and ovoid, whereas arteries generally have a thick muscular wall and are round. The application of gentle pressure will compress a patent vein, but will not affect the shape of an artery. Visualization of full compressibility of a vein also rules out the presence of thrombus at that location. Arteries will exhibit pulsatility, which is generally absent in veins, but care should be taken when using this criteria, as veins adjacent to arteries can appear pulsatile. Utilizing Doppler color flow can distinguish vessels from other round, anechoic structures, but the color itself should not necessarily guide the sonographer, as the flow is determined by the direction of flow in relation to the position of the probe. Measurement of Doppler flow will show a continuous, laminar flow pattern in a vein and a higher-velocity, pulsatile pattern in an artery (Fig. 30.2). Misidentification of the vessel with ultrasound is one of the most common causes of arterial puncture; the combination of these factors aids in correct identification of central veins and increases the chances of successful placement.

Approach

Once the ultrasonographer and machine are correctly positioned and the target vessel is identified, the provider must decide which ultrasonographic view they will utilize to access the vessel. Vascular structures can be imaged in short (transverse), long (longitudinal), or oblique orientations. The transverse approach is an out-of-plane technique in which only one point of the needle is visualized and appears as a hyperechoic dot on the screen (Fig. 30.3A). In this view, vessels are visualized

in cross-section and appear as anechoic circles. This approach has two main advantages. First, it is the least technically difficult method to visualize the vessel and the needle. Second, the short axis provides the advantage of continuous visualization of both artery and vein, which is crucial for avoiding arterial puncture. Using this technique, the needle will be inserted just proximal to the center of the probe and visualized as it passes under the probe's beam (Fig. 30.3B). The longitudinal approach is an in-plane technique in which the entire length of the needle is visualized as it approaches and enters the vessel, which appears as a anechoic tube. The needle is inserted at the proximal aspect of the probe, and its entire length is visualized as it advances from the left to the right of the screen (Fig. 30.4). Significant dexterity is required to maintain alignment of the ultrasound beam and the needle, both of which measure about 1 mm. As the longitudinal approach is more technically challenging for novice ultrasonographers, two methods have been described to overcome these

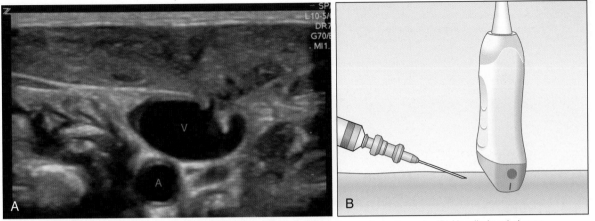

Fig. 30.3 (A) Central vein (*V*) and artery (*A*) in the short axis with needle in the vein. (B) Needle in relation to ultrasound transducer for short-axis approach.

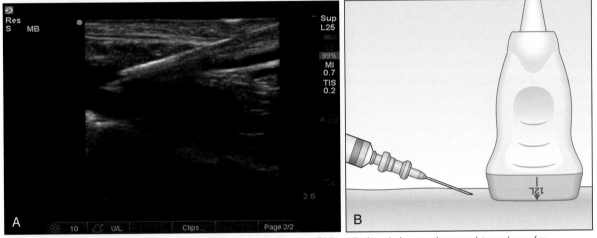

Fig. 30.4 (A) Central vein in the long axis with needle. (B) Needle in relation to ultrasound transducer for long-axis approach.

downsides. The first is the "tilt to follow" method, which is utilized with the transverse visualization. Using this technique, the ultrasonographer continuously fans the probe superiorly and inferiorly as the needle is advanced so that the tip of the needle is continuously visualized as it is advanced. This technique converts the procedure from ultrasound assisted to truly ultrasound guided. The second technique is the oblique approach, which allows a combination of short and long axes, and combines their respective advantages. The probe is rotated 45 degrees to a position between the short and long axes of the vessels. The vein and artery are both visualized but appear ovoid rather than round or cylindrical (Fig. 30.5). The needle is inserted at the lateral aspect of the probe and advanced using an in-plane technique. The needle tip is continuously visualized at the same time that both vessels are visualized, decreasing the chance that the operator will mistake the artery for the vein. A third technique uses an all in-plane approach. The operator obtains a longitudinal (or oblique) view of the vessel while bracing their hand to minimize movement. The proximal end of the transducer is then rocked off the skin, lifting the proximal aspect of the probe off the skin. The needle is then inserted at the seam of the transducer under the footprint of the probe. When the transducer is rocked back to make full contact with the skin, the needle tip will be in view and can be advanced without moving the probe.

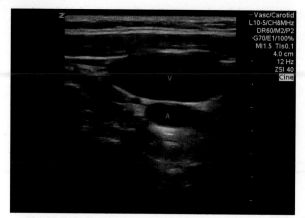

Fig. 30.5 Oblique axis of central vein (*V*) and artery (*A*).

Vessel Depth

Before needle insertion the operator should note the depth of the vessel using the depth markers on the right of the screen. Care should be taken to place the probe gently on the patient's skin, as applying too much pressure can obscure the vessel and make depth measurements inaccurate. If a transverse or short-access approach is taken to access the vessel, a "right triangle" method can be used to insert the needle. The needle should be inserted at a 45-degree angle at a distance proximal to the probe that is equal to the depth of the vessel. For example, if the vessel is 1 cm deep, the needle should be inserted at a 45-degree angle 1 cm from the probe. It can then be estimated that the vessel will be accessed at about 1.5 cm of needle length (the triangle's hypotenuse) (Fig. 30.6). Before the needle is inserted the operator should note how much of the needle will be inserted. This technique is useful in avoiding overshooting the vessel, as the tip of the needle is not always visualized in the transverse view.

Vessel Puncture

As the needle contacts the vessel, the anterior wall will tent inward (Fig. 30.7). When the wall is punctured, the vessel will no longer tent, and aspiration of blood will be noted in the syringe. In a significantly hypovolemic or hypotensive patient, it is possible to puncture the anterior and posterior vessel walls at the same time. In the case of significant vessel overlap, this can result in cannulation of the artery. If the length of the needle is continuously visualized using in-plane techniques, these complications can be avoided. If a short-axis technique

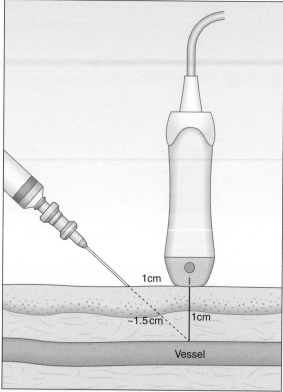

Fig. 30.6 The "right triangle" technique for estimating depth of needle insertion.

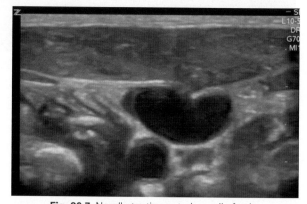

Fig. 30.7 Needle tenting anterior wall of vein.

is employed, care should be taken to continuously visualize the needle tip using techniques detailed earlier.

Complications

Multiple complications are still possible, despite the use of ultrasound guidance. Arterial puncture occurs as a

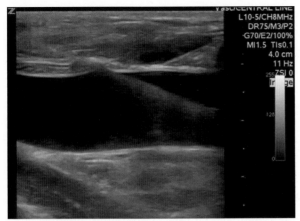

Fig. 30.8 Longitudinal axis of guidewire in vein.

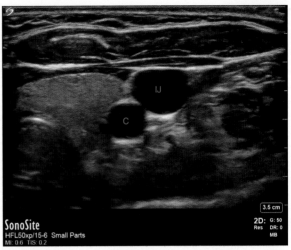

Fig. 30.9 The internal jugular vein (*IJ*) and carotid artery (*C*) in the short axis.

result of many factors, including a failure to visualize the tip of the needle, leading to through-and-through puncture of the vein into the artery and misidentification of an artery for a vein. Ultrasound should be used to visualize the wire within the lumen of the vein before dilation of the vessel (Fig. 30.8). Confirmation of venous placement can also be done after catheter placement by observing turbulent flow in the right atrium after the injection of 5 mL of sterile saline. Echocardiographic evaluation is covered in Chapter 9.

Pneumothorax remains a complication of IJ and subclavian cannulation, although real-time ultrasound guidance has decreased the rate of pneumothorax, as pleural tissue can be identified and avoided. The presence of a pneumothorax can be identified with ultrasound and may be part of the postprocedure process. See Chapter 8 for further description of evaluating for pneumothorax. Hematomas and oozing at puncture sites remain common complications to central line placement, despite ultrasound guidance, particularly in high-risk patient populations, such as those with hemostasis disorders, the uncooperative, and the critically ill.

INTERNAL JUGULAR VEIN CANNULATION

In the traditional approach, external anatomic landmarks approximate the location of the vessel of interest. For IJ vein cannulation, a triangle is drawn between the two heads of the sternocleidomastoid muscle and the clavicle, and the needle is introduced at the apex of the triangle and directed to the ipsilateral nipple to a depth of 1.0 to 1.5 cm. Normal anatomic variation likely

accounts for the reported failure rate of 7% to 19%. The size of the IJ vein greatly depends on the volume status, patient position, and local pathology. If allowable in the context of the patient's clinical condition, the Trendelenburg position or Valsalva maneuver augments venous distention, increases IJ diameter, and can help further distinguish vein from artery in the hypotensive or hypovolemic patient.

The carotid artery is further differentiated by its pulsatility; however, due to the proximity of other structures, the IJ vein can also appear pulsatile. An understanding of anatomic position can also aid in identification. The carotid artery is most often inferomedial (deep) to the IJ vein (Fig. 30.9), but this is not always the case, as the carotid artery is found inferolateral and lateral to the IJ vein in 4.5% and 1% of patients, respectively.

Ultrasound allows for the identification of vessel overlap and can be used to direct the needle from a medial to lateral approach away from the carotid artery toward the IJ vein. Carotid artery and IJ vein overlap can also be decreased by turning the patient's head toward midline. Measurement of the diameter of the vein can also be useful, as an IJ vein diameter less than 7 mm is associated with decreased success and may prompt the operator to evaluate a different site for vascular access.

Accessing the IJ vein can be accomplished using the transverse, longitudinal, or oblique approaches detailed earlier. A step-by-step approach to IJ vein cannulation using ultrasound guidance can be found in Box 30.1.

1. Identify the internal jugular (IJ) vein and carotid artery (CA) with ultrasound
   a. IJ will compress with outwardly applied pressure
   b. CA will be pulsatile
   c. Apply Doppler color flow (see Fig. 30.2A and B)
2. Clean the access site
3. Prepare the sterile field and apply a sterile ultrasound probe cover
4. The nondominant hand operates the probe while the dominant hand controls the needle
5. Confirm successful vessel puncture
   a. Direct visualization of needle in vessel (see Fig. 30.3A)
   b. Aspiration of blood into the syringe
6. Set ultrasound probe aside on a sterile surface
7. Remove syringe from needle
8. Thread wire through needle
9. Confirm wire placement in IJ vein (see Fig. 30.8)
10. Continue central line placement as without ultrasound
    a. Scalpel nick
    b. Dilate vessel
    c. Introduce catheter over wire
    d. Remove wire
    e. Aspirate and flush all ports, apply caps
    f. Suture line in place and apply sterile occlusive dressing
    g. Obtain confirmatory imaging

SUBCLAVIAN VEIN CANNULATION

The subclavian vein offers an important access point for central venous cannulation. Rates of infection associated with subclavian central lines are lower than both femoral and IJ lines. Central lines in place for an extended period are frequently accessed for obtaining samples and infusing medications. Therefore an increased distance from potential sites of contamination, including the groin for femoral lines and the oropharynx for IJ lines, puts subclavian lines at a theoretical advantage in relation to long-term infection. Additionally, subclavian lines offer a good solution for central cannulation in patients wearing a cervical collar or those with trauma or burns to the extremities.

The most significant downside to subclavian central lines is the potential for mechanical complications such as pneumothorax or arterial puncture. The vessel's close proximity to important structures, including the pleural dome and subclavian artery, make the traditionally favored landmark-based technique an unnecessarily risky procedure. Complication rates with landmark-guided placement have been documented as high as 18.8%. Direct visualization of the subclavian vein and surrounding structures with ultrasound provides a potentially safer technique for this procedure. The subclavian vein, as the name implies, lies primarily deep to the clavicle, making ultrasound visualization more technically challenging due to bone shadowing. As a result, adoption of ultrasound-guided placement of subclavian lines has largely lagged behind its use in the IJ and femoral veins. Despite this, multiple techniques, including the supraclavicular and infraclavicular approaches, have been described to overcome this limitation.

Supraclavicular Approach

The right subclavian vein is the preferred site of access due to the lower pleural dome on this side, more linear route to the superior vena cava, and the absence of the thoracic duct. The supraclavicular approach to subclavian central line placement approaches the vessel near the confluence of the IJ and subclavian veins, just proximal to the formation of the brachiocephalic vein (Fig. 30.10).

A potential limitation to the supraclavicular approach is the reduced surface area available to place both the ultrasound probe and the needle. Therefore a linear probe with the smallest possible footprint should be used. Alternatively, the use of an endocavitary probe placed in the supraclavicular fossa can be used to overcome this problem. The ultrasound transducer should be placed medial to the site of needle introduction. To facilitate visualization of the vessel, the probe should be placed in the transverse orientation relative to the neck just superior to the clavicle and tilted anteriorly, effectively obtaining an image deep to the clavicle. The subclavian artery will be visible deep to the subclavian vein (Fig. 30.11). If the subclavian vein is not easily located, the operator can place the probe more superiorly on the neck to locate the IJ vein in the short axis then slowly scan down the neck to locate the confluence of the IJ and subclavian veins (Video 30.1). The subclavian vein will be visualized in the long axis at this point and will be accessed using an in-plane approach. At this position the subclavian vein will be relatively superficial. Using depth markers, the operator will find it located about 1 to 2 cm deep to the

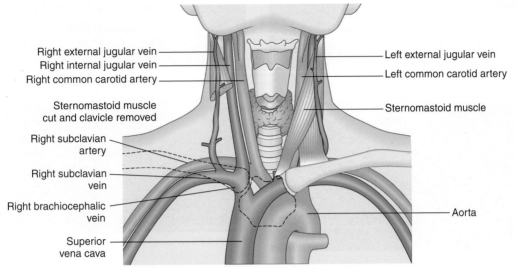

Fig. 30.10 Vessels of the neck and upper chest.

Labels: Right external jugular vein, Right internal jugular vein, Right common carotid artery, Sternomastoid muscle cut and clavicle removed, Right subclavian artery, Right subclavian vein, Right brachiocephalic vein, Superior vena cava, Left external jugular vein, Left common carotid artery, Sternomastoid muscle, Aorta

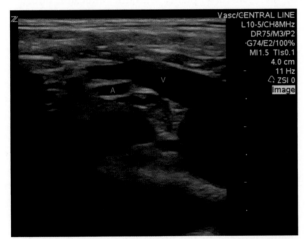

Fig. 30.11 The supraclavicular view of the subclavian vein (*V*) and artery (*A*).

skin. This is important to note, as the lung pleura can be visualized just deep to the vessels as a hyperechoic line. As the in-plane approach will be utilized, the tip of the needle can be directed away from this structure. The needle will be inserted in the lateral-to-medial orientation directed toward the sternal notch. If the probe's indicator is to the patient's left (see earlier for a discussion of this technique), the needle will be seen approaching the vessel from the right upper portion of the screen. After venous puncture, the procedure proceeds as detailed earlier, including visualization of the guidewire within the lumen of the target vessel (see Box 30.1).

Infraclavicular Approach

The infraclavicular approach to the subclavian vein using ultrasound guidance occurs at a point lateral to the traditional landmark-based approach. At this position the vessel is, in fact, the axillary vein before it becomes the subclavian as it courses under the clavicle. The vessel most frequently accessed will be the right axillary vein. The operator will be standing to the right of the patient facing the head of the bed. The axillary vein will be visualized in the short access with the indicator pointed toward the patient's head. On the left side of the screen the clavicle will be visualized as a hyperechoic structure with posterior acoustic shadowing. The axillary artery and vein will be visualized to the right (caudally) of the clavicle (Fig. 30.12). The previously described methods should be used to distinguish between artery and vein. Once the vein is identified and centered on the screen, the probe should be rotated 90 degrees counterclockwise to visualize the vessel in the long access (Fig. 30.13). Care should be taken to continuously maintain the vein in the center of the screen so that the long axis of the artery is not inadvertently visualized. At this point, the indicator will be pointing toward the patient's right. The pleural will be visualized deep to the vein. Insert the needle at the lateral edge of the probe and continuously visualize the entire needle length as it enters the axillary vein. At this point the procedure will proceed as detailed earlier (see Box 30.1).

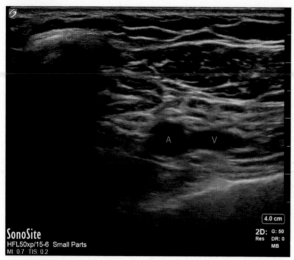

Fig. 30.12 The infraclavicular view of the axillary vein (*V*) and artery (*A*) in the short axis, clavicle (*C*), and pleura (*P*).

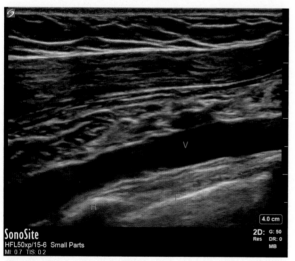

Fig. 30.13 Long axis of axillary vein (*V*), pleura (*P*), and rib (*R*).

FEMORAL VEIN CANNULATION

Obtaining central venous access at the femoral vein offers several advantages over accessing the IJ and subclavian veins. At this location there is no risk of pneumothorax or hemothorax, and the site can be accessed more easily while cardiopulmonary resuscitation (CPR) is ongoing.

Complications associated with this site are most frequently due to inadvertent femoral artery puncture.

For the right-handed sonographer, the right femoral vein is most easily assessed. The linear transducer

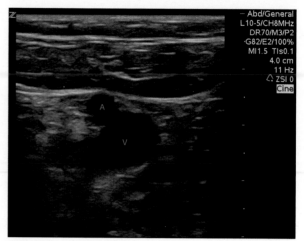

Fig. 30.14 The femoral vein (*V*) and artery (*A*) in the transverse axis.

should be placed just inferior to the inguinal ligament in the transverse plane, with the indicator directed toward the patient's right. Patients' variable anatomy in this area make ultrasound guidance particularly useful. The femoral vein will generally be visualized as an ovoid structure medial to the femoral artery (Fig. 30.14). If the vein is found immediately superficial or deep to the artery, the vessels of the other leg should be visualized to see if the anatomy is more favorable to access. External rotation of the thigh will also decrease vessel overlap by moving the vein in a medial and superficial direction. Placement of the patient in the reverse Trendelenburg position will increase the diameter of the vessel. Once the vessel is definitively identified, it is most frequently accessed using the transverse view while continuously visualizing the femoral artery. Cannulation of the vein should proceed in the previously described steps (see Box 30.1).

PERIPHERAL VENOUS ACCESS

Peripheral IV placement using ultrasound guidance follows the same principles as central access, but the vessels' smaller diameter can make it more technically challenging for practitioners more accustomed to accessing larger central vessels. With proper training and practice, the use of ultrasound guidance for peripheral IV placement can increase first-pass success rates and decrease the use of central venous catheters, particularly in patients with a history of difficult IV access.

Upper Extremity Venous Anatomy

A tourniquet should be applied to the upper arm to facilitate visualization and access of the vein. In selecting a site for venous access, the more superficial veins in the distal arm should be evaluated first, followed by the more proximal veins (Fig. 30.15). In the forearm, the cephalic vein runs on the lateral aspect of the extremity, whereas the basilic vein is more medial and posterior. In the antecubital fossa the cephalic, median cubital, and basilic veins can be visualized laterally to medially. The veins of the distal arm and antecubital fossa are generally very superficial and can often be accessed by direct visualization/palpation. In patients with obesity, chronic illness with multiple previous IVs, or history of IV drug use, ultrasound guidance can be helpful to access these veins. The veins of the proximal arm are deeper and require ultrasound guidance for access in almost all patients. The veins of the proximal arm include the cephalic vein laterally; the basilic vein medially; and the brachial veins, which course adjacent to the brachial artery in the deep compartment of the upper arm. The basilic vein is often a good point of access, as it is usually large and does not run adjacent to an artery in the mid-upper arm. More proximally it runs adjacent to the ulnar nerve and brachial artery. If the basilic vein is not accessible, the cephalic vein will be more superficial in the upper arm on the lateral aspect, but is generally not as large as the basilic. The brachial veins will be found in the deep compartment of the upper arm and offer a good option if the more superficial veins are not accessible. Care should be taken to avoid the brachial artery and median nerve.

Techniques

Sterile technique is not necessary for peripheral access, but the practitioner should take universal precautions to reduce the risk of infection. A waterproof transparent dressing traditionally used to secure a catheter can be applied to the probe over a strip of ultrasound gel to provide a clean interface with the patient's skin and avoid contaminating the puncture site with nonsterile gel. Care should be taken to smooth out the gel under the dressing to avoid artifact from air bubbles. If the vein is less than 1 cm deep, a standard-length catheter of 1 inch can be used. If the vein is deeper, a longer catheter should be used. For deeper vessels a guidewire catheter can be utilized to improve chances of successful placement. The "right triangle" method (see Fig. 30.6) should be utilized when performing ultrasound-guided peripheral IV placement. The needle should be inserted

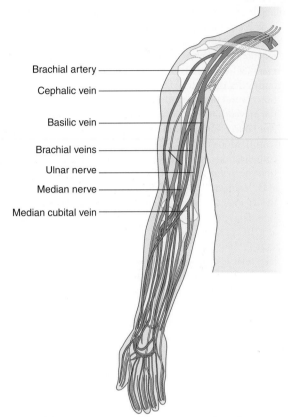

Fig. 30.15 Anatomy of upper extremity veins.

the same distance from the probe as the depth of the vessel at a 45-degree angle and be expected to access the vein at the length of the hypotenuse. Once a flash is visualized, the angle of approach should be decreased and the needle should be advanced 1 to 2 mm along the path of the vessel to ensure that the tip of the catheter is within the lumen of the vein. The catheter should then be threaded over the needle, attached to IV tubing or a syringe, flushed, and secured.

BIBLIOGRAPHY

McNamee J, Jeong J, Patel N. 10 Tips for Ultrasound-Guided Peripheral Venous Access. ACEP Now. http://www.acep-now.com/article/10-tips-ultrasound-guided-peripheral-venous-access/. Updated December 17, 2014. Accessed December 8, 2017.

Mey U, Glasmacher A, Hahn C, Gorschluter M, Ziske C, Mergelsbery M, et al. Evaluation of an ultrasound-guided technique for central venous access via the internal jugular vein in 493 patients. *Support Care Cancer.* 2003;11:148–155.

Milling Jr TJ, Rose J, Briggs WM, Birkham R, Gaeta TJ, Bove JJ, et al. Randomized, controlled clinical trial of point-of-care limited ultrasonography assistance of central venous cannulation: the Third Sonography Outcomes Assessment Program (SOAP-3) trial. *Crit. Care Med.* 2005;33:1764–1769.

O'Grady NP, Alexander M, Burns LA, et al. Healthcare infection control practices advisory committee. guidelines for the prevention of intravascular catheter-related infections. *Am J Infect Control.* 2011;39(4 suppl 1):S1–S34.

Parienti JJ, Mongardon N, Mégarbane B, et al. Intravascular complications of central venous catheterization by insertion site. *N Engl J Med.* 2015;373:1220–1229.

Read H, Holdgate A, Watkins S. Simple external rotation of the leg increases the size and accessibility of the femoral vein. *Emerg Med Australas.* 2012;24:408–413. https://doi.org/10.1111/j.1742-6723.2012.01568.x.

Rezayat T, Stowell JR, Kendall JL, Turner E, Fox JC, Barjaktarevic I. Ultrasound-guided cannulation: time to bring subclavian central lines back. *West J Emerg Med.* 2016;17(2):216–221. https://doi.org/10.5811/westjem.2016.1.29462.

Schofer JM, Nomura JT, Bauman MJ, Hyde R, Schmier C. The "Ski Lift": a technique to maximize needle visualization with the long-axis approach for ultrasound-guided vascular access. *Acad Emerg Med.* 2010;17:e83–e84. https://doi.org/10.1111/j.1553-2712.2010.00784.x.

Sznajder JI, Zveibil FR, Bitterman H, Weiner P, Bursztein S. Central vein catheterization: failure and complication rates by three percutaneous approaches. *Arch Intern Med.* 1986;146:259–261.

Troianos CA, et al. Guidelines for performing ultrasound guided vascular cannulation: recommendations of the American Society of Echocardiography and the Society of Cardiovascular Anesthesiologists. *J Am Soc Echocardiogr.* 2011;24:1291–1318.

Turba UC, Uflacker R, Hannegan C, Selby JB. Anatomic relationship of the internal jugular vein and the common carotid artery applied to percutaneous transjugular procedures. *J Vasc Interv Radiol.* 2005;28:303–306.

31

Nerve Blocks

Arun Nagdev, Chad McCarthy, David A. Martin

INTRODUCTION

Single-injection ultrasound-guided peripheral nerve blocks (USGNBs) are ideal for pain relief from acute injuries and adjunct analgesic for painful procedures. By injecting local anesthetic adjacent to the nerve, both motor and sensory innervation distally can be "blocked." Depending on the efficacy of the USGNB, adjunctive therapies (such as intravenous medications) can be employed to achieve maximal patient comfort. Incorporation of USGNBs into clinical practice allows for a targeted approach to treat pain effectively and reduces the known complications of repeated (or high-dose) opioids.

Emergency physicians have demonstrated the ability to effectively and safely perform USGNBs in the acute setting for multiple indications (fractures, abscess drainage, joint reduction, etc.). Ultrasound guidance may reduce time of block onset and volume of anesthetic required compared with standard nonvisualized/landmark techniques. Ultrasound visualization can also decrease the likelihood of intraneural injections and inadvertent vascular puncture.

Clinicians performing USGNBs should be aware of two uncommon complications that can occur: peripheral nerve injury (PNI) and local anesthetic systemic toxicity (LAST). PNI is defined as persistent motor or sensory deficit and/or pain after the nerve block. The incidence of PNI ranges from 0.5% to 2.4% in the current literature, and the mechanism is not clearly understood in all reported cases. Hypotheses include direct needle trauma, increased intrafascicular pressures from injection, direct cytotoxic effects of anesthetic, or metabolic stress of the anesthetic leading to nerve ischemia.

Patients with underlying peripheral neuropathy are contraindicated from having a nerve block because post-block determination of PNI will be not possible.

Recommendations to minimize PNI include maintaining visualization of the needle tip to avoid direct contact with the nerve fascicle and a deliberate, low-pressure injection technique. Instruct the patient to inform the clinician of radicular pain during the procedure. If the patient reports any symptoms, the procedure should be interrupted, and the patient and needle placement reassessed. Subsequent actions are based on the clinical scenario. These safeguards cannot completely prevent PNI but may minimize the incidence.

LAST can occur with a toxic dose of anesthetic, with rapid absorption of anesthetic, or due to inadvertent intravascular injection. Patients are maintained on continuous cardiac monitoring for these procedures. If a patient develops signs or symptoms of LAST, a hyper-lipophilic solution (20% Intralipid; 1–1.5-mg/kg bolus with continued infusion of 0.25 mL/kg/min) should be infused. Intralipid in 20% should be readily available when performing a nerve block.

There are two commonly used approaches to perform USGNBs: in-plane and out-of-plane. The in-plane technique, in which the transducer is aligned in the long axis of the needle, allows clear visualization of the entire needle. This technique allows confirmation of the needle tip, the nerve, and the injected anesthetic. With the out-of-plane technique, in which the transducer is aligned in the long axis of the needle, the needle will not be visualized in its entirety. In this view, the operator must ensure that the needle tip, rather than the shaft of the needle, is being visualized to prevent misplacement of the needle tip.

There are general preparation steps to be performed for all USGNBs. Single-injection USGNBs are performed with aseptic technique and do not require sterile preparation. Perform skin preparation. Then perform the ultrasound survey to locate the nerve and identify other anatomic structures of interest. Place a skin wheal of rapidly acting local anesthetic at the planned needle insertion site. Clean the ultrasound probe and cover it with a transparent, adhesive dressing or insert into a sleeve. We recommend using sterile gel for the procedure. A blunt tip can be used for nerve blocks but are not required.

Before performing an ultrasound-guided nerve block, the clinician should look up the maximal dose and volume of anesthetic based on the patient's weight. All volumes presented in this chapter are for adult patients. Again, the clinician should not confuse the maximal dose of anesthetic with volumes (as listed in the chapter).

Before injecting the local anesthetic, the patient should be educated regarding the symptoms of local anesthetic toxicity and instructed to notify the clinician immediately if any symptoms are noted. Injecting large volumes of local anesthetic should be performed incrementally. After each injection, the clinician should pause and monitor for signs and symptoms of local anesthetic toxicity. If the patient reports any symptoms, the procedure should be interrupted, and the patient and needle placement reassessed. Subsequent actions are based on the clinical scenario.

FEMORAL NERVE

Indications

The femoral nerve provides innervation to the entire anterior thigh and most of the femur and knee joint, making it an ideal nerve block for hip fractures, proximal and midshaft femur fractures, large anterior thigh wound repairs, and patellar injuries. In patients with a hip fracture, a femoral nerve block gives moderate pain reduction but does not provide complete analgesia to the hip because the obturator nerve, one of the three nerves that innervate the hip, is not blocked by this approach. However, the femoral nerve block can significantly decrease the need for intravenous opioid medications, thereby reducing the risk of adverse effects, including respiratory depression, confusion, and hypotension, especially in the elderly. Although the risk of developing compartment syndrome of the thigh is very rare, we recommend the block be performed after achieving consensus with the consultative service in situations that require it.

Anatomy

The femoral nerve is one of the major branches of the lumbar plexus arising from the first through fourth lumbar ventral rami (L1–L4) before descending toward the lower extremity. The femoral nerve can be identified lateral to the femoral artery, beneath the fascia iliaca and superficial to the iliopsoas muscle at the level of the inguinal canal (Fig. 31.1).

Technique

Place the patient in a supine position. Attempt to externally rotate and abduct the hip, realizing that it is often not possible in the acutely injured patient and may not be needed. Place the high-frequency linear transducer just below and parallel to the inguinal crease. Locate the femoral artery and vein in cross-section, and slowly slide the transducer laterally to identify the femoral nerve. The femoral nerve appears as a hyperechoic, triangular structure below the hyperechoic fascia iliaca and above the iliopsoas muscle (see Fig. 31.1). Slightly fanning the probe in a caudal direction, perpendicular to the trajectory of the nerve, will often allow for better visualization of the nerve. The operator should also locate the fascia iliaca—the fascial covering that covers the femoral nerve. Placing the anesthetic just below the hyperechoic fascia iliaca is key to obtaining an effective femoral nerve block.

Once the femoral nerve and surrounding anatomic structures are identified, a small skin wheal should be made approximately 0.5 to 1 cm lateral to the probe, which will represent the site of needle entry. Perform the preparatory steps discussed earlier. A 20-gauge, 3.5-inch (approximately 8.9 cm) block needle is inserted with direct ultrasound visualization. Advance the needle slowly at an angle parallel to the transducer using an in-plane approach, maintaining the needle shaft and tip in view at all times. The angle of entry will depend on the depth of the target depth of the fascia iliaca. More shallow angles of entry will improve needle visualization. Target the hyperechoic fascia iliaca overlying the iliopsoas muscle 1 to 3 cm lateral to the femoral nerve.

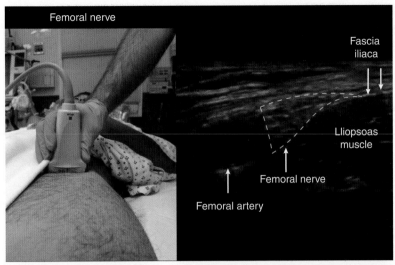

Fig. 31.1 The femoral nerve can often easily be visualized next to the femoral artery and underneath the fascia iliaca.

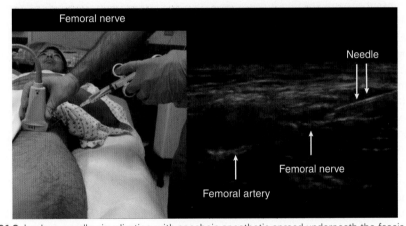

Fig. 31.2 In-plane needle visualization with anechoic anesthetic spread underneath the fascia iliaca.

Once beneath the fascia iliaca, aspirate to confirm the needle tip has not entered a vessel and then slowly inject 3 to 5 mL of local anesthetic in a dose that is appropriate for the concentration of the anesthetic and the weight of the patient. With the needle tip in view, the spread of hypoechoic fluid should be visualized hydrodissecting the potential space below the fascia iliaca and around the nerve (Fig. 31.2). After confirming optimal needle tip location, proceed to inject a total of 20 mL of local anesthetic in a dose that is appropriate for the concentration of the anesthetic and the weight of the patient in 3- to 5-mL aliquots. The most common pitfall is failure to get under the fascia iliaca; therefore anesthetic should be visualized under the fascial plane

with the spread of anechoic fluid. The risk of intravascular and intraneural injection can be reduced by targeting the needle tip to be 1 cm lateral to the femoral nerve and vessels, yet deep to the fascia iliaca. If at any point the spread of local anesthetic is not visualized, intravascular injection should be suspected and the procedure halted.

DISTAL SCIATIC NERVE AND POPLITEAL FOSSA

Indications

The distal sciatic nerve innervates most of the lower extremity, making it an ideal block for fractures of the ankle, distal tibia, fibula, and injuries of the foot. A distal sciatic nerve block does not anesthetize the medial aspect of the lower leg, which is innervated by the saphenous nerve, a distal branch of the femoral nerve. Thus this block is not ideal for superficial injuries of the distal, medial leg. It should also be noted that, although this block is ideal for pain relief for tibial fractures, tibial injuries are typically high-energy and commonly associated with compartment syndrome. As the distal sciatic block may obscure clinical findings of compartment syndrome, it should be performed only after speaking in consensus with consulting services.

Anatomy

The lumbosacral plexus forms the sciatic nerve in the posterior pelvis. As the nerve tracks inferiorly through the posterior thigh, it enters the popliteal fossa bordered by the long head of the biceps femoris superolaterally and by the semimembranosus and semitendinosus tendons superomedially. At the most proximal point in the popliteal fossa, the large sciatic nerve bifurcates into a tibial nerve medially and a common peroneal nerve laterally. The sciatic nerve can be blocked at any location from the proximal, deep gluteal region to the distal, superficial popliteal fossa. The distal location is generally preferred for USGNB, given the ease with which adequate patient positioning can be obtained and anatomic landmarks can be sonographically identified (Fig. 31.3).

Technique

The distal sciatic nerve block at the popliteal fossa is most easily accomplished with the patient in a prone position. This allows easy access to the popliteal fossa and facilitates needle movements in the anteroposterior plane that correlate with images on the ultrasound screen. In patients who are unable to lie prone (e.g., cervical spine immobilization), the affected extremity must be elevated and supported with mild flexion of the knee to fit the transducer between the popliteal fossa and the patient's bed. Needle movements made under visualization of a transducer facing upward will appear reversed in the anteroposterior plane on the ultrasound screen.

When appropriate patient positioning has been achieved, use a high-frequency linear transducer to locate the popliteal artery and vein at the popliteal crease (this may be more easily done with slight flexion at the knee). The tibial nerve is commonly located superficial to the popliteal vein and appears as a hyperechoic

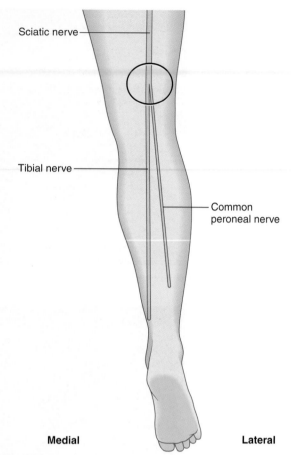

Fig. 31.3 The distal sciatic nerve splits into the tibial and common peroneal nerves just above the popliteal fossa.

"honeycomb." Once the tibial nerve is optimally visualized, slowly slide the transducer proximally. At the cephalad border of the popliteal fossa, the common peroneal nerve should be visualized joining the tibial nerve, forming the distal sciatic nerve (Fig. 31.4). The operator should mark this location and note the depth of the nerve.

In contrast to a femoral nerve block in which the needle is inserted adjacent to the transducer, for a distal sciatic nerve block, we recommend inserting the needle farther away from the transducer on the lateral aspect of the leg. The distal sciatic nerve is often 2 to 4 cm deep to the skin surface, and a steep needle angle from a point of entry just adjacent to the ultrasound probe would prevent clear needle tip visualization. To improve needle visualization, we recommend measuring the nerve depth and entering the lateral leg at a similar depth

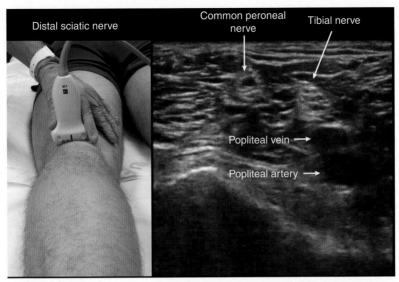

Fig. 31.4 Locate the popliteal artery and vein in the fossa and then note the tibial and common peroneal nerve just superficial.

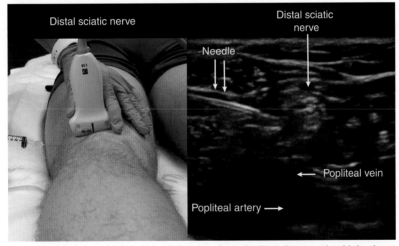

Fig. 31.5 Once the distal sciatic nerve is identified, enter from the lateral approach with in-plane needle visualization. Anesthetic should be placed in close proximity to the distal sciatic nerve.

with a fairly flat angle (parallel to the surface of a linear probe).

After placing a skin wheal at the site of needle entry, advance a 20-gauge, 3.5-inch needle slowly at an angle parallel to the transducer using an in-plane approach. Maintain the needle shaft and tip in view at all times. Target the honeycomb appearance of the sciatic nerve without placing the needle directly into the nerve. Place the needle tip just superficial to the nerve (anywhere from 2–3 mm) to reduce the risk of nerve injury. Gently aspirate to confirm there has been no inadvertent vascular puncture and then slowly inject 3 to 5 mL of local anesthetic in a dose that is appropriate for the concentration of the anesthetic and the weight of the patient. With the needle tip in view, the spread of anechoic fluid should be visualized in real time (Fig. 31.5). For novice sonographers, we do not recommend attempting to inject on the deep aspect of the nerve because of the close proximity to the popliteal vasculature and the increased possibility of inadvertent intravascular injection. If at any point the spread of local anesthetic is not visualized, intravascular injection should be suspected and the procedure halted.

POSTERIOR TIBIAL NERVE

Indications

The posterior tibial nerve is a distal branch of the sciatic nerve. Blocking it above the medial malleolus in the distal leg results in excellent anesthesia for the skin of the sole of the foot and the underlying deep structures. Classic indications for this block include anesthesia for the sole of the foot (repairs, abscesses, foreign body removal), as well as an adjunct for pain during the reduction of calcaneal fractures. The ankle joint itself has multiple innervations and will not be blocked with a posterior tibial block alone.

Anatomy

The posterior tibial nerve runs parallel to the posterior tibial artery, which branches from the popliteal artery at the popliteal fossa and runs down the length of the posteromedial tibia. At the level of the ankle, the posterior tibial artery travels posteriorly and inferiorly around the medial malleolus. The posterior tibial nerve, in turn, travels posterior and inferior to the artery (Fig. 31.6).

Technique

Position the patient with the ipsilateral hip externally rotated and flexed at the knee so that the medial malleolus is well exposed. If this position cannot be tolerated, the patient can be positioned in a lateral decubitus position with the medial side of the foot and ankle exposed. Identify the medial malleolus and posterior tibial artery by inspection and palpation.

Holding the linear probe in a position perpendicular to the orientation of the tibial artery, slide up the leg from the ankle and watch for separation of the posterior tibial artery and posterior tibial nerve. Classically, you should see the nerve posterior to the vascular bundle, but there is a great deal of anatomic variation (Fig. 31.7A).

If an out-of-plane approach is used, whether as a result of patient positioning or provider preference, we recommend inserting a 21- to 25-gauge needle in the middle of the probe at a steep angle. Aim posterior to the posterior tibial nerve bundle and maintain visualization of the needle tip. After puncturing the fascial plane

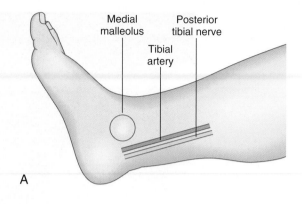

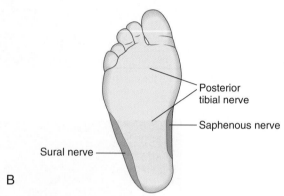

Fig. 31.6 (A) The tibial nerve is just posterior to the tibial artery. (B) The nerve supplies most of the innervation to the sole of the foot.

superficial to both the vascular bundle and posterior tibial nerve, inject a small aliquot of normal saline or local anesthetic to confirm appropriate placement.

For the in-plane approach to the posterior tibial nerve, insert a 21- to 25-gauge needle posterior to the linear probe. This approach will give better visualization when entering the fascial plane that contains the posterior tibial nerve and vascular bundle. Entering posteriorly provides a lower risk of puncturing the anterior vascular structures (Fig. 31.7B).

BRACHIAL PLEXUS: INTERSCALENE NERVE BLOCK

Indications

The interscalene brachial plexus block results in anesthesia to the shoulder and upper arm. The interscalene brachial plexus block has multiple applications, including pain control of proximal upper extremity fractures,

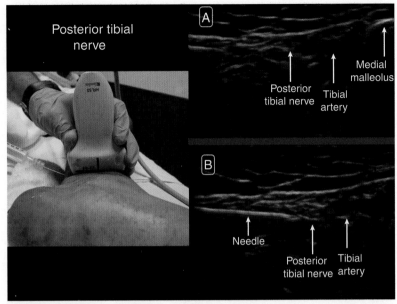

Fig. 31.7 An in-plane approach can be used to gently place anesthetic around the posterior tibial nerve.

large deltoid abscess drainage, pain control and debridement of burns, deep wound exploration, complex laceration repairs, and as an alternative method to procedural sedation for the reduction of shoulder dislocations. Of note, the interscalene block does not reliably provide anesthesia distal to the elbow.

The interscalene nerve block is associated with a risk of transient hemidiaphragmatic paresis due to the close proximity of the phrenic nerve. The use of ultrasound guidance has decreased the rate of diaphragmatic paresis due to the lower volume of anesthetic and increased precision of anesthetic delivery. Although the clinical significance of transient paralysis in unilateral phrenic nerve distribution is debated, caution is recommended when considering an interscalene block in patients with poor pulmonary reserve.

Anatomy

The interscalene nerve block targets the brachial plexus at the level of the roots as they pass through the interscalene groove, lateral to the carotid artery, between the anterior and middle scalene muscles. The interscalene groove is bordered medially by the anterior scalene muscle and laterally by the middle scalene muscle at the level of the cricoid cartilage and below the clavicular head of the sternocleidomastoid muscle (Fig. 31.8). The C5–T1 nerve roots are positioned vertically within the interscalene groove, starting with C5, the most superficial root. Anesthetic placed in this fascial plane commonly does

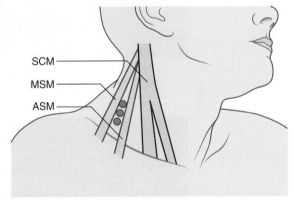

Fig. 31.8 The brachial plexus can be found between the anterior and middle scalene muscles on the lateral aspect of the neck. *ASM,* anterior scalene muscle; *MSM,* middle scalene muscle; *SCM,* sternocleidomastoid muscle.

not track around the inferiorly located C8–T1 nerve roots and therefore does not reliably provide anesthesia for injuries distal to the elbow. The carotid artery and internal jugular vein lie medial to the anterior scalene muscle. The dome of the pleura is located caudally. Risk of iatrogenic pneumothorax due to pleural puncture is low with ultrasound-guided needle visualization.

Technique

Place the patient supine on a stretcher with the head of the bed elevated at approximately 30 degrees, with the patient's head turned toward the opposite side. Place a towel under the ipsilateral scapula to improve needle visualization.

Locate the internal jugular vein and carotid artery in a transverse orientation at the level of the cricoid cartilage using the high-frequency linear transducer (Fig. 31.9). Slowly slide the transducer laterally on the neck until the clavicular head of the sternocleidomastoid muscle is identified. The anterior scalene muscle lies below the sternocleidomastoid muscle. The brachial plexus roots are located in the interscalene groove between the anterior and middle scalene muscles. The C5–C7 roots of the brachial plexus appear as hypoechoic, round or ovoid structures vertically aligned in the interscalene groove, commonly referred to as the *traffic light sign* (Fig. 31.10). Color flow Doppler can be used to differentiate the hypoechoic cords of the brachial plexus from vessels in the anterior neck.

When visualization of the brachial plexus using the former approach is difficult, an alternative approach involves identifying the brachial plexus at the level of

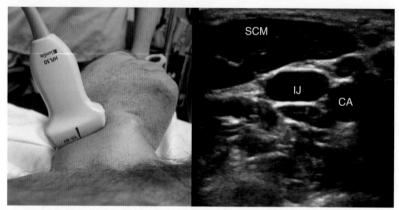

Fig. 31.9 For novice sonographers, locate the internal jugular vein (*IJV*), carotid artery (*CA*), and sternocleidomastoid muscle (*SCM*) first before attempting to locate the interscalene brachial plexus.

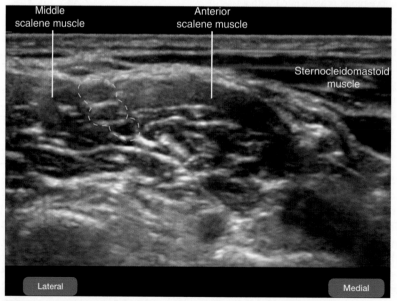

Fig. 31.10 Slide the transducer laterally to identify the interscalene brachial plexus (located between the anterior and middle scalene muscles).

the supraclavicular fossa and tracing the nerve trunks cephalad until the nerve roots are visualized in the interscalene groove. Place the transducer in the supraclavicular fossa parallel to the clavicle and fan the transducer caudally until the subclavian artery is visualized in cross-section (Fig. 31.11). The brachial plexus is identified lateral to the subclavian artery and has a "honeycomb" or "cluster of grapes" appearance at this level. Follow the brachial plexus cephalad until the roots coalesce to form the "traffic light" sign within the interscalene groove.

Once the C5–C7 roots of the brachial plexus and surrounding anatomic structures are identified, a small skin wheal should be made approximately 0.5 to 1 cm lateral to the probe, which will represent the site of needle entry. After injecting a skin wheal at the site of needle entry, a 21- to 23-gauge, 1.5-inch (approximately 3.8 cm) block needle is inserted using a longitudinal (in-plane) approach. The needle tip is advanced through the middle scalene muscle to the lateral border of the deepest nerve root, below the fascial plane. Approximately 10 to 20 mL of local anesthetic in a dose that is appropriate to the weight of the patient and the concentration of the anesthetic is then injected into the potential space between the middle scalene muscle and brachial plexus sheath (Fig. 31.12). With a successful block, local anesthetic tracks in the fascial plane between the middle scalene muscle and the nerve roots. If at any point the spread of local anesthetic is not visualized, intravascular injection should be suspected and the procedure interrupted to confirm proper needle location and assess patient status.

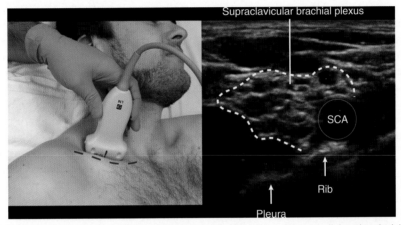

Fig. 31.11 To locate the supraclavicular brachial plexus, place the transducer parallel to the clavicle and note the nerve bundle just lateral to the subclavian artery (*SCA*). The pleura and first rib are commonly visualized.

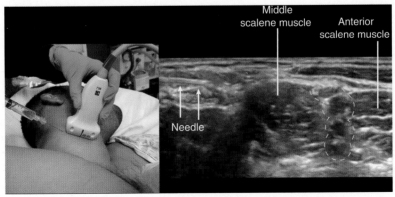

Fig. 31.12 In-plane needle visualization of an interscalene brachial plexus block. Note the needle approaching from the lateral aspect, with the goal to place anesthetic in the interscalene groove.

BRACHIAL PLEXUS: SUPRACLAVICULAR NERVE BLOCK

Indications

The supraclavicular brachial plexus nerve block (SCB) reliably provides anesthesia distal to the level of the midhumerus. The SCB therefore can be used to facilitate reductions of elbow dislocations and distal radius fractures, as well as management of complex wounds of the forearm. The suprascapular nerve branches proximal to the brachial plexus in the supraclavicular fossa; therefore the SCB does not reliably provide analgesia to injuries of the distal clavicle and shoulder. The SCB targets the brachial plexus more distally than the interscalene nerve block; therefore the incidence of inadvertent paralysis of the hemidiaphragm (phrenic nerve palsy) is lower, but still present, when compared with the interscalene nerve block. Given the close proximity of the subclavian artery to the brachial plexus, color Doppler can be used to distinguish the brachial plexus from surrounding vascular structures to avoid intravascular injection of anesthetic. Pneumothorax is a potential, though rare, complication, given the close proximity of the dome of the pleura to the brachial plexus in the supraclavicular fossa; therefore mastery of needle tip visualization is required before incorporating this procedure into practice.

Anatomy

The trunks and divisions of the brachial plexus are compactly arranged within a fascial sheath in the supraclavicular fossa that is superficial to the middle scalene muscle and lateral to the subclavian artery. The subclavian artery is visualized in cross-section as an anechoic, round structure at the midpoint of the clavicle, superficial to the first rib. The brachial plexus at this level can be seen as a bundle of hypoechoic nodules posterior and superficial to the subclavian artery. The hyperechoic pleura lies posterior to the first rib and slides back and forth in accordance with the patient's respiratory cycle (see Fig. 31.11).

Technique

The patient is positioned upright or semi-recumbent with their head facing toward the contralateral side. An SCB should be performed using a longitudinal (in-plane) approach from a lateral-to-medial trajectory. The SCB is a shallow target that can be accessed using a standard 21- to 23-gauge, 1.5-inch (approximately 3.8 cm) needle. Patients with more prominent subcutaneous tissue may require a longer needle, such as 3.5-inch (approximately 9 cm) needle.

Place the high-frequency linear transducer in the supraclavicular fossa in the long axis of the clavicle, posterior and parallel to the midportion of the clavicle, with the indicator facing the patient's right. The transducer footprint is aimed caudally until the subclavian artery is visualized in cross-section as a pulsating, hypoechoic, circular structure that lies superficial to the hyperechoic linear first rib. The brachial plexus will appear as a hyperechoic, honeycomb-like structure lateral to the subclavian artery and medial to the middle scalene muscle. The hyperechoic pleura can be seen posterior and lateral to the first rib and should be avoided.

Once the brachial plexus and surrounding anatomic structures are identified, a small skin wheal should be made approximately 0.5 to 1 cm lateral to the probe, which will represent the site of needle entry. After injecting a skin wheal at the site of needle entry, a needle is inserted using an in-plane approach. The needle is advanced toward the lateral border of the brachial plexus under direct visualization of the needle shaft and tip at all times. A popping sensation is often associated with insertion of the needle into the connective tissue sheath surrounding the brachial plexus. With the needle tip in view, low-pressure injections using small aliquots of 3 to 5 mL of local anesthetic are used to hydrodissect above and below the brachial plexus (Fig. 31.13). A total of 20 to 30 mL of local anesthetic in a dose that is appropriate for the concentration of the anesthetic and the weight of the patient may be used to achieve adequate anesthesia. If at any point the spread of local anesthetic is not visualized, intravascular injection should be suspected and the procedure interrupted to confirm proper needle location and assess patient status.

FOREARM NERVE BLOCKS

Indications

The medial, radial, and ulnar nerves are the three major forearm nerves that supply sensory and motor innervations to the hand. Each of these nerves can be blocked individually or in combination to provide anesthesia for a variety of acute hand injuries. Ultrasound guidance has been shown to result in more effective hand anesthesia than traditional anatomic landmark–based wrist blocks.

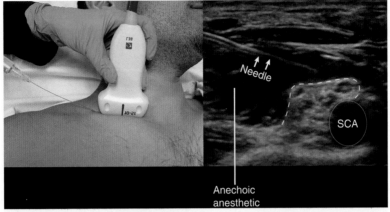

Fig. 31.13 In-plane lateral-to-medial approach to the supraclavicular brachial plexus. Note clear needle visualization and anesthetic deposition around the brachial plexus. *SCA*, subclavian artery.

For major injuries to the hand, such as blast injuries, all three forearm nerves can be blocked. The median and radial nerves can be blocked for injuries involving the thumb, index, long and ring finger, or radial aspect of the hand. The ulnar nerve can be blocked for injuries to the little finger or to the ulnar aspect of the hand (e.g., boxer's fracture). Generally, there is overlap of the distributions of innervation for each nerve; therefore injuries located close to transition zones between sensory nerve distributions may require both nerves to be blocked to ensure adequate pain control. The forearm nerve blocks do not provide anesthesia to the wrist or to the volar aspect of the forearm due to innervation from other nerves, which are missed with the forearm blocks.

Anatomy

The median nerve travels along the midline of the anterior compartment of the forearm between the flexor digitorum superficialis and the flexor digitorum profundus. The median nerve provides sensory innervation to the radial/lateral aspect of the volar hand and the volar surface of the thumb, index, long, and radial/lateral side of the ring finger.

The radial nerve divides into a deep and superficial branch at the level of the cubital fossa, the latter of which is the sensory branch. The superficial branch of the radial nerve travels lateral to the radial artery. The radial nerve provides sensory innervation to the radial/lateral aspect of the dorsal hand; dorsal surface of the thumb; and dorsal surface proximal to the distal interphalangeal joints of the index, long, and radial/lateral side of the ring finger.

The ulnar nerve travels in the anterior compartment of the forearm, deep to the flexor carpi ulnaris muscle

and lateral to the ulnar artery. The ulnar nerve provides sensory innervation to the ulnar/medial aspect of the dorsal and volar hand, including the hypothenar eminence, fifth digit, and ulnar/medial aspect of the ring finger.

Technique

Place the patient in a supine or 45-degree upright position with the upper extremity abducted and supinated and the forearm resting on a flat surface. The median nerve lies along the midline of the forearm between the flexor digitorum superficialis and flexor digitorum profundus. Place the high-frequency linear transducer on the volar surface of the distal forearm in a transverse orientation. Slide the transducer proximally toward the mid-forearm and look for an oval-shaped, hyperechoic structure, classically described as honeycomb-like in appearance (Fig. 31.14). Unlike the radial and ulnar nerve, there are typically no vascular structures surrounding the median nerve, except in rare cases. Differentiation of the median nerve from adjacent tendons and connective tissue in the distal wrist can be challenging due to their similar honeycomb-like appearance. By scanning more proximally along the mid-forearm, tendons will disappear and the nerve will become easier to identify.

The radial nerve lies radially to the radial artery in the ventral forearm. Place the transducer in a transverse orientation over the radial artery on the volar aspect of the distal forearm. Slide the transducer proximally until the nerve separating from the artery in the mid-to-proximal forearm is visualized (Fig. 31.15). Alternatively, find the nerve more proximally in the supracondylar region

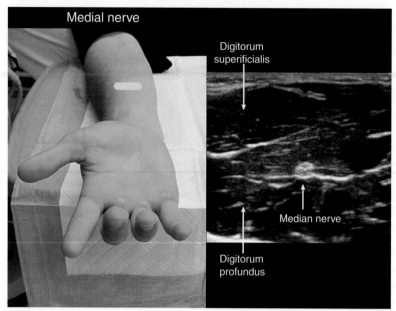

Fig. 31.14 Mid-forearm transverse transducer positioning will allow for clear median nerve visualization. Note the digitorum superficialis and profundus.

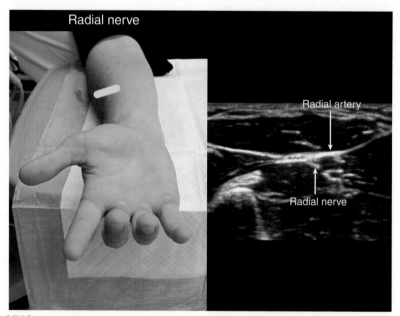

Fig. 31.15 Mid-forearm transverse transducer positioning for the radial nerve. Note that the radial nerve will be just lateral to the radial artery.

above the lateral aspect of the elbow, in the fascial plane between the brachioradialis and the brachialis muscles. The block can be performed at any level between the lateral elbow and distal wrist.

The ulnar nerve lies just medial (or on the ulnar aspect) to the ulnar artery in the ventral forearm. Place

the transducer on the volar surface of the wrist or distal forearm overlying the ulnar artery. Slide the transducer proximally until the nerve separating from the artery in the mid-to-proximal forearm can be visualized (Fig. 31.16).

Once the target nerve has been identified, a small skin wheal should be made approximately 0.5 to 1 cm lateral

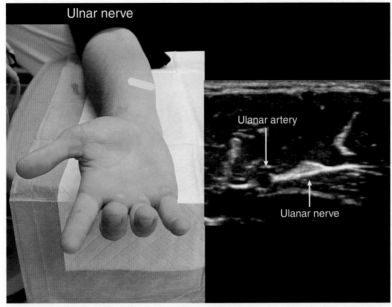

Fig. 31.16 Mid-forearm transverse transducer positioning for the ulnar nerve. The ulnar nerve will be located just medial to the ulnar artery.

to the probe, which will represent the site of needle entry. A 25-gauge, 1.5-inch (approximately 3.8 cm) block needle is inserted using an in-plane approach for all three forearm nerve blocks. To block the median nerve, enter the skin from the side most comfortable and accessible to the operator (Fig. 31.17). To block the radial nerve, enter the skin from a direction radially positioned to the probe (Fig. 31.18). To block the ulnar nerve, enter the skin from the ulnar aspect of the probe (Fig. 31.19). Alternatively, the patient can be positioned with the upper extremity abducted and the elbow supported on a flat surface and flexed at 90 degrees to allow for a more comfortable position to perform an in-plane approach. The needle is advanced toward the target nerve under direct visualization of the needle shaft and tip at all times, taking care to avoid inserting the needle into the nerve sheath. Slowly inject 3 to 5 mL of local anesthetic in a dose that is appropriate for the concentration of the anesthetic and the weight of the patient into the facial plane containing the nerve. Hypoechoic fluid should gradually surround the nerve; however, full circumferential spread is not required. If at any point the spread of local anesthetic is not visualized, intravascular injection should be suspected and the procedure interrupted to confirm proper needle location and assess patient status.

SERRATUS ANTERIOR PLANE

Indications

The serratus anterior plane block can be used to assist with analgesia for procedures in the axillary region (i.e., abscess drainage, thoracoscopy) or for pain relief from traumatic injuries in the lateral or anterior chest wall (i.e., rib fractures).

Anatomy

The lateral cutaneous branches of the thoracic intercostal nerves (T2–T12) branch posterior to the angle of the rib and run anteriorly and posteriorly just superficial to the serratus anterior muscle. These nerves provide cutaneous innervation lateral to the mid-clavicular line. Anesthetic deposited in this plane does not extend to the depth of the thoracic intercostal nerves (between the innermost and internal intercostal muscles). Thus the mechanism by which this block provides pain relief from rib fractures remains somewhat unclear. It has been posited that rib fractures disrupt the normal anatomic planes, allowing for more expansive spread of local anesthetic.

Of note, the long thoracic nerve and thoracodorsal nerve also lie on the surface of the serratus anterior

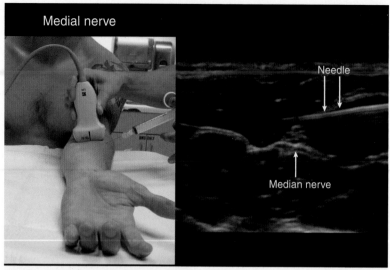

Fig. 31.17 In-plane approach to the medial nerve. Note the needle tip and the median nerve.

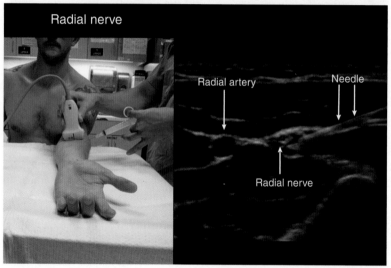

Fig. 31.18 In-plane approach to the radial nerve. Anechoic anesthetic injection will often allow for improved radial nerve visualization.

muscle. The extent to which blockade of these nerves contributes to analgesia is unclear.

Technique

For easiest visualization of the serratus plane, the patient should be placed in a lateral decubitus position with the affected side up. The provider should stand behind the patient and angle the linear probe anteriorly and slightly inferiorly on the mid-axillary line at the level of the fifth intercostal space with the indicator toward the patient's right. The ultrasound should display the

superficial latissimus muscle overlying the serratus muscle. Beneath the serratus muscle, the fourth and fifth ribs may be visualized, separated by the intercostal muscles. Deep to the intercostal muscles, pleura and lung should be visualized (Fig. 31.20A). No nerve bundle is visualized in this procedure.

After the serratus plane has been visualized and the fourth rib brought into view, create a small skin wheal posterior to the probe and introduce a 20-gauge, 3.5-inch (9 cm) needle primed for injection of 30 to 40 mL of dilute anesthetic in a dose that is appropriate for the

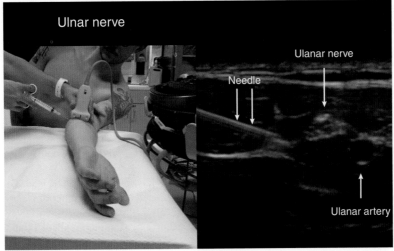

Fig. 31.19 Hypersupination of the forearm will allow for easier access to the ulnar nerve. Again, note the in-plane approach with clear needle visualization.

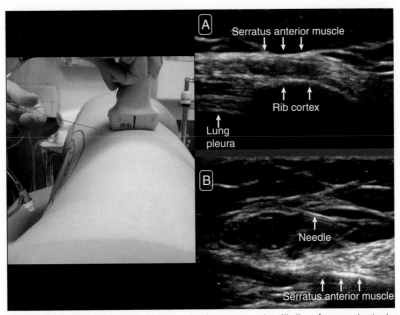

Fig. 31.20 For the serratus anterior plane block, an in-plane approach will allow for anesthetic deposition just above the serratus anterior muscle.

concentration of the anesthetic and the weight of the patient. Angle the needle in such a way that the fourth rib can act as a "backstop" to prevent accidental disruption of the pleura. Introduce the needle so that it can be placed in the fascial plane that lies on top of the serratus anterior muscle. Anechoic anesthetic fluid should be gently placed into this potential space, allowing clear visualization

of the fluid tracking above the muscle. We recommend introducing a small amount of normal saline or dilute anesthetic to confirm adequate placement of the needle. Fluid should be observed dissecting broadly on top of the serratus anterior muscle (Fig. 31.20B).

Of note, many different ultrasound-guided approaches to this fascial plane have been described.

The authors' experience is that the posterior approach (proceduralist standing behind the patient with insertion of block needle posterior to transducer) with injection of anesthetic above the serratus muscle offers the simplest and safest approach with no appreciable difference in anesthesia provided.

CONCLUSION

USGNBs can be a great addition to the current practice of a multimodal approach to pain management in the emergency department. Clinicians can learn regional anesthesia and integrate these techniques into clinical practice to actively manage acute pain.

BIBLIOGRAPHY

Beaudoin FL, Haran JP, Liebmann O. A comparison of ultrasound-guided three-in-one femoral nerve block versus parenteral opioids alone for analgesia in emergency department patients with hip fractures: a randomized controlled trial. *Acad Emerg Med.* 2013;20(6):584–591.

Blanco R, Parras T, McDonnell JG, Prats-Galino A. Serratus plane block: a novel ultrasound-guided thoracic wall nerve block. *Anaesthesia.* 2013;68(11):1107–1113.

Cornish PB, Leaper CJ, Nelson G, Anstis F, McQuillan C, Stienstra R. Avoidance of phrenic nerve paresis during continuous supraclavicular regional anaesthesia. *Anaesthesia.* 2007;62(4):354–358.

Guideline for ultrasound transducer cleaning and disinfection. *Ann Emerg Med.* 2018; 72(4):e45–e47.

Hartmann FVG, Novaes MRCG, de Carvalho MR. Femoral nerve block versus intravenous fentanyl in adult patients with hip fractures - a systematic review. *Braz J Anesthesiol.* 2017;67(1):67–71.

Herring AA, Promes SB. Bringing ultrasound-guided regional anesthesia to emergency medicine. *AEM Educ Train.* 2017;1(2):165–168.

Hogan QH. Pathophysiology of peripheral nerve injury during regional anesthesia. *Reg Anesth Pain Med.* 2008;33(5):435–441.

Hussain N, Goldar G, Ragina N, Banfield L, Laffey JG, Abdallah FW. Suprascapular and interscalene nerve block for shoulder surgery: a systematic review and meta-analysis. *Anesthesiology.* 2017;127(6):998–1013.

Jeng CL, Rosenblatt MA. Intraneural injections and regional anesthesia: the known and the unknown. *Minerva Anestesiol.* 2011;77(1):54–58.

Kakazu C, Tokhner V, Li J, Ou R, Simmons E. *Br J Anaesth.* 2014;113(1):190–191.

Liebmann O, Price D, Mills C, et al. Feasibility of forearm ultrasonography-guided nerve blocks of the radial, ulnar, and median nerves for hand procedures in the emergency department. *Ann Emerg Med.* 2006;48(5):558–562.

Marhofer P, Harrop-Griffiths W, Kettner SC, Kirchmair L. Fifteen years of ultrasound guidance in regional anaesthesia: part 1. *Br J Anaesth.* 2010;104(5):538–546.

Marhofer P, Harrop-Griffiths W, Willschke H, Kirchmair L. Fifteen years of ultrasound guidance in regional anaesthesia: part 2—recent developments in block techniques. *Br J Anaesth.* 2010;104(6):673–683.

Mayes J, Davison E, Panahi P, et al. An anatomical evaluation of the serratus anterior plane block. *Anaesthesia.* 2016;71(9):1064–1069.

Melton MS, Monroe HE, Qi W, Lewis SL, Nielsen KC, Klein SM. Effect of interscalene brachial plexus block on the pulmonary function of obese patients: a prospective, observational cohort study. *Anesth Analg.* 2017;125(1):313–319.

Neal JM, Barrington MJ, Fettiplace MR, et al. The Third American Society of Regional Anesthesia and Pain Medicine Practice Advisory on Local Anesthetic Systemic Toxicity: executive summary 2017. *Reg Anesth Pain Med.* 2018;43(2):113–123.

Neal JM, Bernards CM, Hadzic A, et al. ASRA practice advisory on neurologic complications in regional anesthesia and pain medicine. *Reg Anesth Pain Med.* 2008;33(5):404–415.

Renes SH, Rettig HC, Gielen MJ, Wilder-Smith OH, van Geffen GJ. Ultrasound-guided low-dose interscalene brachial plexus block reduces the incidence of hemidiaphragmatic paresis. *Reg Anesth Pain Med.* 2009;34(5):498–502.

Ritcey B, Pageau P, Woo MY, Perry JJ. Regional nerve blocks for hip and femoral neck fractures in the emergency department: a systematic review. *CJEM.* 2016;18(1):37–47.

Sohoni A, Nagdev A, Takhar S, Stone M. Forearm ultrasound-guided nerve blocks vs landmark-based wrist blocks for hand anesthesia in healthy volunteers. *Am J Emerg Med.* 2016;34(4):730–734.

Tirado A, Nagdev A, Henningsen C, Breckon P, Chiles K. Ultrasound-guided procedures in the emergency department-needle guidance and localization. *Emerg Med Clin North Am.* 2013;31(1):87–115.

Toles K, Nagdev A. Trick of the trade: patient positioning for ultrasound-guided ulnar nerve block. *ALiEM.* 2016. https://www.aliem.com/2016/01/trick-of-the-trade-patient-positioning-for-ultrasound-guided-ulnar-nerve-block/.

Tran DQH, Elgueta MF, Aliste J, Finlayson RJ. Dia-phragm-sparing nerve blocks for shoulder surgery. *Reg Anesth Pain Med*. 2017;42(1):32–38.

Unneby A, Svensson O, Gustafson Y, Olofsson B. Femoral nerve block in a representative sample of elderly people with hip fracture: a randomised controlled trial. *Injury*. 2017;48(7):1542–1549.

Walker KJ, McGrattan K, Aas-Eng K, Smith AF. Ultrasound guidance for peripheral nerve blockade. *Cochrane Database Syst Rev*. 2009;(4):CD006459.

Wroe P, O'Shea R, Johnson B, Hoffman R, Nagdev A. Ultrasound-guided forearm nerve blocks for hand blast injuries: case series and multidisciplinary protocol. *Am J Emerg Med*. 2016;34(9):1895–1897.

INDEX

A

A-lines, in lungs, 99, 100f
AAA. *See* Abdominal aortic aneurysm
Abdomen
    focused assessment with sonography, 161–173
    lower, 241–257
        pediatric, 248
    ultrasound-guided resuscitation for, 156
Abdominal aorta, 232–240.e1
    anatomy of, 232, 233f
    differential diagnosis in, 233b
    evaluation of, 156
    pathology for, 235–238
        abdominal aortic aneurysm, 235, 235t, 236f
        aneurysmal leak or rupture, 235–236, 237f, 237t
        aortic dissection, 237–238, 238f
        endovascular aortic grafts, 238, 239f, 239t
        intramural and intraluminal thrombus, 236–237, 237f
    sonographic findings of, 232–233, 234f–235f
    ultrasound technique and tips for, 233–235
Abdominal aortic aneurysm (AAA), 235, 235t, 236f
Abdominal pain
    acute
        acute pancreatitis causing, 203–204, 204f, 204t
        chronic pancreatitis, 206, 206f
        subacute pancreatitis causing, 204–205, 205f
    in pregnancy, 293–294
Abdominal/peritoneal pregnancy, 289
Abnormal volume status, basic echocardiography of, 112
Abscess
    amebic, 177
    appendiceal, 247
    liver, 177, 179f–180f, 196

Abscess *(Continued)*
    peritonsillar, 40–47, 54f
        anatomy of, 41–42, 42f
        aspiration, 45–46, 45f–46f
        clinical considerations of, 41
        insertion locations, 46f
        intraoral ultrasound evaluation, preparation and technique for, 43–44
        pitfalls/common mistakes of, 47
        ultrasound findings of, 44, 44f–45f
        ultrasound-guided drainage of, 45–46
Absorption, 6, 6f
Acalculous cholecystitis, acute, 194–195, 195f, 195t
Achilles tendon rupture, ultrasound of, 327–328, 328f
Acoustic enhancement, 28–29, 29f
Acoustic impedance, 2–4, 5f
Acoustic intensity, 24
Acoustic power, 24–25
Acoustic shadowing, 28–29, 29f
Acoustic streaming, 267
Acute abdominal pain
    acute pancreatitis causing, 203–204, 204f, 204t
    chronic pancreatitis, 206, 206f
    subacute pancreatitis causing, 204–205, 205f
Acute acalculous cholecystitis, 194–195, 195f, 195t
Acute and chronic deep venous thrombosis, 312–318
    clinical correlation of, 312–314
    imaging in, 314–316, 315f, 317f–318f
    normal anatomy of, 314, 314f
    pathology of, 315f–316f, 316–318, 318t
Acute appendicitis, 249f–250f, 256
Acute calculus cholecystitis, 191–194, 194f, 194t
Acute cholecystitis, 293–294

Acute flank pain, 212–217, 214t
    hydronephrosis, 212–215, 214f–215f, 214t
    pyelonephritis, 217, 217f–218f
    renal stones, 215–217, 216f
Acute infectious cystitis, 220, 221f, 222t
Acute pancreatitis, 203–204, 204f, 204t
Acute renal insufficiency, 219–220
Acute right heart strain, chronic *versus*, 111
Adenoma, pleomorphic, 53f
Adenomyomatosis, 189–191, 192f
Adenopathy, 54–56
Adnexal torsion, 274–276, 275f
Agency for Healthcare Research and Quality (AHRQ), 347
Air bronchograms, 103f
ALARA. *See* As low as reasonably achievable (ALARA) concept
Aliasing, 18–19
Alobar holoprosencephaly, 91f
Amaurosis fugax, 69
Amebic abscesses, 177
American College of Emergency Physicians (ACEP), 347
Amniotic fluid, 293
Amniotic fluid volume, 292
Anaplastic thyroid cancer, 51–52, 52f
Aneurysmal leak or rupture, 235–236, 237f, 237t
Anterior chamber (AC), of eye, 59
Aorta
    abdominal, 232–240.e1
        anatomy of, 232, 233f
        differential diagnosis in, 233b
        evaluation of, 156
        pathology for, 235–238
            abdominal aortic aneurysm, 235, 235t, 236f
            aneurysmal leak or rupture, 235–236, 237f, 237t
            aortic dissection, 237–238, 238f
            endovascular aortic grafts, 238, 239f, 239t

Note: Page numbers followed by "f" indicate figures, "b" indicate boxes, and "t" indicate tables.